PSYCHIATRIC NURSING

ETHICAL
STRIFE

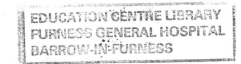

PSYCHIATRIC NURSING

ETHICAL
STRIFE

Edited by Philip J. Barker

PhD, RN, FRCN, Royal Victoria Infirmary, University of Newcastle, UK

and Ben Davidson

*BA joint hons, RN, Pathfinder Mental Health Services
NHS Trust, London, UK*

ARNOLD

A member of the Hodder Headline Group

LONDON • NEW YORK • SYDNEY • AUCKLAND

First published in Great Britain in 1998 by
Arnold, a member of the Hodder Headline Group,
338 Euston Road, London, NW1 3BH
http://www.arnoldpublishers.com

© 1998 Arnold

Whilst the advice and information in this book is believed to be true and accurate at the date of going to press, neither the authors nor the publisher can accept any legal responsibility or liability for any errors or omissions that may be made.

British Library Cataloguing in Publication Data
A catalogue record for this book is available from the British Library

Library of Congress Cataloging-in-Publication Data
A catalog record for this book is available from the Library of Congress

ISBN 0 340 62523 6

Publisher: Clare Parker
Production Editor: James Rabson
Production Controller: Priya Gohil
Cover designer: Julie Martin

Typeset in 10/12pt Palatino by J&L Composition Ltd, Filey, North Yorkshire
Printed and bound in Great Britain by J W Arrowsmith Ltd, Bristol

DEDICATION

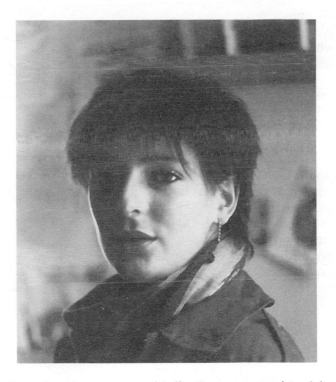

This book is dedicated to the memory of Sally Cameron, my friend for 15 years, who was born in Leeds and who died in London in 1996, aged 35. Sally nurtured living things skilfully; her relationships abounded with love and awareness; and an inspirational, almost other-worldly perceptiveness suffused her writing. May Sally's spirit, as it re-emerges in this book, call forth a new vista and ethic of mental health care.

Ben Davidson

The front cover shows a reproduction of a lino print by Liz Davies accompanied in its original form by the following:

And you will crumple my body like a leaf of paper
burn it, bury it,
toss it in the air.

What use have I for it
with its severed head,
one leg
no arms
feet without toes?

If I stretch my arms
or breathe in deeply the air
I am filled with germs
and fragments of missiles.

If I take off my blood-stained rags
I fear you will crumple my body like a leaf of paper
burn it, bury it,
toss it in the air.

I am scared to death
for this wretched and vulnerable vehicle
all it harbours even
is tainted with anger at your anger
which will pursue me
even as I carry my bag of jewels
across the seven bridges
to the far stars.

Liz Davies
(1968)

CONTENTS

EDITORS' PROFILES

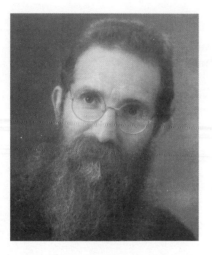

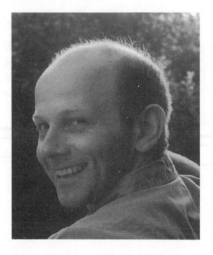

PHIL BARKER

Phil Barker, PhD, RN, FRCN, is Professor of Psychiatric Nursing Practice in the Department of Psychiatry, University of Newcastle, UK. In his clinical practice he is most involved with people in depression and psychosis. He has wide-ranging research interests, but is mainly interested in human questions: what is personal meaning in mental distress, and why do people need psychiatric nurses?
E-mail: P.J.Barker@newcastle.ac.uk

BEN DAVIDSON

Ben Davidson, BA (joint Hons), RMN, co-ordinates the User Employment Project at Springfield Hospital in Tooting, South London, UK, supporting the paid employment of people with a history of serious mental health problems in clinical posts within the Trust. He lives in a small community in East Dulwich, South East London with 6 friends and his 9-year-old son Jack, whose care he shares with Jack's mother who lives nearby. He is training as a group psychotherapist with the Institute of Group Analysis and his hobbies include paragliding, playing guitar and writing.
E-mail: Ben_Davidson@compuserve.com

AUTHORS' PROFILES

JOSEPH H. BERKE

Joseph H. Berke, MD, is the Director of the Arbours Association and the Arbours Crisis Centre in London, where he also has a private practice as an individual and family psychotherapist. His forthcoming books include *Even Paranoids Have Enemies: New Perspectives on Paranoia and Persecution* (co-editor and contributor), Routledge, and *Psychoanalysis and Kabbalah* (with Stanley Schneider), Jason Aronson Inc.

KARLA BOYCE

Karla Anne-Marie Boyce, BSc (Hons), RMN, MSc, is a Trinidadian who has been living in the UK for the last 11 years. She works as a staff nurse in central London on a ward run along therapeutic community principles with a group-work focus.

JOY BRAY

Joy Dean Bray, MA, RGN, RMN, RNT, ENB650, is employed as a Senior Lecturer at Homerton College, Cambridge. She lives with her family in a small village outside Cambridge. She is currently registered for a part-time PhD at Essex University, investigating acute in-patient psychiatric nursing from both psychoanalytical and sociological perspectives. She has an abiding interest in all aspects of group work, in particular the effects of organisational dynamics on the individual in the workplace.

JAMES BROWN

James M. Brown, BA, MA, MSc, is a Senior Lecturer in Philosophy at the University of Ulster at Coleraine in Northern Ireland. He is interested in formal and informal logic, epistemology, philosophy of science, and especially theoretical and applied ethics. He is the author of articles in philosophy and nursing journals and co-author with A. Kitson and T. McKnight of *Challenges in Caring* (Chapman and Hall, 1992). He has the support of his wife and three daughters and is fond of jazz.

SALLY CAMERON

Sally Cameron was born in Leeds in 1961. Her last year at Keele University was overshadowed by the diagnosis of a severe illness, but she graduated in 1983. Moving to London, she worked as a psychiatric nursing auxilliary until her illness forced her to retire. It was then that she started writing short stories, a number of which have been published during the time the current text has been in preparation. She also created and tended a community garden which won a European-wide competition as an oasis in the midst of the squalor of London's East End, and she took up (informally) a post of housing co-op 'counsellor in residence'. Sally's sudden death on 10 June 1996 was devastating to her family, her many close friends and all who knew and loved her.

PETER CAMPBELL

Peter Campbell, BA (Hons), is a freelance writer and trainer and lives in Cricklewood, North-West London. He is a mental health system survivor and has been in regular receipt of mental health services for thirty years. He was a founder member of Survivors Speak Out and of Survivors' Poetry and has been involved in action to change attitudes and practice towards people with a mental illness diagnosis since the early 1980s. He is a cartoonist and performing poet and supports Hendon AFC.

BRENDA CURZON

Brenda Curzon, BSocSc, RN, is completing a MA (Social Policy) at Massey University, New Zealand. Her thesis 'The Crisis in Auckland's Mental Health Services during the 1980s', reflects her interest in the impact of Social Policy on health. She lectures in the department of social sciences at Manukau Institute of Technology, Auckland, and practises in a variety of settings. Brenda has two children, Richard and Anna, and lives with her husband in the Waitakere Ranges. Her interests include: surfing the Net, growing roses, cryptic crosswords and creating great food. E-mail: ajmac@iconz.co.nz

JOHN DANIEL

John Daniel, RGN, RMN, Cert. Counselling, is a secular Carmelite who has worked in Calcutta for the Red Cross, in various nursing specialities in the UK, and as a Social Worker in Toxteth, Liverpool during an extensive period of social and political upheaval in the 70s and 80s. He gave up work 4 years ago due to fatigue caused by the HIV virus but has recently started another career in writing and public speaking, also sitting on the co-ordinating committee of Catholic Aids Link.

VINCENT DEARY

Vincent Deary lives in London with his daughter and extended family. He is a cognitive behavioural therapist, working with Chronic Fatigue Sydrome. He trained at the Maudsley, gaining a diploma in CBT and an RMN. Long before that he studied medicine, then psychology. He is from Carluke in Scotland.

PARAMABANDHU GROVES

Paramabandhu Groves, BA, MB, BS, MRCPsych, is a senior registrar in psychiatry at the Maudsley Hospital, London. He is training in core process psychotherapy at the Karuna Institute in Devon and works as a psychotherapist at Bodywise, a Buddhist complementary health centre in East London. He was ordained into the Western Buddhist Order in 1990, lives in a community and teaches meditation and Buddhism at the London Buddhist Centre.

EIBHLÍN INGLESBY

Eibhlín Inglesby, MA (Theology), SRN, RNT, has recently commenced doctoral research in the field of spirituality and mental illness in the department of Religious Studies at the University of Newcastle, where she is an assistant lecturer. She lives in Sunderland with her husband and two daughters and is an enthusiastic runner and Irish set dancer.

RICHARD LAKEMAN

Richard Lakeman, BN, RCpN, is employed as a nursing lecturer at the Eastern Institute of Technology, Taradale, New Zealand. He lives in Hastings with his partner Claire and two children, Amelia and Silvana. His practice experience includes roles as group facilitator and staff nurse in various psychiatric care facilities including day hospital, acute, intensive care and continuing care units. He is interested in how nurses can use the Internet to facilitate global communication and share resources. E-mail: rlakeman@xtra.co.nz

ED MANOS

Ed Manos has worked with the Collaborative Support Program, New Jersey for nine years. Currently he is Supervisor of Maintenance for Butterfly Property Management which provides housing for people with an experience of mental illness. He is also an Adjunct Instructor at the University of Medicine and Dentistry, New Jersey where he lectures in psychosocial rehabilitation.

HUGH MCKENNA

Hugh McKenna, RMN, RGN, D.Phil, BSc(Hons), DipN (Lond) Adv Dip Ed RNT, is a senior lecturer and co-ordinator of nursing research in the School of Health Sciences at the University of Ulster in Northern Ireland. He has a particular interest in quality appraisal in mental health care and in the theoretical basis for nursing. His outside interests include travel, playing and listening to music and reading biographies. He is married to a nurse, and has two children Saoirse and Gowain, and they live 5 miles north of Belfast.
E-mail: HP.McKenna@Ulst.ac.uk

STEVE MELLUISH

Steve Melluish, BSc (Hons), MSc, is employed as a Clinical and Community Psychologist by Nottingham Community Mental Health NHS Trust, and lives in Nottingham with his partner and daughter.

JIM MOOREY

James Moorey, BA (Hons), MSc., Dip. Psych., C. Psychol., has trained as a clinical psychologist and as a psychoanalytic psychotherapist. He is employed as a Research Fellow in the Department of Psychiatry at Manchester University. He is currently completing a PhD on psychoanalytic epistemology, and working on a randomised controlled trial of psychotherapy with treatment-resistant out-patients.

PETER MORRALL

Peter A. Morrall, PhD, MSc, BA (Hons), PGCE, RGN, RMN, RMMH, has a background in medical sociology and mental health nursing. Formerly of the University of Teesside, he is now employed as a senior lecturer in the School of Healthcare Studies at the University of Leeds, with a specific responsibility for co-ordinating sociology teaching, and developing health and social science research. Peter has travelled extensively, is a 'born-again motorcyclist', and lives in York.
E-mail: hcspam@Leeds.ac.uk

VIC NOVAK

Vic Novak is a teaching fellow at the University of Stirling, Department of Nursing, Highland Campus, Inverness. His interests are mental health, in particular the interpersonal aspects of nursing. His past experience as a charge nurse in an addiction unit led to an interest in group therapy and individual counselling. His leisure interests are golf and fishing.

BILL REYNOLDS

Bill Reynolds is Senior Lecturer at the Department of Nursing, University of Stirling, Highland Campus, Inverness. His interests are mental health, empathy and interpersonal relations in particular. His research interests tend towards clinical research and patient outcomes. His wife is Margaret, his daughter, Iona, and the cat is called Tizer. He likes football and would like to see his country (Scotland) join the other nations of the world as a free and independent country.
E-mail: w.j.reynolds@stirling.ac.uk

JEFFREY SCHALER

Jeffrey Schaler, PhD, is an adjunct professor of justice, law and society at American University's School of Public Affairs, Washington, DC; an adjunct professor of psychology at Montgomery College, Rockville, Md; and teaches psychology at John Hopkins University, Baltimore, Md. A psychotherapist since 1973 and third-degree black belt in Korean martial arts (1988), his hobbies now include long-distance swimming. He lives in Silver Spring, Md. E-mail: jschale@american.edu

DAVID SMAIL

David Smail works part-time as an NHS Clinical Psychologist, having retired in 1993 from his post as Head of Clinical Psychology Services in Nottingham. He holds the honorary post of Special Professor in Clinical Psychology at the University of Nottingham. He has thought and written about psychological approaches to treatment for many years, and his most recent book, *How to Survive Without Psychotherapy*, was published by Constable in 1996. His principle hobby over the past five years has been collecting grandchildren.

CHRIS STEVENSON

Chris Stevenson, RMN, BA (Hons), MSc, PhD, is a lecturer in psychiatric nursing practice in the Department of Psychiatry, University of Newcastle, and is course director for a master's programme in psychiatric and mental health nursing. Her research interests are in family meetings in psychiatric settings and in defining why people need psychiatric and mental health nurses. She combines her career with a busy family life and horse-riding in the Northumbrian countryside.

DAWN THIBERT

Dawn Thibert, BA (joint Honours), Diploma in Innovations in Mental Health Work, is employed as the project manager of the Community Care Officers Team by Lambeth Social Services, London, lives alone in South London and enjoys travelling.

GARY WINSHIP

Gary Winship, MA, DipGpPsych, RMN, ENB616, is a Nurse Psychotherapist with the West Berkshire NHS Trust. He trained and worked at the Maudsley for 14 years. He is a co-opted Council member for the Association of Psychoanalytic Psychotherapists in the NHS (APP), a member of the Fabian Society and a full member of the Group Analytic Society. He is currently studying for a PhD.

FOREWORD

Defining and treating psychiatric illness are not necessarily closely related to trying to understand it. 'Mental health', indeed, is the field *par excellence* where professional interest and cultural prejudice clash head-on with the truth of personal anguish. No wonder that ethical strife is one of the principal outcomes for those whose task it is to clarify the meaning of their own role as helpers.

What is encouraging about this book is the honesty with which the authors – most of them psychiatric nurses – engage in the task of trying to make ethical sense of their professional activity. You will not find in these pages the kind of dogmatic assertion and confident clinical pronouncement so typical of orthodox psychiatry, but rather the reflections – even confessions – of people who are desperately aware of the ethical conflicts within their role. The authors try by every means available to develop a wide-ranging critique of the moral and intellectual framework in which they find themselves while staying true to their own and their patients' experience of unhappiness, confusion and despair.

Some things quickly become obvious: our ideas and practices in the field of mental health are inextricably bound up with the socio-political setting in which they occur. Nobody is in a better position to know this than psychiatric nurses, who are forced to live with the problems in ways which are more easily avoided by their colleagues in, for instance, medicine and psychology. Ideology is in this way constantly challenged by experience. Not, of course, that being forced into such close proximity with those our society damages and excludes necessarily generates honesty or even compassion, but for those who manage to hold onto their moral and mental integrity, part of their *striving* to understand makes it almost impossible to deny that the suffering of those with whom they work is shaped, as for the rest of us, by the world we all live in. Some of those writing in these pages are even brave enough to underline the fact that there is really no significant distinction to be made between nurse and patient by revealing their personal knowledge of distress.

There are not any easy answers to the questions raised in this book. Maybe there are not any answers at all of the kind we might hope to find. The contributors to this volume cast their nets widely, borrowing from philosophy, psychology, religion, their own experience of confusion and pain, to try to get to grips with the conflicts and dilemmas of their role. The result is not always tidy, but tidiness isn't the point. In a culture where intellectual endeavour has become a market commodity like any other, and in which leading thinkers adopt the role of 'celebs' whom others are expected to admire rather than engage with, it is refreshing to come across the living grappling with ideas to be used as tools rather than as blunt instruments for the enforcement of assent. Rather than treating their moral and philosophical mentors merely as fodder for academic debate, the authors here pay them the compliment of having something to say about the social world which might help us in our efforts to understand it: the *strife* involved is not only between competing systems of ideology and explanation, but a feature of the struggle to understand *per se*. There is here none of the spuriously uniform professional gloss of the official textbook, but a series of profoundly serious attempts to delineate – one might say, after the depredations of the last two decades, almost to excavate – a human and humane approach to so-called madness.

David Smail
Special Professor in Clinical Psychology
University of Nottingham

PREFACE

If history is to be believed, people have suffered from problems with their 'mental health' for as long as there has been language to express their fears and anxieties. As this text is being edited, the Bethlem and Maudsley Hospital in London prepares to celebrate its 750th anniversay of caring for people with 'mental health problems'. Formerly, the religious orders were responsible for much of that history at the Bethlem, and their brethren, the Celtic monks of Northumbria, were caring for similarly dispossessed peoples as far back as the ninth century. As a new millennium approaches, society continues to wrestle with the same question posed by our religious forebears: 'What is right and fitting in the name of care of the "mentally ill"?'

This link with the past is not merely an academic reference point, but is historically meaningful to us. Ben Davidson trained and worked as a psychiatric nurse at the Bethlem and Maudsley, while Phil Barker became the UK's first professor of psychiatric nursing at Newcastle, in the old Kingdom of Northumbria. We feel a sense of kinship with our professional ancestors, continuing the tradition of 'psychic healing and spiritual rebirth'. We also feel we have been handed the baton of philosophical enquiry by them. It remains, of course, unclear exactly *who* has been handed *what* by *whom*.

This is a book about ethics. Ethics is traditionally understood as something elevated, if not beyond the ken of psychiatric nurse practitioners. This is the great lie of the common understanding of philosophy. Ordinary people wrestle with moral decisions on an everyday basis. This is the truth and reality of ethics. We, the editors, are ordinary psychiatric nurses, who, occasionally, feel an extraordinary sense of vocation, which may not be so dissimilar from that of our ancestral brethren. In that sense, we believe that it is both our honour and our responsibility to continue the tradition they began one thousand years ago. This is no grandiose gesture: all nurses are obliged to confront ethical dilemmas on a daily basis, as were their ancestors. In so doing, few, if any, stop to question whether or not they have the intelligence or education to make ethical decisions. Decisions have to be made and nurses make them. This book is a celebration of the doubts and anxieties and, occasionally, misplaced convictions of such ordinary nurses. We, as editors, have rarely doubted the legitimacy of our role as everyday moral philosophers. One of our aims in publishing this book has been to encourage our colleagues to recognise that the baton of ethical enquiry is being passed, metaphorically, down the ages to them also.

Phil Barker and Ben Davidson
1996

ACKNOWLEDGEMENTS

The editors would like to acknowledge the part played by the following in bringing this text into being:

PHIL BARKER

I thank my wife, Poppy, and my daughter, Charlie, for their continued support in helping me to find the path; and my late father, Joe Barker, for first introducing me to the concept of morality.

BEN DAVIDSON

Thanks to Maureen Crooks, my fiancée during most of the period this book was in preparation, for the first encouragement, for continued practical and financial support, and for her love. Gratitude also to my older sister Liz Davies, from whose experience and vision emerged in early years my interest in the link between mental health/ illness, interpersonal politics and spirituality.

1

THE ETHICAL LANDSCAPE

Phil Barker and Ben Davidson

A PHILOSOPHICAL CANVAS: SKETCHES OF CONSIDERED EXPERIENCE

There are few decisions in life which are not, in some way, ethical. Although *ethics* is usually defined narrowly in terms of professional conduct or life or death decision-making, more mundane actions also have an ethical dimension. None the less, we are often encouraged to think that there is a limited range of ethical problems 'out there' waiting to confront us: abortion, euthanasia, capital punishment, etc. It seems more likely, however, that it is *ethicists,* ordinary, ethically-minded people with ordinary, active consciences, who *determine,* or even *construct,* ethical dilemmas. The times we live in project changing scenarios which are judged by the voices (and pens) of such ethically-minded people inhabiting them. The more ethically-minded people there are, the more ethical dilemmas there are likely to be. That said, there are some principles of human conduct which have endured down the ages, and which provide the basis for all ethical argument, if not ethical decision-making. Some of these enduring principles prompt the emergence of *ethicists* today, and remain the focus of much debate as to what is 'right' or 'wrong' conduct. Of course, there are also powerful interests exerting an influence on current ideology of 'right' and 'wrong', to some extent quite independently of what ethicists might say and ominously lurking behind their views.

This book aims to address some of the ethical issues which confront psychiatric nurses in the course of their practice. We began this book with the assumption that ethics as *applied within* and *to* psychiatric nursing was primarily an issue *for* psychiatric nurses. Ethics is the business of every psychiatric nurse. As a result, all of the nursing contributors are either practitioners of psychiatric nursing, or have been closely connected with the practice of psychiatric nursing. Non-nursing contributions come from people who might have a better view of psychiatric nurses 'at work', and from people who have been in receipt of psychiatric nursing practice. In every case, however, the ethical issues emerge from the experience, perceptions and 'personal philosophies' of the contributors.

When this book was proposed a reviewer believed that it was an impossible project since neither of the editors, and apparently none of the other contributors, were 'proper philosophers'.[1] The view was taken that ethics was a complex branch of moral philosophy, possessing many specific theories and intricate arguments which could only be explicated by a professional philosopher. We did not dispute that view then, nor do we challenge it now. We restate the sentiments of that critical reviewer simply because they exemplify what this book is *not* about. We have no intention of addressing ethics as an arcane subject, intelligible to only a limited audience, and open to review and disputation by an even more limited audience. Although we aim to recognise the historical lineage of ethical enquiry, this is not a book about ethics in a philosophical sense. Everyone needs to make moral judgements as part of everyday life. These require each of us to consider, at some level, our moral position. What is the 'bottom line' beneath which we shall not allow our standards to fall? These are, by definition, ethical standards; and the 'bottom line' is our moral cut-off point. Our intention was that this would be a book of ethics in psychiatric nursing, which would prove useful to psychiatric nurses as they approach the everyday business of psychiatric caring. If we draw an analogy with representation in art, this book is no more than a sketch of the ethical territory. The sketches which will emerge in the subsequent chapters will, none the less, be based on the ethical reality which derives from the world of mental health care, of which our contributors have some genuine knowledge.

ETHICAL CONTEXTS

Professional and philosophical backdrops

Nursing ethics was once viewed as, at best, an offshoot of medical ethics and, at worst, a set of rules about manners and morals which were often indistinguishable from a professional etiquette.[2] Thus, nursing ethics was 'largely about doing your duty and that duty was largely obvious . . . summed up in the demand for "implicit, unquestioning obedience", and in the requirements of conventional respectability' (Thompson *et al.* 1983; p. v). As nursing has developed its professional stance, the need to clarify the nature of the ethical issues involved in the conduct of the profession has increased. Burnard and Chapman (1988) recognised that terms like 'profession' and 'ethics' were difficult to define. Efforts to define the moral basis of nursing by asserting that 'ethics is caring' or 'to act ethically is to care . . . for ourselves and others' were viewed by Burnard and Chapman as tautological, offering no practical or realistic guide to action. Such assertions remind us of Hare's view that the 'language of morals is one sort of prescriptive language' (Hare, 1952; p.1). The statement that 'caring *is* good' appears simple, but we remain uncertain not only of what we might mean by 'good', but also what might be meant by 'caring'. It was one of our requirements that authors should confront these uncertainties, albeit in very specific contexts.

The uncertainty over language, especially apparently simple terms, is part and parcel of the ethical landscape. Burnard and Chapman noted how Cambell (1979)

---

[1] We believe that all people who have the capacity to think critically about their own life and that of others are involved in some kind of philosophising.

[2] When PJB was a student nurse in 1970 one lecture was devoted to the 'proper conduct of the nurse' which included such 'rules' as 'nurses should not read nursing or medical text books on buses as this draws unnecessary attention to their calling'. Meanwhile, the ethical code of the International Council of Nurses was not 'taught' but 'required reading'.

had acknowledged that the original Greek and Latin words from which *ethics* and *morals* were derived, meant much the same thing - '*that which is customary or generally accepted*'. Despite this unanimity, Cambell tried to use the word 'morals' to describe that which was studied by 'ethics'. Such tautology demonstrates the basic truth of our reviewer's concern; even philosophers find it difficult to say *exactly* what they mean when discussing 'morals' and 'ethics'. Such difficulties should not, however, deter us from exploring the ethical territory of psychiatric nursing. We hope our example will serve as a model for other practitioners – who may not be philosophers – to examine their understanding of the meaning of such terms, and associated issues.

A science of ethics?

Ethics or moral philosophy, both in relation to nursing and elsewhere, may be distinguished from everyday decision-making by the extent to which it involves a systematic consideration of human values. Most, if not all of the authors represented here will consider, carefully and systematically, the influence of various theories of human conduct on their own thinking. Many will also consider the meanings of moral terms – such as 'goodness' or 'rightness' – as applied to the conduct of their professional affairs. We have narrowed the focus of those affairs specifically to that of psychiatric nursing practice. We required each author to consider how a life situation came to be an ethical problem *in the light of their practical experience*. As noted, this practical focus is the hallmark of the book. It is not so much a book 'about' ethics, as a book *of* ethics: deriving from the lived experience of the authors; the antithesis of what might be called an academic appraisal. That said, we challenged the authors to present what might be passed on as a 'systematic study' of their human values; eschewing personal opinion in favour of a considered set of values.

Ethics has long been promoted as a science of human conduct. Locke's *Essay Concerning Human Understanding* (1690) classified ethics as the second of the three divisions of the sciences: 'that which man himself ought to do, as a rational and voluntary agent, for the attainment of any end, especially happiness' (Locke, 1964: 442). Locke recognised that ethics involved the exercise of a skill: 'the skill of right applying our own powers and actions for the attainment of things good and useful'. We are often deceived into thinking that ethics is an intellectual activity pursued only by academics within a delimited academic community. Locke emphasised that this was not the case: 'this is not bare speculation and the knowledge of truth; but *right*, and a conduct suitable to it' (ibid., p.442, emphasis added).

Almost exactly a century ago, Muirhead (1892) drew a clear comparison between ethics and other sciences: 'there are those sciences which have to do primarily, not with facts in space and time, but with judgements about those facts . . . . It is judgement in the latter sense that ethics has to do. It deals with conduct as the subject of judicial judgement, not with conduct merely as a physical fact' (p.17). Muirhead promoted ethics as a science on the grounds that it aimed to explain moral imperatives, not merely describe them or define them within the context of some personal moral outrage, or expression of divine will. 'Theft is wrong', Muirhead argued, not (simply) because it is personally offensive, or offends some theological code, but because it showed 'disregard for other people's property [which] is inconsistent with that system of mutual relations which we call social life' (p.25).

Old questions and new challenges

Muirhead's view is particularly apposite since he saw his own age (the 1890s) as 'a time of moral and political unrest, resulting in a new demand among large numbers of the educated classes to understand the meaning of the moral code under which they live, and the institutions which support it' (p.10). His list of 'contradictions' and 'seemingly irreconcilable antitheses which . . . harass and perplex our age' reads like a catalogue of our contemporary crises:

> 'the field of religion, the opposition between faith and reason, science and religion, authority and private judgement . . . the antithesis between the individual and the state . . . on the one side are asserted 'the rights of man', on the other 'the duties of citizenship'. *Man versus State is the cause célèbre of the century.*'
>
> (p.10, emphasis added)

One hundred years later, we assume that the ethical challenges we face are somehow a function of global capitalism or are the *dénouement* of the twentieth century, as the millennium approaches. On reflection, we may only be facing age-old human problems which appear different, given the social context within which they arise.

This concern with the 'contradictions and antitheses' which perplex our age was evident also fifty years ago when the philosopher C.E.M. Joad described the collapse of the influence of religious values, and the effect this had on the youth of the day: 'Once the practice of virtue [was] identified with pleasing God . . . it is notorious today that heavenly rewards no longer attract and infernal punishments no longer deter with their pristine force; many people are frankly derisive of both' (Joad, 1942, p.209). One could be forgiven for assuming that Muirhead's and Joad's concern would mean that by the end of the century civilisation would have collapsed completely. Although the ethical status of (at least) Western society may be in a parlous state, interest in ethics – in its broadest applied sense – has, paradoxically, probably never been greater: from ecological concern for the planet, through concerns about factory farming, to concerns involving the effect of the media on 'young minds'.

Secular and religious pedigrees

As editors, we recognise that ethics is a form of inquiry closely related to other disciplines: anthropology, psychology and sociology, notwithstanding the close, and often direct, relationship with various religions. Indeed, much of what we accept as being 'right and fitting', in an ethical sense, is influenced greatly by the Judaeo-Christian ethic of our Western civilisation. However, we recognise that even the body of ideas about 'how people should live' which stems from a religious orientation, is multidimensional in character. Such ideas follow some kind of thread from Lao Tzu and Buddha (along with the Old Testament prophets) in the fifth and sixth centuries BC, the *axial age*, as Jaspers has called it, through Christ and Muhammad to the present. Although we might not always acknowledge it, our 'personal ethics' are as likely to be a function of Taoism, Buddhism or Islam – or any other creed – as a function of Judaism or Christianity. In our multi-cultural, post-modern society, this is increasingly so. Moreover, the possibility that anyone might develop a code of ethics which is *not* influenced by these traditions, seems most unlikely. We may think that we are facing new ethical problems, or are devising new principles to guide our practice, but our moral philosophy may be no more than further revisions of the thoughts of the many previous ethicists.

Ethics and religion have long been intertwined. If moral philosophy occupies a different intellectual space from religion, it follows a similar chronology: Also beginning around the fifth century BC, with Socrates, secular ethics is characterised, arguably, by as many schisms and factions as the many religious traditions.

Much of our moral philosophy derives from Greek thinkers who seem to have captured the mood of their contemporary culture. Plato presented the belief that justice and goodness were objective things, which existed beyond our everyday experience. Aristotle upheld the view that virtue was a natural phenomenon, and that we could acquire moral virtues – and, thus, happiness – by practice, in much the same way as we develop skills. These Greek philosophies were adopted by the Romans – especially Stoicism, who developed the belief that people should refrain from self-interest (and hedonism) and should promote the common good of humanity as part of their duty under providence.

In the 2000 years since, ethics has been shaped and re-shaped: from the Chinese philosophers who believed that the natural compassion of human beings was corrupted by adverse natural conditions; to those who represent the increasing challenge to a dominant masculine view of ethics, arguing that the moral sense of women is quite different from that of men. The common thread linking all these views of human conduct, down the ages and across civilisations, is the pursuit of some 'standard' which will apply irrespective of the situation in which people find themselves.

As noted, the assumption that ethics might provide us with a 'rule' or 'law' is linked to the many theological perspectives on human conduct. However, although theology may offer us further perspectives on *what* is right conduct, it does not reveal to us in a sufficiently compelling way *why* this is so. His interest in a science of ethics gave Freud some cause to challenge religious principles in this respect:

> Religion is an attempt to master the sensory world in which we are situated by means of the wishful world which we have developed within us as a result of biological and psychological necessities. But religion cannot achieve this. Its doctrines bear the imprint of the times in which they arose, the ignorant times of the childhood of humanity. Its consolations deserve no trust. Experience teaches us that the world is no nursery. The ethical demands on which religion seeks to lay stress need, rather, to be given another basis; for they are indispensable to human society and it is dangerous to link obedience to them with religious faith.
>
> (Freud, 1995, p.788)

Freud was evidently concerned that mere obedience to a Supreme Will would prevent us from ever internalising the kind of ethical code which humanity needed to develop, perhaps even to survive: 'Ethics is to be regarded as a therapeutic attempt – as an endeavour to achieve, by means of a command of the super-ego, something which has so far not been achieved by means of any other cultural activities.' (Gay, 1995, p.15)

THE SHAPING OF MORAL CONDUCT IN CONTEMPORARY CULTURE

Ethics can appear to be a fairly simple business: ethics is about how we ought to live. What makes an action right, rather than the wrong thing to do? What should our goals be? Having posed such simple questions, a flood of frustrating – and arguably even more fundamental questions – is begged: 'What do you mean by ethics anyway? Where do ethics come from? Will it ever be possible to find a rational way of deciding why we should do this rather than that?' The unresolved nature of such *meta-ethical* questions seems not to deter our expectation that ethics will provide some guidance for moral conduct. And yet the emerging ethical agenda is predicated on the recognition that ethics cannot be realistically imposed: we cannot make people moral either by decree of God or by Act of Parliament. In the 1960s organised religion began its slow decline in support and popularity. Ironically, the 1960s saw the relationship with a godhead re-defined in a dramatic and revolutionary manner.

Religious codes and relationships

Ethics has become more, rather than less, of a problem since Freud's day. We often assume that our societies are making progress and, especially as a result of our technological sophistication, we are in a better position to make ethical decisions. The opposite may well be the case. As Zohar (1990) has observed:

> People are not on the whole more self-realized or self-fulfilled than they were when Freud began his work. If anything, loneliness and alienation – alienation both from self and from others – are more of a problem of our time than of Freud's, as is the narcissism which underpins much of it.
>
> (p.140)

Our relations – with ourselves as much as with each other – have grown more, rather than less complex. These complexities may render it more difficult to decide what is 'right' or 'wrong' in terms of ethical conduct, in relation to ourselves and others. Bloom (1988) saw the development of 'relationships' between people – rather than old-fashioned 'love' – as one example of the growing complexity of 'self and others' which was the distant outcome of the popularisation of psychotherapy. People no longer are ruled by the view of marriage as a sacrament. In Bloom's view this kind of development emerged from the 'belief that by becoming more "inner-directed", going further down the path of the isolated self, people will be less lonely' (p.125). Somewhat pessimistically, Bloom believed that people have, however, in so doing, lost the capacity for friendship – as exemplified by Aristotle in *Ethics*. Friendship, like love, 'requires notions of soul and nature that, for a mixture of theoretical and political reasons, we cannot even consider' (pp.125–6).

The social, economic and political changes which have occurred since the 1960s have led to the further disintegration both of religion and also of the 'natural laws' which facilitated the co-existence of men and women. Nothing certain has taken its place.[3] If the established church was to survive, it had to adapt to these circumstances, and if possible capitalise on them. In 1963 the Bishop of Woolwich, John Robinson, published a highly controversial book, *Honest to God*, which relocated the sacred

---

[3] This view is relevant to the discussion throughout this book. Many of the authors may be trying to establish a kind of ethical certainty which simply is not possible. It is this *search* for ethical certainty which may, however, be the true ethical project and which, within the context of psychiatric nursing, may need to be seen as the core of our moral order.

within the sphere of *personal relations*. Robinson promised salvation by arguing that God was not something which was 'out there' but, rather, was something to be realized by a commitment to relationships involving love between individual human beings. Robinson's thesis, though provocative for the time, was hardly new. His argument derived from existential theologians – such as Bonhoeffer and Tillich – who had echoed Martin Heidegger's idea of the 'Divine' as 'the ground of Being: not a projection "out there", but a divinity manifest in every particular "thou" encountered through love, the unconditional element in all our relationships, and supremely in our relationships with other persons' (cited by Waugh, 1995, p.66). Robinson's reframing of the concept of the 'godhead' within the context of human relations led, indirectly, to the development of a spiritual rebirth within Christianity in England which remains a source of conflict. By relocating God within people Robinson shifted, perhaps unwittingly, the ethical framework also. No longer was it acceptable to simply follow rules of morality laid out in some ethical catechism. It was expected that people would explore the true meaning of 'good' and 'right' within their worldly relationships with others. From that point, ethics – as a theological event – appeared to join forces with moral philosophy in the fertilisation of a human science.

Psychotherapy, nursing and power

Psychiatric nursing is about healing within relationships. Perhaps there is a continuum in the work we do – at one end we keep people from harming themselves and others, sometimes against their will and using medication and restraint, as we judge that the social, interpersonal and intra-psychic effect of compromising their autonomy in this way is a lesser evil than the social, interpersonal and intra-psychic damage which would result from allowing them free reign. We believe it is the *right* thing to do. At the other end of the spectrum we contribute to the manifestation of the sacred in our personal relations with patients. But always it is the relationship which is the main medium of our effectiveness, or lack thereof. However, there are other forces at work in our sphere of activity, operating through our relationships with patients, and serving interests at odds perhaps with either the patient's or society's at large.

In *A Clockwork Orange*, Anthony Burgess addressed the concept of free will and the ethical limits of social engineering. His 'antihero', Alex, commits acts of pornographic violence to the accompaniment of Beethoven's sublime music. When Alex is, ultimately, 'reclaimed and rehabilitated' through aversion therapy he loses his violent instincts. He also loses his capacity to respond to art. In effect he becomes a 'nonperson'. Although Burgess's critique appeared to be focused on behavioural engineering, he had confessed also to a grave concern over the (British) welfare state's appropriation of Anna Freud's adaptive ego psychology. This emphasised adaptation and independent ego-functioning, and was a stark contrast to the received wisdom of the Freudian unconscious, with its intractable irrationality. The welfare state could – within ego psychology, as well as through employment of more behavioural methods – remedy any lapse in efficiency of personal identity. Such beliefs represented to Burgess 'a serious assault on human freedom and a dangerous denial of decent ethical limits upon social engineering' (Waugh, 1995: 146). Scenes from *One Flew Over the Cuckoo's Nest* (Kesey, 1973) may also spring to mind in relation to the psychic manipulation that can be effected through our role. When we sharpen our ethical focus on psychiatry and the care and treatment of people in mental distress, power and control emerge as critical characteristics.

Notwithstanding the contribution of psychiatric nursing to the secular and religious quest to explore and heal our relationships, it appears there is inevitably some manifestation of power, some furtherance of powerful interests, in our relationships with patients that demands further scrutiny. One may think not. Nurses are, after all, bound by a professional code which prohibits certain actions and activities. However, we would distinguish such a code of conduct from the kind of ethical problems which are the subject of this book. A compulsory morality, concerning itself largely with 'dramatic ethics', might be seen as equivalent to no morality at all. Nurses who act 'ethically' towards their patients only for fear of criticism or penalty and only concerning themselves with ethics at all in relation to such dramatic issues, might be regarded as having no professional morals. If ethical conduct does not arise freely and universally, as a function of choice and awareness, to what extent is it in any way 'ethical'?

Acting skilfully: the ethical thread

In this respect, it may be instructive to consider the framework for ethical practice offered by Buddhist philosophy. The point of practising ethics is, for a Buddhist, the development of wholesome states of being and relating with each other in the world – 'ethical' is a rough translation of *kusala*, which, more literally, means *skilful*. By practising *skilful* conduct, *emotionally vibrant* and *psychologically integrated* states of mind arise, which can occasion higher (meditative) states of consciousness. On the basis of refining these meditative (or spiritual) states, there arises, in turn, a receptivity to transformative visions of things as they really are, transcendental wisdom.

It may help to view this schema from a step further back. According to Buddhist thought, the three stages of human evolution (Ethics, Meditation and Wisdom) follow on from the evolutionary processes of biology that have brought us this far. On the basis of development in our psycho-physical organism, consciousness arises: we transcend the biological and move into a psychological realm. On the basis of development in our psychological organisation (consciousness), self-awareness arises, transcending the psychological realm and moving into something uniquely human. At this stage (and beyond) the individual has to work actively to achieve further development, the biological processes of psycho-physical being taking us only so far on the continuum of human evolution. It is claimed that individual endeavour, which takes over from biological development at this point in the schema, can make use of tools such as psychotherapy,[4] ethical conduct and meditation practice. One stands back and actively reflects on the processes of denial, projection etc. and their outcomes in terms of one's conduct, in order to act ethically and with self-awareness, and one then has to work at sitting and calming the mind rather than following distractions, in order to allow the stillness and peace with oneself to develop that will occasion meditative awareness. All of which serves to cultivate and prepare the ground for the arising of 'higher' states of consciousness still. This adds up to a sort of hierarchy of biological, psychological, ethical, aesthetic and spiritual refinement and transcen-

---

[4] Szasz (see Chapter 2) characterise 'psychoanalysis . . . with all its variations [as] conversations based in secular ethics'.

dence (all of which is seen as a platform from which to develop, or from which can arise, wisdom. None of the states described are ends in themselves.)

Although it may seem odd for the editors thus to promote such a specific system of thought, the reader is invited to consider the way this ethical system is shaped. There is neither divine injunction from God–Creator, nor any more local imperative from social, ideological or psychological sources. Morality is not imposed through domination by an over-developed super-ego in any form. Acting a particular way through fear, or submission, would not be skilful. In a devotional chant used daily by many Buddhists around the world, the merits of the 'three jewels' are enumerated. In singing the praises of the Dharma, the teachings, one quality ascribed to the Buddha's teachings is *ehipassiko*, which, translated, means 'of the nature of a personal invitation'. Which is to say, the ethical and other teachings of Buddhism are offered in the spirit of 'come and try it out for yourself, reflect, measure it against your own experience and see if it doesn't help'. It may well be that by following certain guidelines, after suitable reflection and readiness to 'own' the form of conduct prescribed, it is found that living this way helps, brings happiness, well-being, harmony; in short, it feels right and is good. This is a view of ethics and its place in a hierarchy of human evolution that appears to be gaining ground. It is far removed from a view which confines ethics to the letter of a rule book and allows the operation of power to influence or even determine our relationships, and it is a view which we would endorse.

SO WHAT'S THE POINT?

The dawning of a new age

Having set out a framework for ethical enquiry, the content of that enquiry needs to be addressed. We would argue that many of our contemporary ethical concerns are classic in character, addressing similar questions to those posited down the ages. These questions have, however, been reframed by a period of social and intellectual upheaval which began with the post-war cultural revolution of the 'Beat Generation', which soon was overtaken by the economic and cultural affluence of the 1960s.

Although associated mainly with literary life in the USA, the 'Beats' came to represent the generation of disaffected, yet committed, post-war youth who recognised the need for a major overhaul in the values of their times and the institutions which supported those values. The term 'beat' probably meant both 'beaten' and 'beatified', since many of the writers of the period 'felt crushed by the outmoded values of society, yet elevated by headiness of their own revolt' (McLeish, 1994). These American writers were a cultural echo of the 'Angry Young Men' in Britain who attacked the Establishment, not merely in thought and utterance, but in a social way (by letting us hear the voice of what one critic called 'the bright working class') (McLeish, 1994). The beat generation spawned that new phenomenon, the 'teenage culture'. For the first time young people found a public voice which challenged the canons of taste and morality of the day. By the end of the 1950s the boat was well and truly rocking and there was never any question of turning back.

With the 1960s began a process of dismantling and re-building on an unprecedented scale: this applied to intellectual traditions as much as to architecture. The wild optimism of the 1960s was only one side of the coin, the reverse being the fast-rising crime rate, the emergence of football hooliganism, race riots and political scandals, all of which continued through subsequent decades. The flirtation with drugs which began in the 'counterculture' of the 1950s and 1960s would also become the basis for a national drug problem completely detached from the idealistic consciousness-raising of the late 1960s 'flower children'. The generation which followed, especially the 'yuppies' of the 1980s, appeared to be founded on a wholly materialistic base, and occupied a moral and spiritual vacuum.

Glyn Jones (1996) would argue that history shows that all civilisations which rejected their spiritual and religious traditions in favour of materialism and 'science', ultimately collapsed under the weight of their 'empty' hedonism.

As the millennium approaches there is, however, a virtual renaissance of interest in spirituality – both religious and secular in character. Coupled with the growing awareness of ethical issues as diverse as politics, farming and child-rearing, perhaps the anticipated death of the post-modern society is premature.

Madness and reality

The 1960s also marked a critical phase in the development of the concept of mental health, presaging the beginning of the 'therapy era' and the more widespread influence of psychoanalysis as a method for interpreting both people and society. Psychoanalysis seemed able to provide what religion had once offered: 'a means of charting and making safe [life's] unknown terrain in existential and universal terms. It provided a means to dismantle the hell which was now oneself and other people, and thereby supplied a faith arrived at authentically through struggle and doubt' (Waugh, 1996, p.67). Thirty years on psychoanalysis appears to have lost its place within the 'church' of psychiatry, having been displaced by neuroscience and a re-invigorated biomedical model of mental illness. Psychoanalysis has been relegated to a world of private practice or 'fringe medicine' and probably has had most impact within the arts. Where psychological models are allowed entry into the field of mental health care they represent a largely positivist set of idealistic therapies: shaping and re-modelling people in variants of the marriage of behaviourism and ego psychology which so appalled Burgess in *A Clockwork Orange*.

However, those who have wished to exorcise completely the ghost of psychoanalysis have found that the task was not a simple one. We remain haunted by the concern that 'mad' behaviour may, after all, be a reflection of distress experienced either at the hands of others directly, or the effects of a 'mad' world, indirectly. Freud had originally recognised that some forms of 'psychopathology' were a consequence of childhood sexual abuse. When his colleagues could not tolerate the idea that fathers would sexually molest their children, he experienced a crisis of confidence, bowed to peer pressure and abandoned his 'seduction theory', replacing it with the notion that such 'memories' were no more than Oedipal fantasies (Masson, 1985). Ironically, in the 1990s, as we experience an epidemic of child abuse – both physical and sexual – we are faced with a reprise of Freud's confrontation with his peers. Now, however, the opposition is represented by parents – and their advocates – who charge therapists with cultivating, perhaps unwittingly, a 'false memory syndrome': encouraging children to recall episodes of sexual abuse which never happened.

The 1960s also saw the rise to prominence of a psychoanalyst and psychiatrist who appeared to have intellect and personality in sufficient measure to take up the Freudian mantle. R.D. Laing presented what we would regard as an almost self-evident hypothesis, that madness – in its most severe forms – was a function of relationships with the world, especially the parental world. His theory was easily distorted and translated into the tabloid psychology, which, despite clear disavowals on his part, he was ever after associated with, that 'families drove their children mad'. However, in the counterculture of the 1960s – when the 'teenage culture' began to grasp power for the first time – whether true or not, this was a liberating idea, and Laing was elevated almost overnight to the status of a guru and revolutionary visionary. Thirty years on Laing is dead, his memory is sadly vilified and his ideas misrepresented. Ironically, a popular theory of interpersonal relations which has been applied to schizophrenia – *expressed emotion* – acknowledges that families which are highly critical or suffocatingly supportive can provoke (unwittingly) psychotic crises (Leff *et al.*). This is evidently no more than a sanitised version of Laing and Esterson's original thesis (Laing and Esterson, 1964).

The ethical dilemma facing psychiatric nursing

From an ethical perspective, even if Laing was 'right' could we ever live and work with that version of reality? Ordinary people may have great difficulty in accepting unusual experiences, like psychosis, as a representation of 'reality'. Susan experiences tactile hallucinations and hears obscene voices shouting at her. Even if we could understand that these are part of her coping with the experience of childhood sexual abuse at the hands of her father from the age of 7, we may feel compelled to argue that there must, nevertheless, be something further *wrong* with her. It is just not right that she experiences the world in that way, when there *are* no voices or tactile sensations so far as anyone else is concerned. It just isn't reality!

Arguably though, it is not simple generosity to take the view that maybe she is right; that she should be free to experience her world in that way. Perhaps her most real knowledge of the world conveys a poetic accuracy to her 'psychotic' experience. We should not be surprised, however, that her experiences disrupt her career, or that her fragmented experience frightens us into treating the phenomena she witnesses (and treating Susan herself) as somehow alien. The inner world, with its subjective perspective, remains a largely uncharted territory. This is the realm of intuition and psychic experience, where religion and spiritual development surface and grow. Our increasing reliance on 'science' and our commitment to objectivity, have reduced our familiarity with the power of our own reflective awareness. Increasingly, the pathway into this world – via aesthetics, art, poetry – is diminished, as is our confidence in our own ethical sense. There is a big world 'inside there' where people like Susan find themselves thrown by their experiences, and where they may end up losing themselves. Although metaphorical, such places are no less real.

Our concern with empiricism as the dominant discourse within mental health care has largely ruled out a great deal of enquiry into such areas of human experience. It is little wonder that the experience of 'being human' is increasingly re-defined as a biological (neuroscientific) event. European philosophy – especially existentialism and, more recently, post-modernism – which once promised a methodology to unravel some of the mysteries of human experience, appears to have drifted so far into the poetic and arcane that many of us find it hard to fathom and impossible to follow. There is a danger that psychiatric nursing will lose the thread of human enquiry, personified originally by the pioneering work of Peplau, who explored the context of the nurse–patient relationship with people in psychosis; and later by Altschul, who described, in more general detail, the nature of the bonding which took place when nurse first met patient.

Much of the early promise of psychological explanations of madness appear unfulfilled. Laing charted his own chaotic course from early work in traditional mental hospitals, through the Kingsley Hall experimental therapeutic community, progressing through his phenomenological critique of psychoanalysis to psychedelia, to spend a year in contemplation in a Buddhist monastery in Ceylon. His quest for understanding took him from guru status to an extended period as an alcoholic outsider, appearing fitfully on television chat shows. There is a danger that the only 'new voice' in the last half of the century of psychiatry may be buried, along with his ideas and ideals. More importantly for us, there is a danger that the most significant voices in psychiatric nursing history, namely Peplau and Altschul, may be buried, metaphorically, along with him. In our view, any such burial would not only be premature, but would represent an attempt to deny the importance of the enquiry into the human conditions which represent 'madness' in its truest forms.

Attempts by Klein and others from the analytical psychotherapy schools to provide an 'interior' account of the structure of experience, often meander into such implausibility and convolution that the efforts of critics, like Masson (1992) to discredit the entire enterprise of psychotherapy have found widespread favour. We should not forget, however, that Masson's popularity may also be a reflection of the abuse of power for which psychotherapy and psychiatry deserves to be castigated (Szasz, 1961; 1996). The widespread popularity of the psychotherapeutic critique also may reflect the genuine difficulties encountered in attempting a plausible, scientific, falsifiable account of the subjective universe. This should, however, come as no surprise. Our increasingly 'scientific' culture largely denies the very existence of an interior universe. Wittgenstein – a deeply religious man – characterised the nature of the problem: 'there is something further . . . you can't say it; . . . the most essential part of . . . experience . . . cannot be described . . . it is this idea which plays hell with us' (Wittgenstein, 1953, para 304). This difficulty should not, however, deter us from attempting to develop an approach which might allow us to acknowledge the validity and uniqueness of individual experience, if not also help us to appreciate further how a subjective reality might be the starting-point for the development of a new understanding of, and relationship with, 'mental illness'.

If the experiential significance and spiritual potential of psychiatric crisis, and the power-ethic problems identified earlier are to be taken seriously, one might view them as the defining moral dilemmas of psychiatric nursing practice. They are certainly the two main ethical themes emerging from the chapters that follow.

CONCLUSION

Sprigge (1988) acknowledged that philosophers were 'as bad at reaching agreement with each other on the nature of moral judgement (or anything else) as humans in general seem to be on what is right and wrong, or rather much worse' (p.5). We agree that any 'philosophy' may, by allowing us an 'insight into one aspect of things tend to blind us to other aspects'. In that sense, some contributors to this book will appear to disagree with others. At this stage of our professional development, this can only be a good thing. Our quest for ethical understanding involves not only asking 'how should we live?' but also 'how can we help others live?' and also 'should we help others live?' It is hardly surprising if different people's responses conflict.

Psychiatric nursing has come of age in this final quarter of the century, having begun to realise its own value as a therapeutic medium and, as nurses increasingly work alone in community settings, finally recognising that it might become an autonomous mental health promotion medium. It is clear that psychiatric nursing has changed more in the past quarter century than it changed in the preceding two hundred years. Those changes have brought new freedoms and, in their wake, the likelihood of new dangers and restrictions. Nurses can no longer rely on the institutional psychiatrist for support and guidance. In many residential settings the programme is 'nurse-led' and in the community, where much of the care is being re-located, the nurse is responsible *and* accountable. More and more nurses are described as 'therapists' in their own right; many more are case managers, which often means managing, independently, the care of the most distressed and disadvantaged people in the community. Those who still work in teams in hospital settings are likely to be responsible for people with highly complex problems, since only the most distressed or vulnerable people receive hospital care. The challenges faced by nurses, often against a background of diminishing resources, if not also a 'hospital closure programme' culture, are considerable indeed. For many of today's nurses, deciding 'how they should live' and what, exactly, is the meaning of 'good' and 'right' in nursing terms, is likely to become a process of career-long inquiry.

We hope that the contributors in this book will, at the very least, chart some of the dilemmas, a taste of which we have offered above, which face the discipline. The range of ethical problems in psychiatric nursing is wide and there are few, if any, clear-cut answers. Readers will, doubtless, be reassured to learn that their dilemmas are not only shared by others, but tax the minds of even those who have tried, systematically, to find an answer to such problems. In the final analysis, however, we expect readers to arrive at their own appreciation of 'goodness'. By following the vague and often meandering path through this text, we hope that readers may find some of the answers which brought them to this book in the first place. More, importantly, we hope the reader will gain a clearer sense of the meaning of ethical strife.

REFERENCES

Bloom, A. 1988: *The closing of the American mind.* London: Penguin.

Burnard, P. and **Chapman, C.M.** 1988: *Professional and ethical issues in nursing: the code of professional conduct.* Chichester: John Wiley.

Cambell, A.V. 1979: Plato. Apology 3A. In *Moral dilemmas in medicine.* Edinburgh: Churchill Livingstone.

Freud, S. 1995a: Lecture XXXV: The question of a Weltanschauung. In P. Gay (ed.), *The Freud reader.* London: Vintage, 788.

Freud, S. 1995b: Civilisation and its discontents. In P. Gay (ed.), *The Freud reader.* London: Vintage, 740.

Glyn Jones, A. 1996: *Holding up a mirror: how civilizations decline.* Century.

Hare, R.M. 1952: *The language of morals*. Oxford: the Clarendon Press.

Joad, C.E.M. 1942: *Guide to modern thought*. London: Faber & Faber.

Laing, R.D. and **Esterson, A.** 1964: *Sanity, madness and the family*. Harmondsworth: Penguin.

Locke, J. 1964: *An essay concerning human understanding*. Ed. A.D. Woozley, Glasgow: Collins.

McLeish, K. 1994: *Key ideas in human thought*. London: Bloomsbury.

Masson, J.M. 1985: *The assault on truth: Freud's suppression of the seduction theory*. London: Penguin.

Masson, J. 1992: *Against therapy*. London: Collins.

Muirhead, J.H. 1892: *The elements of ethics*. London: John Murray.

Rhees, R. (ed.) 1968: Wittgenstein's Notes of Lectures on 'Private experience' and 'Sense Donton', *The Philosophical Review* **77**, 271–320.

Sprigge, T.L.S. 1988: *Rational foundations of ethics*. London: Routledge.

Szasz, T. 1961: *The myth of mental illness*. New York: Hoeber-Harper.

Szasz, T. 1996: The case against psychiatric power, paper presented to conference 'The Construction of Psychiatric Authority,' University of Newcastle, 18 June 1996.

Thiroux, J.P. 1980: *Ethics, theory and practice*. Glencoe, CA.: The Glencoe Publishing Co.

Thompson, I.E., Melia, K.M. and **Boyd, K.M.** 1983: *Nursing ethics*. Edinburgh: Churchill Livingstone.

Waugh, P. 1995: *Harvest of the sixties: English literature and its background – 1960 to 1990*. Oxford: Oxford University Press.

Wittgenstein, L. 1953: *Philosophical investigations*. Oxford: Blackwell.

Zohar, D. 1990: *The quantum self*. Flamingo: London.

Part 1

Social Relations

Although the common assumption is that mental illness[1] is located in people's heads, virtually everything which is the business of psychiatry goes on between people. And much of what goes on between staff and patients[1] is often little more than a distant echo of what went on between the patient and other significant people in his life:

> Psychiatric patients expect to be controlled, manipulated, used and derogated or belittled, and in general seen as largely worthless. . . . Each staff member who does confirm these expectations, wittingly or unwittingly, reinforces the expectations and convinces the patient that subsequent persons will likewise reinforce them.
>
> (Peplau, 1994 pp. 91–2)

Peplau's observation acknowledges not only the translatory power of interactions between people where one is – or is presumed to be – helpless, but also what might be understood in a wider context to represent the essentially social nature of mental health care and treatment.

In Part 1 the contributors address the roots of our 'working ethics' in our social relations. The assumption that probably lies behind all of the following chapter is that any psychiatric disorder is itself, essentially, a social construct. But this assumption is merely alluded to, not discussed in any formal sense, as it has been addressed by many other authors whose work is used as philosophical anchors. The following eight chapters explore the ramifications of the way in which psychiatric illness is socially constructed. Specifically, they delineate ethical issues for mental health and psychiatric nursing care emerging at a macroscopic level and from a broad societal perspective.

The chapters contribute to the further development of ethical critiques from two main ideological perspectives on psychiatry which emerged in the 1960s. The first of these perspectives, explored in chapters 2 to 5, focuses on issues of power and its abuse, as well as related economic and social factors, which underpin people's alienation and distress. The thrust of these chapters is that since abuse of power has been defined by various authorities, especially Illich (1975; 1977) and Szasz (1972), as a characteristic feature of all medical services and one of the critical characteristics of psychiatry, there is considerable potential within our professional practice for further exploitation of vulnerability and mis-handling of power over people. This is, of course, of the utmost importance to us as workers in this field. The way power is manifest in our relationships, through our institutions, interwoven with our professional status is an ethical concern that demands particular and immediate scrutiny. Both naturally occurring (i.e. interpersonal) power and also power which is legally constructed are implicated.

Chapter 2 concerns principles of justice and democracy. The constitutional and ethical status of psychiatry as an organ of state is explored and its legitimacy in this respect called into question. Chapter 3 examines the way in which we participate in this organ of state as 'front-line' workers. Professional notions of care are compromised by the legal powers and the

---

[1] Throughout the book a number of different terms will be used to describe people and whatever ails them. We begin here by using the traditional terms since, presumably, the conventional naming of states and people associated with such states represents a starting-point for ethical enquiry.

social mandate bestowed on psychiatric nurses to control. Chapter 4 examines the nature of professionalised mental health care in relation to these themes. All workers in the 'psyche industry' have a duty to scrutinise the operation of their professional and personal interest as in probable conflict, at some level, with the interests of their patients. Chapter 5 seeks to define an ethically sound role for psychiatric nurses. A framework is set out for psychiatric nursing practice which may avoid some of the aforementioned ethical pitfalls.

The next four chapters develop this Part's second focus, which is more of an ethical opportunity than an ethical hazard. Chapters 6 to 9 offer an overview of the way in which individuals struggle to reconstruct and make sense of their experience. While accounts and details of such struggles are left to Part 2 of the book, here the process of developing personal meaning for psychiatric disorder is explored in general terms, as a powerful tool in facing adversity and an important aspect of individual growth. Endorsement is thus given to consideration of the spiritual aspect of psychiatric experience and the pastoral component to psychiatric nursing care, framing breakdown as potential breakthrough and the healing process as a pilgrimage through adversity. The thrust of these chapters is that we have an ethical obligation to work in this way and promote healing through participating with clients in a political, social and emotional reconstruction, certainly, but also offering a spiritual recon-struction of their experience.

Chapter 6 considers the emergence, meaning and ethical basis of the 'anti-psychiatry' movement. It is possible to create an institution whose ethos is one of shared pilgrimage and where care and healing are promoted, rather than control and treatment. Chapter 7 examines the notion of 'pilgrimage' in more detail. There is a theoretical basis and further practical implications of using creative symbolism and religious imagery in effecting growth from crisis. Chapter 8 explores hurdles at a personal level that need to be overcome in order to do so. There may be a form of psychopathology associated with being a psychiatric nurse or working in an allied profession that should be understood and journeyed through if one is to help others on their journey. Chapter 9 concludes this section with an account of the position in which the preceding analysis leaves us. Politically, professionally, socially and spiritually, what does it mean to take an ethical stand?

Our aim in this Part has been to transcend the traditional polarisation of such 'political' and 'personal' perspectives. The ethical analyses offered recognise the contribution of political, economic and interpersonal issues to the construction and 'colouring' of experiences conven-tionally described as 'mental illness'. They also acknowledge the existence and importance of an 'inner world', accessible to introspection and representing the subjective reflection of individuals' spiritual struggles. We, as editors, wish to emphasise the complementary nature of such socio-political and spiritual perspectives.

References

Illich, I. 1975: *The expropriation of health*. London: Calder Boyars.
Illich, I. 1977: *Limits to medicine*. London: Penguin.
Peplau, H.E. 1994: Psychiatric nursing: the nurse's role in preventing chonicity. In O'Toole, A.W. and Welt, S.R. (eds), *Hildegard E. Peplau: selected works: interpersonal theory in nursing*. London: Macmillan.
Szasz, T.S. 1972: *The myth of mental illness*. St Albans: Paladin.

2

FREEDOM, PSYCHIATRY AND RESPONSIBILITY[1],[2]

Jeffrey Schaler

Part I commences with a treatise on political philosophy. An odd opening for a text on psychiatric nursing ethics? Consider the assertion by Szasz (1970, p. 179) that 'Organized medicine is now as much a part of the American government as organized religion had been of the government in fifteenth-century Spain.' The point is that the connection between psychiatry and state, psychiatry *as an organ of state*, is a profoundly undemocratic, not to say unconstitutional development. Jeff Schaler develops this argument methodically and plainly, so that there should be no doubt in the reader's mind by the end that something hugely surreal has taken place in our experience, if we believe that mental illness as defined by psychiatrists is any more 'real' than the energy channels in Chinese acupuncture theory or the chakras in Eastern mysticism and yoga. The only difference between these three sets of hypothesised phenomena is that psychiatry is backed up by force of law and the power of the state.

If you are feeling a little overwhelmed by the craziness, the frenetic energy and the insensitivity of people around you and sense that you need to protect yourself from their influence, you may choose to go to a yoga teacher for some sort of guidance. When the teacher gives you some advice based on an idea that you are particularly susceptible to malevolent influences in the ether, you may decide that you don't really believe in all this. If you doubt the potential for psychic transmission and prefer to avoid thinking about the opening of chakras around your third eye, there is not that much your yoga teacher can do about it. However, if your experience becomes a little more exaggerated, and you come before a psychiatrist who can't think what to do about the situation but decides you may be at some risk with these ideas, you may not be wise to assume that you are free simply to take his advice or leave it.

It should be clear that the power within psychiatry to deprive people of their freedom is by no means *necessarily* good. Which is not to say that people should not, on occasion, be so

---

[1] One of three lectures presented at the Institute for Humane Studies Liberty and Society Seminar, The First Amendment and Beyond, Babson College, Babson Park, Massachusetts, July 24 1996.

[2] This article originally appeared in *Psychnews International*, volume 1, issue 4 (July, 1996) and is reprinted here by permission. To subscribe to Psychnews International, send the following command to 'listserv@listserv.nodak.edu': 'subscribe psychnews yourfirstname yourlastname.'

deprived. Neither have we made any claims so far as to what structures might (or indeed should) take the place of institutional psychiatry as an organ of state to protect people from being harmed by someone out of control, or to protect such people from harming themselves. Nor, indeed, have we said what might be best to help such people calm down. To such matters, the contributors will return in due course. For now, let us begin at the beginning, and set the debate in context with a little political philosophy and consideration of the issues of freedom, psychiatry and responsibility.

Congress shall make no law repecting an establishment of religion, or prohibiting the free exercise thereof.

Amendment I, The Constitution of the United States

In examining the consequences of state-sanctioned psychiatry in society today, it is instructive to compare Thomas Jefferson's thoughts about religion and the state with Thomas Szasz's thoughts about medicine and the state (Szasz, 1963; 1965; 1987). Jefferson was an advocate of the establishment and free exercise clauses, which guarantee freedom *from* and *of* religion, respectively. Both were written to protect individuals from a despotic state in unique ways. Szasz has proposed a new constitutional amendment, extending those guarantees to medicine: 'Congress shall make no law respecting an establishment of medicine, or prohibiting the free exercise thereof' (Szasz, 1970, p. 179).

Jefferson considered 'the constitutional freedom of religion the most inalienable and sacred of all human rights' (7 October 1822). With James Madison, he sought to protect society from the deprivation of liberty that would result from a theocratic state. Szasz considers freedom of thought and action the most inalienable and sacred of all human rights. He warns against the deprivation of liberty caused by a therapeutic state, i.e., a state entangled with the institution of medicine.

'To Jefferson . . . the institution of the Church . . . was the enemy of freedom and the ally of obscurantism' (Padover, 1970, p.43). To Szasz, institutional psychiatry, i.e., state-sanctioned psychiatry, is the enemy of freedom and the ally of obscurantism: 'Organized Medicine is now as much a part of the American government as Organized Religion had been of the government in fifteenth-century Spain' (Szasz, 1970, p. 179).

> 'Jefferson's critical attitude did not extend to the ethical teachings of religion, which he accepted, but to its political alignments and aspects, which he rejected. Religion was a menace to a free society when it was either an instrument of the State, as with Lutheranism in Prussia, or when it used the State for its sanguinary purposes, as in Inquisition-ridden Spain. There was sufficient historical evidence to prove that the partnership of Church and State had always led, and perforce must lead, to tyranny and oppression. 'In every country and in every age,' Jefferson said, 'the priest has been hostile to liberty. He is always in alliance with the despot, abetting his abuses in return for protection of his own.' So long as the Church was woven into the same fabric as the State, a self-governing commonwealth based upon justice and freedom was a fool's illusion. What Jefferson wanted, and ultimately achieved, was liberty – liberty, fully protected by the law, to believe or not believe whatever a man saw fit' (Padover, 1970, pp. 43–4).

Note that Jefferson supported liberty to believe or not believe whatever a man saw fit, including religious beliefs. Jefferson was interested in protection of *any* and *all* beliefs.

Szasz's critical attitude does not extend to the ethical teachings of psychoanalysis *per se*, which he accepts (with all its variations, i.e. the conversations based in secular ethics called 'psychotherapy'), but to its political alignments and aspects, which he rejects. Institutional psychiatry (as opposed to contractual psychiatry) is a menace to a free society when used as an instrument of the state. There is sufficient historical evidence to prove that the partnership of psychiatry and the state has always led, and perforce must lead, to tyranny and oppression. In every country and since psychiatry's invention, the institutional psychiatrist has been hostile to liberty.

So long as institutional psychiatry is woven into the same fabric as the state, an autonomous, free society based on the Rule of Law is a fool's illusion. What Szasz wants is liberty fully protected by the law, liberty to believe or not to believe whatever people see fit, and the liberty to act responsibly in relation to others

Had Szasz been alive in Jefferson's time he'd have written and spoken out against the theocratic state. If Jefferson were alive today, he would write and speak out against the therapeutic state. Jefferson is a hero; Szasz is (for the time being) a heretic.

PSYCHIATRY IS THE NEW CHURCH

Today, institutional psychiatry is the church Jefferson criticised so passionately. Religious concepts of good and evil have been replaced with psychiatric concepts of mental health and illness. An unconstitutional alliance exists between medicine and the state, and criticism of that alliance is discouraged, if not punished.

Institutional psychiatry is the enemy of freedom in a least three specific ways: (1) innocent persons are regarded as guilty, deprived of liberty and forcibly committed to psychiatric 'treatment' for 'mental illness'; (2) guilty persons are regarded as innocent by reason of insanity and committed to a psychiatric facility for treatment of mental illness; (3) persons accused of a crime are deprived of their constitutional right to due process (the Fifth and Sixth Amendments) when they are diagnosed as mentally incompetent and meet the actual legal criteria for competency to stand trial (when those accused meet the legal criteria for competency, they understand the charges brought against them, are able to assist counsel with their defence and understand the proceedings of the court). The legal, psychiatric circumvention of constitutional protections against these assaults on individual liberty is the working of the Rule of Man masquerading as the Rule of Law. These assaults are discriminatory. The law is applied to support bias and partiality.

Psychiatric and religious diagnoses are threats to liberty only when the state is involved, i.e. when they exist as formal, not informal, sanctions. If separation of state and medicine were to occur, in the same way separation of church and state now exists, the use of institutional psychiatry to deprive persons of liberty and responsibility for their behaviour would be impossible. Psychiatric diagnoses are moral judgements disguised as medical ones. The separation of medicine and state would no more destroy psychiatry than the separation of church and state has destroyed religion. People would still be free to find meaning in psychiatry and psychotherapy, just as they now find meaning in any number of diverse religious beliefs and practices. Problems arise when people do not want to abide by the dictates of psychiatry and religion and are coerced into doing so.

The authority of religious institutions was unchallenged in the past because opposition could be punished by the state. Also, the leaders of these institutions convinced people they knew more about the purpose and meaning of life than anyone else. They used mystical language to intimidate people into obedience, e.g. the fear of something bad happening if religious teaching was not obeyed. A symbolic world, i.e. heaven, hell, etc., was reified. Religious rhetoric obscured social control. Recognising the tactic, Jefferson and Madison constructed an invisible wall of separation between church and state to safeguard against such abuse.

What people often fail to recognise is how institutional psychiatry is now used in similar ways. During the Inquisition, denying the existence of witches was viewed as a 'sign' of being a witch. Today, denying the existence of mental illness is viewed as a 'sign' of mental illness. As Karl Kraus wrote: 'The psychiatrist unfailingly recognizes the madman by his excited behavior on being incarcerated' (Szasz, 1976, p. 127). The church, in a theocracy, can punish a person for heresy because the state enforces such religious diagnoses. When church and state were separated by the First Amendment, the power to enforce religious diagnoses was rendered harmless. *Mutatis mutandis*. Institutional psychiatry can punish a person for medical heresy because the state has the power to enforce such psychiatric diagnoses. The individual is no match against the power of the state. If medicine and state were separate, the power to enforce such psychiatric diagnoses would be rendered harmless.

It is important to remember that religious belief is just one category of belief. Jefferson was very clear about this. The Constitution protects *any* belief. Freedom of religious belief and practice is the right to believe *whatever* one chooses to believe, and to act on that belief in any way, as long as such action does not infringe upon the freedom of others.

The free exercise clause protects the right of belief – especially the right to atheism. The establishment clause protects against state endorsement of, i.e. entanglement with, religion. The state must remain neutral in matters of personal belief. It must not condone or reject any particular belief system or behaviour based on that belief system. In other words, the state must stay out of the individual citizen's head. Yet institutional psychiatry is used by the state to get 'inside' a person's head.

Many people believe God is more real than mental illness. Denying the existence of mental illness is no different from atheism. Belief is belief, whether it be belief in God, aliens, Satan, etc. Beliefs cannot be protected on the basis of validity. If that were the case, mental illness would be considered more real than God. (The idea of mental illness is a historically new phenomenon. The idea of God is a slightly older one.) While all beliefs are heretical to some, under our Constitution a person cannot be deprived of liberty on the basis of any beliefs.

LITERAL VERSUS METAPHORICAL CONDITIONS

We can understand more about how a therapeutic state deprives people of liberty by examining the situations in which involuntary treatment, i.e. medical treatment without one's consent, is *not* considered unconstitutional. There are three situations in which medical treatment may be administered without consent. The first is when a person is literally unconscious. For example, a person is in an accident and is rendered unconscious; medical treatment is administered because the person is literally incapable of giving consent. To wait for the person to regain consciousness (if ever) could result in more serious injury or death.

The second situation occurs when a person is literally a child. For example, a child is sick and needs a blood test or throat culture, but the child objects to medical tests and treatment. Medical procedures are administered despite the child's objections because the child is viewed as incapable of understanding the consequences of treatment refusal. An adult, in contrast, can refuse medical treatment for life-threatening illness.

The third situation occurs when a person is literally contagious with an infectious disease, for example, a student at a university is diagnosed with contagious meningitis. In such a case, a person can be quarantined and treated without consent for the protection of others.

In each of these three situations, literal signs (objective symptoms) and sometimes accompanying symptoms (subjective signs) are an integral part of treatment without consent. Rarely is treatment administered without consent solely on the basis of symptoms alone. In the first case, the person is incapable of responding to requests for consent. In the second case, the person is incapable of understanding the consequences of refusal. In the third case, the person is treated to protect others. If the person did not pose a literal threat to others, he or she would not be treated without consent.

Institutional psychiatrists pervert similar situations to justify social control measures. They do so by calling metaphorical conditions literal ones, e.g. mental illness. Moreover, all diagnoses and treatment of mental illness are based on symptoms, not signs. With real diseases it is the other way around. This is the institutional psychiatric version of religious obscurantism.

Let's use the involuntary commitment procedure as an example to explore further the justifications used by institutional psychiatrists. When people exhibit abnormal behaviour, and theoretically constitute a threat to themselves, they may be committed to a psychiatric facility against their will. The institutional psychiatrist, supported by a judge, asserts that these individuals do not know what they are doing, i.e. they are acting unconsciously. They are not literally unconscious but metaphorically unconscious. People cannot 'act unconsciously'. 'Acting unconscious' (not pretending to be unconscious) is an oxymoron.

A second justification used by institutional psychiatrists is claiming that mentally ill persons are like children. 'Being a child' is different from 'being like a child'. Because persons designated as mentally ill act like children, institutional psychiatrists argue they are incapable of understanding the consequences of refusing treatment. Thus, they are committed to psychiatric treatment despite their objections. But an adult labelled mentally ill is not a literal child. He or she is a metaphorical child.

A third justification used by institutional psychiatrists to commit persons to a mental hospital is to claim the persons labelled mentally ill are a threat to others. That's the metaphorical equivalent of being literally contagious. Yet no matter how bizarre people's behaviour, their behaviour is not literally contagious. It's contagious only in the metaphorical sense. If people are a literal threat to others, that's a matter for the criminal justice system. Moreover, people cannot be deprived of liberty on mere grounds of suspicion. That's why the Constitution guarantees due process of law.

In each of these three examples, the institutional psychiatrist literalises a metaphorical condition (the means) in order to justify deprivation of liberty (the end). One irony here is worth noting. One of the criteria used to diagnose a person as psychotic is his or her failure to discriminate between symbolic and real, i.e. the metaphorical and the literal. If institutional psychiatrists are incapable of recognising the difference between metaphorical and literal unconsciousness, metaphorical and literal children, and metaphorical and literal contagions, then they've met their own criteria for psychosis! If they recognise the difference, on what basis do they have the right to deprive people of liberty when they have broken no law?

In each of these three examples, a diagnosis is made on the basis of the beliefs a person holds concerning self and others, as well as the expression of those beliefs. Again, from a constitutional point of view, the accuracy of those beliefs is irrelevant. People are free to believe in and express their belief in God; to deny the existence of God; and to act on the basis of those beliefs. Moreover, freedom of religion is not contingent upon a physiological correlate. Neither should freedom of belief and thought be. People should not be deprived of liberty because a physiological component to mental illness is hypothesised.

LIBERTY AND RESPONSIBILITY

Responsibility and liberty are positively correlated. The more we expect people to be responsible for their behaviour, the more we increase liberty. The inverse is also true. We deprive people of liberty when we claim they are not responsible for their behaviour. Concurrently, the more we assert that people are not responsible for their behaviour, the more we treat people as if they were unconscious, as if they were children or as if they had a contagious disease. Each of the three justifications for involuntary commitment by institutional psychiatrists, i.e. deprivations of liberty, is a claim regarding personal responsibility.

Another way of viewing involuntary commitment is by examining the imposition of 'right' belief systems. When the state deprives a person of liberty because of mental illness, the state, through its agent the institutional psychiatrist, is making a law respecting an establishment of religion and prohibiting the free exercise thereof. It establishes a religion when it rewards 'right' beliefs and punishes 'wrong' beliefs. It prohibits 'the free exercise thereof' when it deprives a person of liberty of thinking and expressing beliefs in heretical ways. When people make certain and unacceptable claims about self and the world, it prohibits the free speech based in those beliefs.

CONCLUSION

The Constitution was written for all men, women and children – not legal, medical or religious experts. It is, like death, a great equaliser. As such, it should be applied in an impartial manner, respecting the diversity of beliefs as beliefs, regardless of whether those beliefs are religious or not. That's the Rule of Law. A therapeutic state interprets the Constitution to support bias and partiality. It discriminates between mentally healthy and mentally ill citizens. That's the Rule of Man. The only way to safeguard against such despotism is to interpret the Constitution as it was intended to be interpreted. Religion masquerading as medicine has no place in the state.

REFERENCES

Padover, S.K. 1970: *Jefferson*. New York: Mentor.

Szasz, T.S. 1963: *Law, liberty and psychiatry: an inquiry into the social uses of mental health practices*. New York: Macmillan.

Szasz, T.S. 1965: *Psychiatric justice*. New York: Macmillan.

Szasz, T.S. 1970: *The manufacture of madness: a comparative study of the Inquisition and the mental health movement*. New York: Harper & Row.

Szasz, T.S. 1976: *Karl Kraus and the soul doctors*. Baton Rouge, LA: Louisiana State University Press.

Szasz, T.S. 1987: *Insanity: the idea and its consequences*. New York: John Wiley & Sons.

3

SOCIETY, DISTURBANCE AND ILLNESS

Richard Lakeman and Brenda Curzon

Notwithstanding the objections in the previous chapter, psychiatry is charged by the state to control the behaviour of people who are, as a result of their 'mental illness', a danger to themselves or others. Such people are 'held', often against their will, in psychiatric institutions. Richard Lakeman and Brenda Curzon here explore nurses' compromised positions against a backdrop of barely compatible pressures and influences, professional, legal, social and political, if they try to offer care rather than enforce control. The chapter focuses on the construction of dangerousness, balancing intrapsychic and social interpretations of what makes people violent, and asks to what extent is 'dangerousness', in any event, 'in the eye of the beholder'. Clinical case study material illustrates the particular challenges faced by nurses in a prison setting, but the institutional difficulties for any nurse trying to care rather than control are underlined.

INTRODUCTION

More often than not, deviant behaviour attributable to mental disturbance is benign in nature, but sometimes it poses a real danger to the physical safety of self and others. For some the conceptualisation of unusual experience/behaviour as dangerous is automatic. Societies are challenged by such unusual phenomena. They pose a challenge to social order, the predictability of daily life. Prejudice and fear surface, as do calls for containment and control. Nurses who choose to work with the dangerous individual are faced with numerous ethical dilemmas in daily practice. They are faced with sometimes paradoxical mandates to care and control, in environments that are often not conducive to caring or therapy. A matrix of organisational, political, legislative, social and ideological pressures impinge on and shape each personal encounter, challenging the ideals of nursing. This chapter considers the issue of care and control. It suggests how such a dilemma has arisen and causes ongoing ethical strife for nurses and society.

Mental illness and mental health public policy have over the last few years become a regular feature of discussion in the popular press in New Zealand. In 1992 the Mental Health Act was rewritten to support the compulsory treatment of people in the least restrictive environment. People can now only be forced to receive treatment if their mental disorder gives rise to a seriously diminished capacity to care for themselves or their behaviour poses a serious danger to themselves or others. Large, rural psychiatric hospitals are being closed to free resources for community care.

Over the last two decades smaller acute psychiatric facilities have been built with the objective of providing short periods of respite, stabilisation and treatment when needed. The bulk of care and treatment is provided by community teams. Sheltered accommodation in the community with varying levels of supervision is offered to people who are unable to manage living independently. These changes have occurred against a backdrop of under-resourcing, public fear, resistance, and a string of tragic events involving 'psychiatric patients' that have effectively overshadowed any positive benefits to either society or individuals from these changes.

A perusal of a local newspaper illustrates the extent of public concern over recent and pending changes in the mental health system and how strongly dangerousness is seen to be associated with mental illness. Recently a man captured the nation's attention and ultimately a fatal bullet, after breaking into a sports store and shooting indiscriminately at passers-by. Shortly before his death it was disclosed that he had been treated for schizophrenia for some twenty years or more. In recent weeks, family members and the Salvation Army had spoken to the community psychiatric nurse involved about the need for secure treatment due to disturbing changes in the man's mental state. There were no facilities available (short of a prison cell) in the immediate vicinity, even had the nurse and the psychiatrist judged that the man posed an immediate danger to others.

A psychopaedic hospital is closing in a nearby town and residents are being relocated to smaller, family-like, sheltered accommodation. The tragedy outlined above has added more fuel to the already brightly burning fire of community resistance to the move. Parents of residents at the hospital talk of their fears that their children will not get the support and supervision they need in the community, and staff are reported to warn about the risks of releasing residents, 'who include paedophiles, sociopaths and arsonists' (Martin, 1995). The newspaper warns that Health authorities who have failed to provide adequate care and prevent seriously mentally disturbed people committing violent crimes may face legal action (Guyan, 1995a; p.1).

Dangerousness is an emotive issue, with public perception of the mentally ill as being violent, influencing the acceptance of people with mental illness in the community. In the same newspaper, Guyan (1995b) cites figures from police national headquarters, which she claims reveal that 13 of the 'worst murders' between 1992 and 1994 were committed by people with psychiatric conditions. Violence by some people with mental illness adds to the stigma and fear associated with mental illness, effectively making victims of the non-violent majority. Bowler (1995), a resident of a psychopaedic hospital for 17 years stated in a letter to the editor entitled 'Let inmates have their say', 'I don't think it's true what they're saying about the people in there. They are not all bad. I would like to see them have a chance'.

The assessment and labelling of someone as dangerous, whether justified or not, are moral judgements with far-reaching implications and consequences for that person. These might include the deprivation of personal freedom and sometimes compulsory treatment for a mental disorder. This is often justified as being in the best interests of the patient or society. The labelling of someone as dangerous is also of a socio-political judgement. If dangerousness is taken only as a prediction of the likelihood of an individual to cause serious physical violence to another, then the rights or good of the individual must still be weighed against the rights or good of society. Psychiatry has a legally sanctioned mandate to identify and treat those whom are deemed dangerous because of a mental disorder. It is arguable, however, whether much violence can be attributed to mental disorder or, indeed, whether anyone can accurately predict most violent behaviour.

Health professionals have been shown to be poor in their predictions of future dangerousness. Bootzin and Acocella (1984 p. 557) claim that 'every study of predictions of dangerousness has yielded far more false positives than negatives'. That is, health professionals are far more likely to falsely identify someone as dangerous than falsely identify someone as benign. This assertion stems from a large number of research studies since the 1960s which followed the course of patients released by court order from maximum security psychiatric facilities into civil hospitals or the community against psychiatric advice. Within a 4-year follow-up only 20 per cent of a group of 1000 such people known as the 'Baxstrom' patients were assaultive to others and only 3 per cent of the released patients were readmitted to maximum security facilities (Fisher, 1995, p. 39). It is from studies such as these that the conclusion has been drawn that for every one person that health professionals correctly identify as dangerous they incorrectly identify four or more others. It is likely that given the shift of focus of mental health legislation towards patient rights that much fewer clearly non-dangerous people are compulsorily detained today. However, the perception of large numbers of dangerous people at large in the community appears to be of greater concern to the public and ensures that pressure is maintained on health professionals to identify, detain and control dangerous individuals.

The concepts of power and control pervade psychiatry, psychiatric treatment and indeed society in general. Szasz (1994) argues that the issue of power is inherent in all psychiatric treatment, that a covert function of psychiatry is social control. Stuart and Sundeen (1987, p. 219) suggest that this idea is supported by the various behavioural disorders that justify commitment e.g. drug addiction and sexual offences. They suggest that assessment of dangerousness is highly subjective and that the underlying issue is one of nonconformity in ways that offend others. Indeed it may be argued that mental illness itself is a highly subjective phenomena. Conrad and Schneider (1980) point out that the various approaches to managing deviant behaviour throughout history have largely been to control those that did not conform to society's dominant values and posed a threat to the established social order. Both criminal justice and mental health systems perform social control functions. They have a responsibility to protect society from fearful events (Fisher, 1989, p. 13). The standard of dangerousness to self or others has increasingly become the criterion which is used to justify social control in the interests of protecting society.

The responsibility of predicting future violence is one which nurses and clinicians cannot shirk. It has been estimated that at least half of all health professionals will be assaulted during their careers (Blair and New, 1991) so such predictions become a matter of personal safety. The possibility of legal action should the health professional fail to predict future violence also provides further incentive to refine the decision-making process. The nurse faces the challenge of having to work in close proximity, and often for long periods of time, with people who have been labelled as dangerous.

Some settings such as prisons, by their very nature, constitute high levels of restrictiveness, together with a climate of suspicion and mistrust. Research into the nature, causes and effects of violence, has the potential to lead to improved interventions to reduce violence, greater precision in the prediction of violence and a reduction in the negative consequences of violence. Research will have served the nurse well if it assists in the assessment of the individual's antecedents of violent behaviour, and leads to interventions which reduce risk while facilitating therapy in the least restrictive environment.

THE RELATIONSHIP BETWEEN MENTAL ILLNESS AND VIOLENCE

A great deal of research attempts to show the relationship of violence to mental illness. Monahan (1992) concluded that the presence of mental illness is a modest but significant risk factor for violent behaviour. However, the studies in this area are plagued with inconsistencies which make generalising from the results difficult. For example, in most western countries, including New Zealand, danger to self or others is a main criteria for commitment, or compulsory treatment. Studies on the incidence of violence in the mentally ill, based on samples of committed patients are flawed because people may be labelled as mentally ill because they are violent, whereas the benign individual may avoid being labelled, or more likely avoid inpatient treatment despite having similar cognitive, affective or perceptual disturbances.

Studies of violent behaviour after discharge from hospital are inevitably confounded with the eligibility criteria for admission, the nature and length of treatment given, the eligibility criteria for discharge and the degree of support offered after discharge. Lack of consensus on what constitutes violence and mental illness, as well as the lack of comparative statistics on the prevalence of violence in well people and those not selected for hospital treatment, make determining the true incidence of violent behaviour amongst the mentally ill almost impossible.

Despite these problems, there is some consistency among findings related to the relationship between some signs of mental illness and violence. There appears to be a significant relationship between drug and alcohol abuse or dependence and likelihood of violence (Morrison, 1994). Diagnosis such as schizophrenia and bipolar affective disorder are more commonly found in people with a history of violent behaviour. But by far the single greatest predictor of violence is a past history of violence (Blomhoff, Seini and Früs, 1990).

Recent research suggests that current psychotic symptomatology is predictive of violence. When such factors as alcohol abuse were controlled for in a comparative study between psychiatric patients and those never hospitalised, the only variable that accounted for differences in the rates of violence was current psychotic symptoms (Monahan, 1992). That is, when a person was experiencing such symptoms as hallucinations and delusions they were more likely to be violent than a non-hospitalised group. However, when not actively experiencing such symptoms, the risk of violence was not appreciably higher than a demographically similar group in their home community.

The results of empirical studies allow people to make estimates of the likelihood of future violence based on the presence or absence of symptoms of mental illness. The inherent assumption in all such studies is that violence is a function of individual pathology. While useful for determining the probability of violent behaviour in groups, such measures are crude and inaccurate predictors of violence when applied to individuals (Gunn, 1982). After all, the majority of people who experience symptoms of mental illness are not in fact violent.

Some violence, however, may be a function of individual pathology. Garza-Trevino (1994) reviewed numerous studies on neurobiological factors which contribute to aggressive behaviour. Damage to certain centres of the brain such as the limbic structures, temporal lobes, and frontal lobes have been found to be associated with aggressiveness and rage. Homicidal, suicidal and impulsive behaviour has been associated with deficiency or dysregulation of serotonin. Other factors such as endocrine dysfunction and brain injury may contribute to paraphilias and sexual aggression. For some medical conditions the link between neurobiological factors and violence is clear (Bear and Fedio, 1977).

Testosterone levels are correlated with increased violent behaviour in humans as well as in other species. According to Kalat (1992, p. 433) the highest incidence of violence, as measured by crime statistics, is in men 15 to 25 years old, who also have the highest serum testosterone levels of any age group. Testosterone levels may contribute to a predisposition towards violence but clearly other factors are involved – not every young man is violent. A belief that aggression and violence are a result of biochemical or structural abnormalities in the brain is a comfortable position because it implies a lack of individual, or societal responsibility for violent behaviour, and the promise of a cure in the form of a biological treatment. While aggression and resulting violence do arise from biological factors in some individuals, at this time biological explanations can at best only partially account for some violence by those with mental illness.

Might there be then, a specific cluster of symptoms that is optimally predictive of latter violence? Lowenstein, Binder and McNiel (1990) examined the relationship between symptoms at admission and later violence. They concluded that patients who showed higher levels of thinking disturbance, hostile–suspiciousness, and agitation–excitement (as measured at admission by the Brief Psychiatric Rating Scale) were at greater risk of becoming assaultive during hospitalisation. Blomhoff, Seim and Friis (1990) found that after history of violence, a high level of aggression at referral but an absence of anxiety at admission were the best predictors of later violence. It will be no great surprise to find that aggression and agitation are linked to violence. These terms are to varying degrees synonymous with menace and violence and are not in themselves indicative of mental illness. Hallucinations and delusions, on the other hand, are often considered a feature of psychotic illness.

Schizophrenia is considered by many to be a biological disorder and has long been associated with violence, although we know that statistically the likelihood of a schizophrenic individual being violent is less than someone with a drug or alcohol dependency problem (Swanson *et al.*, 1990). Junginger (1995) undertook a study examining compliance with command hallucinations, one symptom which people with schizophrenia may experience. Junginger (1995) reported that patients who were able to give an identity to a hallucinated voice, or who identified less dangerous commands, were more likely to comply with the command hallucination. Those that experienced command hallucinations were at risk of dangerous behaviour. Significantly, as individuals reported less dangerous command hallucinations and a greater degree of non-compliance with commands when in hospital, the authors also concluded that the 'level of dangerousness resulting from compliance with command hallucinations may be a function of the patient's environment' (ibid. p.912).

This study is interesting in that it suggests some aspects of the environment have a moderating effect on symptoms which many believe arise from a biochemical disturbance. In this case the hospital environment appeared to have a positive effect on symptoms, which has far-reaching implications for hospital-based assessment of dangerousness based on command hallucinations. As Junginger (1995, p.914) proposes, 'it may be the post-hospital environment that determines the dangerousness of command hallucinations and thus the potential for violent or criminal behaviour'. Violence cannot be merely a function of individual pathology in these cases but rather as Davis (1991) suggests, it is a result of a complex interaction between various factors.

CONTROLLING: A RESPONSE TO, AND PRECIPITANT OF VIOLENCE.

It has been suggested that violence is a reaction to the situation in which a patient finds himself and more often than not is a symptom of disturbance in the hospital itself rather than a symptom of a patient's mental state. Many of the large asylums have been closed down. Some features of these institutions such as the ethos of control still persist in many otherwise enlightened treatment settings. The notion that the mentally ill are out of control and that violence is a symptom of individual pathology leads to the natural conclusion that people need to be controlled. Mechanical and chemical restraints and use of seclusion are overtly controlling practices that arise from these beliefs. In a small number of cases such interventions may be justified but the ethos of control permiates many settings in more subtle ways such as in the use of language and subtle coersion.

Morrison (1990, p. 33) undertook a 9-month study in an inpatient unit in which the the key concept which emerged from the data was a 'tradition of toughness' amongst the staff who worked there. She identified the main values of the unit as being derived from the medical ideology with its emphasis on control and safety, which in turn led to norms of behaviour such as enforcing the rules, controlling and restraining patients and showing strength rather than facilitating therapy. Much of the violence observed was linked to the tradition of toughness and the patently unprofessional nursing care that arose from this tradition. The model arising from the data was used to explain why some violence occurred and why some staff were victims of violence. Morrison (1990, p. 35) concluded that, 'Policies and enforcing the rules aimed to control patients inevitably lead to violence through the process of confrontation and escalation of the violent situation'. Watson (1991) came to similar conclusions in his phenomenological study on the experiences of adults hospitalised with acute mental illness which they consider contributed to the stress of coping with mental illness. Watson (1991, p.14) suggests that controlling practices might in fact 'provoke the very behaviour they are designed to contain'.

Roper and Anderson (1991) in their study examining the interactions between staff and patients on a psychiatric ward also found that the concept of control was pervasive. Patient violence was conceptualised as a loss of control requiring the application of external controls. They found that controlling through denial of requests and using the ward structure to maintain control were typical practices which led to patient violence. However, the question remains as to why controlling practices lead to a violent response in some individuals and a submissive response in others. Further research by Morrison (1994) suggests some possible answers.

Morrison (1994, p. 249) found that 'the primary characteristic which seemed to differentiate violent from nonviolent persons was the presence of an exploitive style with others, i.e., using others for self gain'. The violent individual used coercion and violence to get what they wanted, whereas the non-violent person was not at all exploitive and used an interactional style which she labelled 'accommodation'. Morrison proposed that such styles of communication are learned through the process of social modelling and reinforcement.

The theoretical assumptions underpinning Morrison's (1994) explanatory model are based on a theory of coercive family processes influenced by Bandura's (1973) analysis of aggression using social learning theory. The major assumption of the social learning view is that 'man is neither driven by inner forces nor buffeted helplessly by environmental influences. Rather psychological functioning is best understood in terms of continuous reciprocal interaction between behaviour and its controlling conditions' (Bandura, 1973, p. 43). Such an approach attempts to explain how 'patterns of behaviour are acquired and how their expression is continuously regulated by the interplay of self-generated and external sources of influence' (ibid.: 43).

Violence, then, may be used in a purposeful way by people to get what they want. Someone who characteristically exercises a coercive interactional style might not surprisingly respond violently when placed in a controlling environment. Sheridan *et al.*, (1990) examined precipitants of patient violence leading up to the use of physical restraints in a psychiatric inpatient setting. They found that violent behaviour was more likely to relate to external situations such as enforcement of rules by staff, denial of privileges or conflicts with other patients than to internal psychiatric symptoms such as delusions or hallucinations. Of 73 violent episodes only eight occurred after internal events only. Such findings tend to challenge the popular notion that the mentally ill person is typically out of control and a victim of internal symptoms which lead to uncontrolled violence. Morrison (1993a) argues that violence is primarily a social problem and only a very small number of violent incidents may be accounted for as symptoms of mental disorder.

NURSES: CO-CREATERS OF DANGEROUSNESS?

A colleague recently asked, 'If a person is violent in a controlled setting, what are they likely to do in an uncontrolled setting?' A considerable body of research suggests that it may be the controlled setting which precipitates much violence. Research alone does not provide a sound enough basis on which to make predictions about future dangerousness of most individuals.

Health professionals must consider that their response to those they perceive as dangerous may play a part in creating dangerousness. Dangerousness is not an empirical reality, but rather a social construction although the effects of the label are tangible. Controlling practices, in response to the label of dangerousness may precipitate or provoke violence in predisposed individuals. The person then has a history of violence which may be viewed as justification for previous and future controlling practices. The label of dangerousness adheres to an individual long after any empirical evidence of dangerousness subsides. The distance that others place between themselves and others they perceive as dangerous may engender a sense of alienation in those labelled that may, for some, become one of the multitude of antecedents which contribute to violence.

Those with mental illness are often perceived as unpredictable, frightening and different (Levey and Howells, 1995). This may contribute to the stigma associated with mental illness and the perception of those with mental illness that they are indeed different from others. Mulvey and Lidz (1995) point out that clinical decision-making takes in the conditional nature of violence e.g. one person may be violent when intoxicated while another is likely to be violent in an emotionally charged home environment. It is likely that the effect of perceiving oneself as being different and separate from others is a condition that may predispose some people towards violence. Combine this factor with a coercive style of relating to others and a highly controlling environment and violent behaviour may be reinforced, or be the only means available to get one's needs and wants met. Could it be that at least some of the violence associated with active psychiatric symptomology is due to an interaction of individual factors and others' response to what is seen as unpredictable and frightening behaviour?

Many actions might attempt to be justified under the umbrella of maintaining social safety including social control. Forensic nursing can be a particularly challenging area for nurses as many clients of forensic services have been prejudged as dangerous and such institutions have a mandate to protect society, provide compassionate care and maintain the personal safety of all who work within the institution. These conflicting demands are a source of ethical strife for nurses working in these areas. While care without coercion does happen, a multitude of pressures impinge on health providers to control certain groups identified as dangerous. What part do nurses play in co-creating dangerousness and what effect does being labelled as dangerous have on nursing care?

In the case study below it is readily apparent that the nurses' perceptions of those in their charge as being 'dangerous prisoners' adversely affected the care provided and arguably reduced the individuals to non-person status. The elasticity of the concept of dangerousness is also apparent in the differences in perceptions between the nurse educator, students and prison nurses. How moral can nursing care be if controlling has primacy over caring and care is withheld in order to punish?

CASE STUDY: WHEN CONTROL HAS PRIMACY OVER CARE.

This case study is about the prison nurses' role conflict as I perceived it and was eventually caught up in. The context of my experience was that of a Nurse Educator, supervising registered nurses who were completing the clinical component of a forensic psychiatric nursing course at a prison complex of both maximum and medium security.

Those incarcerated in prisons experience the full force of the justice system whilst doing their 'time' and have no expectations of any other treatment from the prison officers and administration. The custodial role of the guards is contrasted by other professionals working in prisons and, of these, nurses are an important group.

Confidentiality is closely identified with the nursing profession and is so integral to my nursing practice and teaching that it is incomprehensible to me that nurses should violate it. Context, however, is a powerful moderating factor and the prison environment with its own culture, rules and regulations proved to have such an effect for the prison nursing staff.

I had been aware of previous legislative changes relating to prison nursing staff that had been made in order to comply with the United Nations standard minimum rules for the treatment of prisoners. These respectively raised nursing staff levels and created an occupational class of nurses who had no custodial function. It was therefore surprising that the prison nurses we met had become part of the prison establishment with the associated punitive ethos.

The prisoners, who knew we were nurses, seemed at first to be wary of our 'new faces' and did not interact or communicate beyond a polite greeting. The reason for their behaviour soon became obvious as their relationship with the (prison) nurses was observed. Power was a salient factor in this relationship as they practised their own particular form of nursing that included: lack of confidentiality, withholding drugs, delaying medical referrals and ignoring medication orders. Three nurses in particular created strong impressions.

'The nurse counsellor'

One nurse had developed an interest in counselling, although unfortunately not enough of an interest to pursue any training or education in this area. She was a genial and friendly person, who showed me her office with pride and told me she always had the door open during sessions with her 'clients' and a prison officer posted outside. A very large poster was positioned by the door giving the ground rules for counselling; these included no 'aggro', no shouting, standing or swearing. Considering the limited literacy and vocabulary of some prisoners, and that for some English was a second language, it is a wonder any sessions ever got 'off the ground'. Everything said was reported back to those in charge, so why would the prisoners go through this (humiliating) charade? Apparently, it was important to demonstrate that one had made an effort to learn and improve one's behaviour and life skills whilst in prison for the parole board hearings. Attendance at 'counselling' sessions was a way of doing this.

'The nurse with the X-ray vision' or 'supernurse'

My experience with this nurse began with her lecture to me about how the men were always making up injuries and illness. However, I was unprepared for the total rejection of their complaints as she would just look at them and say 'no, nothing wrong' or words of similar effect. The men rationalised her behaviour in their own way by attributing it to her 'x-ray vision'. They laughingly told me that if they went with a sore nose, she would just look hard at it and say 'No, that's alright'. This assessment practice was used for whatever the problem was, from stomach ache to football injuries. It seemed that this nurse was able to assess and diagnose without touch and that she was always right. One Monday morning one of the men attended doctor's clinic with a dislocated shoulder, injured whilst playing football on Saturday morning. The doctors are a phone call away and seemed willing to attend when called but this nurse had decided that the injury could wait until the clinic on Monday morning and that's what happened.

The 'psychiatric drugs are only attention seeking' nurse

The contribution of a nurse who had very definite ideas about psychiatric drugs and the reasons the men took them literally took my breath away. I attended an admission session of a man who had been transferred from another prison. The usual practice of having a prison officer present appeared humiliating for this man and as I was beginning to explain my presence to him I was interrupted and told that I 'didn't need to do that', and it 'didn't matter what he thought'. His medical chart was a catalogue of attempted suicide and self-mutilations and in large writing the psychiatrist from the other prison had noted the 'cocktail' of drugs that he was on, and why it was important for him to stay on them as they seemed to be effective. With a triumphant smile she said, 'Well, he won't get them here, they only take them to get attention'. This breathtaking statement was followed by a proud explanation that her monthly reports to the head of the prison included an exact description of how many drugs had been given. I inquired about these drugs. 'Two paracetamol' she said. 'What, for each man, as an average, is that what you mean?' I gasped. 'No, for the whole prison,' was the answer. I had of course no way of verifying this statement but I believed her, when one considered the other nursing practices observed. Withholding nursing care appeared to be used to further 'punish' the men.

'COMPROMISED NURSES' OR A 'COMPROMISING SITUATION'

The compromised position of these prison nurses and consequently myself and my students was not an enviable one. The pressures and influences they were subject to, and which affected their nursing practice reflected powerful forces at work. Obviously the isolation they experienced as a small group of Caucasian, professional women within a hostile and male-dominated environment created difficulties for them. The issues of 'dangerousness' and 'fear' appeared to undermine their nursing practice as they were used as the reason for violating confidentiality, withholding nursing care, medication and advocacy. The symbiotic relationship they had with the prison officers also related to the 'dangerousness' and 'fear' issues with the guards protecting the nurses and the nurses co-operating with prison rules.

My participation in life-skills workshops, anger management groups and drug and alcohol meetings provided an opportunity to get to know the men without the prison officers being present. These sessions were always held in the Chapel and the prison officers reluctantly remained at the glass doors looking in. I felt quite safe in these groups despite the fact that I was always the only female and frequently the only Caucasian person there. One particular group had all killed a significant female in their lives, but I felt my personal safety was never an issue. However, when I was around the nurses I not only felt unsafe but was careful of what I said and to whom, whilst feeling sad that nursing was given such an image. It should be noted that at that time the mentally ill population of the prison was demonstrable.

To create a level of safety I used strategies to communicate with the men that involved interaction during activities such as sports, artwork, fitness sessions and gardening. These served two purposes: it was difficult to be overheard in such contexts and the men developed confidence in myself and my students. The value of such 'safe' interaction became apparent when a man disclosed to me his fears and anxieties related to his inability to control his anger. He was concerned that his family may be unsafe unless he got help, but if he asked for it it would be difficult to get parole. His problem identified the issues of concern I had about the lack of confidentiality in the prison, without the help he obviously needed he would some day go home and be unsafe and even dangerous to his family. The subsequent demand from the prison officers to divulge the conversation to them was startling: 'We want to know because he never speaks to anybody'. My statement that the conversation was private was met with the explanation that the men had no right to confidential communication. This therefore meant that the nurses had no right to confidential communication either. The authorities were used to getting information from nurses about what the men disclosed to them and this was confirmed when I asked the nurses.

Exposure to these 'incidents' and the nurses involved reaffirmed my commitment to the 'caring' imperative of nursing at a personal level. It reinforced for me, the value of continuing professional education and the need for constant vigilance to avoid slipping into the crevasses of expediency, utilitarianism and other systems' agendas. However, the question needs to be posed: what is the role of the nurse under such circumstances, do the prison authorities define it, as I believe happened in this experience, or do nurses maintain their professional autonomy and risk their safety?

CONCLUSIONS

The first part of this chapter exposed some of the pressures on nurses, and indeed the mental health system to control those whom are perceived as dangerous to society. To many violence is seen as a symptom of sickness. It was highlighted that this stance is extremely problematic in that it does not account for the multitude of social, environmental, psychological and social interactional factors which at the very least contribute to violent behaviour. It suggests a biological cure for violent behaviour that has not been forthcoming in most cases and an imperative to control the violent individual until they are able to regain self-control through treatment, or cure of the underlying disease. It is to a large extent this conceptualisation of violence as a symptom of mental illness that brings many psychiatric nurses into contact with the dangerous patient and which leads to the ethical strife experienced by nurses involving a struggle to both care and control.

Brenda Curzon's case study of her experiences working as a nursing lecturer inside a prison reflected this struggle. For the nurse working in such settings the mandate of the institution is clearly to control. The inmates are viewed as dangerous, manipulative, untrustworthy and unworthy of the dignity afforded to ordinary citizens. Not surprisingly, such a perception will lead to behaviour on the part of the nurse which bears no approximation to care. Such behaviour may go unchallenged and may even be rewarded by the institution. The nurse becomes a tool in the process of punishment and control, and in this process ceases to be a nurse in any sense but name. The nurse in such a situation has lost touch with the philosophical basis on which the discipline of nursing is founded – that which acknowledges the innate uniqueness and worth of every human being and makes no judgements about the deservedness of nursing care.

A prison is an extreme example of a controlling environment where the primary objective is to control. Nurses working in forensic units and even in community settings may experience similar pressures to control those whom they care for. For them the dilemma that arises may be more acute. Society demands quality nursing care as well as containment of dangerousnness. The cost of not identifying someone as dangerous who later harms another, will weigh heavily on their professional reputa-tion and may have dire consequences for victims. The nurse who works in these less restrictive situations requires a sound knowledge of the conditional nature of violence and all its antecedents and a sound philosophical basis of care.

Even in such controlled institutions as prisons, nurses may provide good nursing care, if the caring function of the nurse has primacy over the controlling function of the institution. Brenda's narrative, however, highlights the ethical dilemmas faced by such groups of nurses. The difficulty in maintaining a degree of confidentiality and facilitating trusting relationships in an environment of mistrust provides a stark illustration of their struggles. For some the pressures may be overwhelming, leading to the complete subjugation of caring.

The nurse who is informed by a sound knowledge base and a philosophy of care will recognise that dangerousness ought not to be an arbitrary label; that one's danger to another is conditional on a multitude of factors not merely the passing of time, containment in a secure environment or treatment with medication. Such a nurse will also recognise that the nurse's response to people labelled as dangerous may be crucial to the individual's well-being at that moment and influential on their future well-being and behaviour. The nurse will recognise that where a degree of control is required to be imposed on another, that it must be done in a way that maintains dignity and does not further reinforce a sense of alienation in the individual. Treating people fairly is not the same as treating all people the same and she or he will challenge institutional practices that effectively disempower and limit choice. The nurse will strive towards understanding the individual rather than relying on labels as the guide to their behaviour. These are but some of the ideals of nursing which when combined with societal, institutional and political pressures, create so much ethical strife for the psychiatric nurse.

REFERENCES

Bandura, A. 1973: *Aggression: a social learning analysis.* New Jersey: Prentice Hall.

Bear, D.M. and Fedio, P. 1977: Quantitative analysis of intricately behaviour in temporal lobe epilepsy. *Archives of Neurology* **34**, 42–8.

Blair, D.T. and New, S.A. 1991: Assaultive behaviour: know the risks. *Journal of Psychosocial Nursing* **29**(11), 25–9.

Blomhoff, S., Seim, S. and Friis, S. 1991: Can prediction of violence among psychiatric inpatients be improved? *Hospital and Community Psychiatry* **41**(7), 771–5.

Bootzin, R.R. and **Acocella, J.R.** 1984: *Abnormal Psychology: current perspectives*. 4th edn. New York: Random House.

Bowler, M. 1995: Let inmates have their say (Letter to the editor). *Sunday Star-Times*, 1 Oct, C4.

Conrad, P. and **Schneider, J.W.** 1980: *Deviance and medicalisation: from badness to sickness*. St Louis: C.V. Mosby.

Davis, S. 1991: Violence by psychiatric inpatients: a review. *Hospital and Community Psychiatry* **42**(6), 585–90.

Fisher, A. 1989: The process of definition and action: the case of dangerousness. PhD dissertation, San Francisco: University of California.

Fisher, A. 1995: The ethical problems encountered in psychiatric nursing practice with dangerously mentally ill persons. *Scholarly Inquiry for Nursing Practice* **9**(2), 193–208.

Garza-Trevino, E.S. 1994: Neurobiological factors in aggressive behaviour. *Hospital and Community Psychiatry* **45**(7), 690–99.

Gunn, J. 1982: Defining the terms. In J.R. Hamilton and Freeman, H. (eds) *Dangerousness: Psychiatric Assessment and Management*. Oxford: Alden Press, 7–11.

Guyan, C. 1995a: Families may sue over lack of care. *Sunday Star-Times*, 1 Oct, A1.

Guyan, C. 1995b: Police warn of tragedy with patients. *Sunday Star-Times*, 1 Oct, A1.

Junginger, J. 1995: Command hallucinations and the prediction of dangerousness. *Psychiatric Services* **46**(9), 911–14.

Kalat, J.W. 1992: *Biological Psychology*. 4th edn. Belmont, CA: Wadsworth, Inc.

Levey, S. and **Howells, K.** 1995: Dangerousness, unpredictability and the fear of people with schizophrenia. *Journal of Forensic Psychiatry* **6**(1), 19–39.

Lowenstein, M., Binder, R.L. and **McNiel, D.E.** (1990). The relationship between admission symptoms and hospital assaults. *Hospital and Community Psychiatry* **41**(3), 311–13.

Martin, Y. 1995: Shooting alarms parents of Templeton patients. *Sunday Star-Times*, 1 Oct, A3.

Monahan, J. 1992: Mental disorder and violent behaviour: perceptions and evidence. *American Psychologist* **47**(4), 511–21.

Morrison, E.F. 1990: The tradition of toughness: a study of non-professional nursing care in psychiatric settings. *Image: Journal of Nursing Scholarship* **22**(1), 32–8.

Morrison, E.F. 1993a: Toward a better understanding of violence in psychiatric settings: debunking the myths. *Archives of Psychiatric Nursing* **7**(6), 328–35.

Morrison, E.F. 1993b: The measurement of aggression and violence in hospitalised psychiatric patients. *International Journal of Nursing Studies* **30**(1), 51–64.

Morrison, E.F. 1994: The evolution of a concept: aggression and violence in psychiatric settings. *Archives of Psychiatric Nursing* **8**(4), 245–53.

Mulvey, E.P., and **Lidz, C.W.** 1995: Conditional prediction: a model for research on dangerousness to others in a new era. *International Journal of Law and Psychiatry* **18**(2), 129–43.

Roper, J.M. and **Anderson, N.L.R.** 1991: The interactional dynamics of violence, part 1: an acute psychiatric ward. *Archives of Psychiatric Nursing* **5**(4), 209–15.

Sheridan, M., Henrion, R., Robinson, L. and **Baxter, V.** 1991: Precipitants of violence in a psychiatric inpatient setting. *Hospital and Community Psychiatry* **41**(7), 777–80.

Stuart, G.W. and **Sundeen S.J.** 1987: *Principles and Practice of Psychiatric Nursing*. St Louis: C.V. Mosby.

Swanson, J.W., Holzer, C.E., Ganju, V.K., and **Tsutomu Jono, R.** 1991: Violence and psychiatric disorder in the community: evidence from the epidemiologic catchment area surveys. *Hospital and Community Psychiatry* **41**(7), 761–70.

Szasz, T. 1994: Psychiatric diagnosis, psychiatric power and psychiatric abuse. *Journal of Medical Ethics* **20**, 135–8.

Watson, P. 1991: Care or control: questions and answers for psychiatric nursing practice, *Nursing Praxis in New Zealand* **6**(2), 10–14.

4

THE ETHICS OF PROFESSIONALISED CARE

Jim Moorey

Individual nurses and clinical teams, then, should try to maintain standards of quality and develop healing relationships with their clients, remaining aware of the matrix of constraints and pressures on them. But there may be something greater even than the formidable forces detailed in Chapters 2 and 3 in the way of professional healing for the mentally ill.

Many of us working in this field come to a point of suspecting that, in truth, the very nature of our status as professional carers compromises our ability genuinely to care for patients. What, after all, are we doing when we help them work on 'their problems'? Certainly, we can take care to ensure that we work in a non-pathologising way. But can we ever be careful enough, to the extent that we avoid completely any level of collusion with the message that patients are, somehow, wrong? Jim Moorey may not feel comfortable, in these circumstances, taking the optimistic view and the easy way out; but he does show how it is possible to develop to a very great extent, in principle and in practice, one's awareness of the ideological nature of our professional interactions, avowing that, if nothing else, we can at least maintain a level of ethical scrutiny, self-doubt and honesty in the work we do.

INTRODUCTION

The role of the expert nowadays is to articulate the consensus of people with power. Power can of course be exercised in both benign and malign ways, but the exercise of power always requires justification. On examination, however, such justification is often lacking. While power in a crude form is easy to identify, and in most cases easily shown to be illegitimate, in its more subtle manifestations the operation of power may be elusive, even at times invisible. Invisible, that is in its source and operation, but not in its effects. The writer who has done most to make visible the operation of power, and in particular to elucidate the crucial relationship between power and – what can be regarded as the special currency of the expert – knowledge, is of course, Michel Foucault. Much of what follows in this chapter is influenced by his perspective, but I hope I have avoided the irony of being dominated by it.

In this chapter I will outline some of the more notable features of the formation of professions, and highlight some of the central ethical issues such features raise, especially in the field of 'mental health'. My goal is not to give an exhaustive analysis of the issues, but to raise questions and encourage reflection.

THE TERRITORY OF PROFESSIONALISED CARE

In a figurative sense 'territory' refers to a sphere, region, or domain, over which some form of influence or control is claimed or exerted. The territory of professionalised care is probably best illustrated by considering examples. The following brief accounts will help map out the territory, and introduce some of the questions explored later.

Carlton

Carlton was in his late teens, the youngest of a large family from Moss Side, a working-class area of Manchester, a place with a nationwide reputation for violence. He was of Afro-Caribbean descent. Like the rest of his family he was unemployed. Carlton was brought to the psychiatric unit by the police, who thought his loud and belligerent behaviour was more likely to be signs of madness than criminality (his mother told me she was glad the police thought he was mad: 'At least the doctors don't break your ribs'). Carlton believed malevolent forces were trying to control him. Voices gave him orders but he ignored them. He was unkempt and dirty, he did not like to wash, he did not want to be a 'whitewashed grave'. He thought being employed was equivalent to slavery, that cannabis brought more knowledge than books, and that money was evil. He heard voices, but preferred them to his mother's nagging. He also thought words were cheap, and violence natural. He spoke contemptuously of 'the white world' that he believed was trying to control him, resenting what he called 'legalised white violence', and the 'chicken-shit goodwill' of 'concerned white liberals'. Much of his speech was difficult to follow (although his mother thought he was rather more articulate than usual). Carlton was very angry, swore at the consultant psychiatrist and punched one of the nurses ('for asking stupid questions'). Carlton was considered to be 'schizophrenic' and 'a danger to himself and others'. He showed no gratitude towards staff for their efforts to confine and medicate him.

Carlton is, of course, like many others who enter the orbit of 'mental health' professionals, and his will be a familiar picture to many who work in this field. Carlton's behaviour, beliefs and experiences would be regarded by many as in some way the responsibility (the 'territory') of certain professionals. But many people, including the professionals involved in Carlton's 'care', strongly objected to him. The gulf between staff and patient was not simply that between sane and insane. What is it that Carlton provokes in us, that underlies our desire to intervene? What exactly is it about him that we want to change? What do we want to control?. When Carlton enters our world, is he expected to learn our language and values – to use our words, verbalising frustration rather than striking out, for example? Is persuading him to do so part of the treatment? Or the conditions of treatment? Is it possible to adopt a framework in which Carlton's violence is seen positively – as it was in his 'subculture'? How do we answer Carlton's mother's question: 'He's been surrounded by violence all his life. What else do you expect him to do?' Must violence on the part of someone in Carlton's position (i.e., not a soldier, policeman or someone else with 'appropriate authorisation' [!]), necessarily be either criminal or pathological? Carlton's aggressiveness and lack of cleanliness provoked much more upset and debate than his hallucinations, which didn't seem to bother anyone, least of all Carlton. Are 'mental health' professionals in the 'business' of cure, care or control? Carlton's beliefs, his experiences and behaviour are all regarded as legitimate areas for investigation and assessment, and perhaps, control and intervention. Different professional groups laid claims to various areas of Carlton's life and behaviour. Psychiatrists, nurses, social workers, psychologists, occupational therapists staked their relative claims. On occasions these varying professional claims came into conflict with each other. But whose interests should be paramount in this situation? And, in such situations, whose interests usually do prevail?

Clare

Clare was 40 when she was referred by her GP to the department of Clinical Psychology. Her GP described her as 'depressed and agoraphobic'. Clare had married when she was 31, and given birth to her son, Mark, when she was 36. Within weeks of Mark's birth Clare began to develop what would normally be regarded as typical symptoms of depression and agoraphobia. Clare's GP prescribed antidepressants, which alleviated her depression sufficiently for her to continue to care for Mark, although she would not leave the house unaccompanied. Gradually she became more withdrawn and unable to enter shops or walk in the street. She would only leave the house if she could be driven to her destination. Clare's husband, David, had been a research chemist until shortly after their marriage. He had changed his occupation to a managerial post in a pharmaceutical firm. His new job involved a great deal of evening and weekend work, as well as regular trips abroad. After about a year in his new job David was obliged to take a post in a different city. Clare did not want to move, she enjoyed her secretarial job, and wanted to remain close to friends and relatives. However, she felt obliged to acquiesce: 'David's career obviously had to come first, so we moved'. Soon after moving Clare became pregnant. Her husband and parents were delighted. Clare kept telling herself how fortunate she was, but her feelings were saying something else. At times, as she reflected on her past she wept. Being an only child, having everything she thought she had wanted, being unhappy, her mother's protectiveness, a car accident when she was 10, being bullied at school, trying to please others. She wept also when she realised she hated her life. Her own thoughts and feelings began to terrify her.

Again, this is a familiar situation and doubtless even with such a brief sketch of Clare's situation, hypotheses about what is 'wrong' will be suggested. But here we might pause to ask some general questions about our perception of Clare. Is there really anything 'wrong' with her? In so far as there is a problem, where should it be located? Is there something wrong with Clare's 'inner world'? Or in her 'object relations'? Or is it her history of 'conditioning' that is at fault? Does the problem lie in her 'cognitive schemas'? Perhaps we should locate the problem in her network of relationships. Or perhaps in her role expectations. Perhaps the problem stems from issues of gender and power. Or perhaps her 'being – in – the – world' is essentially inauthentic . . . Obviously we can interpret Clare's situation in a multitude of ways. And of course the way we respond, the help we offer – our 'intervention' – will be justified in terms of our conceptualisation of the problem(s) and the source of the problem(s). But the point I want to emphasise here is that the particular framework we adopt represents a bid for control or influence over aspects of Clare's life, which may to a large extent be a reflection of professional, rather than rational or moral commitments.

By the time Clare began therapy she had seen a male GP, a male consultant psychotherapist and a male counsellor. Now she was seeing a male psychologist. What has already been set in train by this process? What assumptions have already become attached to Clare, as a recipient of professionalised care? What can professional health care workers really offer Clare?

Albert

Albert described himself as 'a survivor'. He was 78; had been raised in an orphanage where he had suffered physical and sexual abuse, and had survived four years as a prisoner-of-war in Burma and Thailand during the Second World War. He had witnessed the suicide of his daughter, and his son's death from cancer. He had worked hard all his life, for many years in various parts of the construction industry and, later, sweeping streets. At various times in his life Albert had been a heavy drinker. There had been times when he had beaten his wife, Joan. Once, so badly that the cuts above her eye, and on her nose and ear, needed stitches. Albert had also sexually abused his daughter, Kate, a 'terrible thing', as he said. But he managed to keep this secret from his wife.

Albert had been told that Joan had Alzheimer's disease when she was 68. Albert was then 70. At the time he didn't know what that meant. Over the following six years the struggle to look after Joan, with minimal support, took its toll. As Albert put it, 'It nearly finished me off'. As he watched Joan's deterioration, there were times when he would become so angry and frustrated that he would shout at her, and sometimes hit her. Often he would sit for hours and cry. He felt he had done his best to care for her through those years, but with no family or friends who could help, it was difficult. He had hoped for more support from professional and voluntary agencies, and felt very bitter at the meagre help that was provided. 'You work and pay taxes all your life, you go to the other side of the world to fight when they tell you to, and at the end, when you need help, they throw you on the scrap heap.' When Joan died, Albert seemed to give up. At first he tried to avoid spending time in his flat because he sensed Joan's presence there, which frightened him. But the cold outside, and the gangs of teenagers who taunted him, eventually drove him back to what he called his 'dungeon' (his council flat). The flat was dark and damp. The bedroom windows needed to be repaired but Albert had lost the will to go through the long routine of repeatedly badgering the council until they responded. Because the flat was so cold and damp Albert felt more comfortable in bed. He would stay there for days, only venturing out to get his pension and buy alcohol, which he preferred to food. Eventually Albert was seen by a psychiatrist who considered him to be suffering from 'depression associated with unresolved grief after the death of his wife'.

Again as we reflect on Albert's experience how should we regard what has happened to him? Is Albert ill? Who should help? Who, if anyone, is responsible for

Albert's condition? Albert's problems will be seen as legitimate territory for a whole range of professionals. His material, physical, psychological and spiritual welfare may all be eyed knowingly by different groups of experts, eager to diagnose, prescribe and treat. However, rather than pursue the multiple explanations of Albert's difficulties, reflect on the following point. The figurative use of the term 'territory' used here, while conveying some aspects of the situation we are considering, is in other respects very misleading. We are considering the lives of real people – both professional care providers and those who receive such care. Apart from our response as professionals – which may be quite rigidly constrained according to the framework we have been more or less successfully inducted into – we respond as people. Sympathy or condemnation, fear or contempt, impatience or concern, boredom or fascination, sorrow or indifference. There is inevitably a personal response, which we may, for the sake of our discussion, distinguish from a professional response. It may be quite common that what we actually feel conflicts sharply with what we consider we ought to feel, as members of a particular profession. And it may be just as common for us to attempt to justify what is actually a personal response by clothing that response in professional garb: this is easily done when the role is as elastic as that of 'mental health' professionals. The 'territory' of professional care is unavoidably an interpersonal 'field', which is shaped by the beliefs and desires of the people involved, the persons occupying their respective roles. In particular this area is one in which various forms of interest emerge and conflict.

POWER AND PROFESSIONS

A startling characteristic of advanced industrial societies is the extent to which the division of labour has led to the creation of professions. Sociologists interested in this phenomenon have attempted to answer three fundamental questions: What exactly is a profession? What functions do professions serve? And, how do professions develop and acquire their status? We will not dwell on the problem of defining a profession other than to note suggestions have ranged from providing lists of the characteristics of professions to the rather more helpful notion that a profession is a structure for controlling an occupation. The other two questions, however, are of direct concern to us, and are explored in the following sections.

The function of professions

Concerning the function of professions there has been a marked difference of opinion. Durkheim (1957) saw the growth of professions as a positive aspect of industrial societies because they contributed to 'stability'. He considered the professions to be a precondition for consensus. The function of professions was seen in terms of their contribution to social cohesion and resistance to dramatic or radical change. Similarly, Carr-Saunders and Wilson (1933) saw the professions as among 'the most stable elements in society'. They are explicit in seeing the function of professions as employing knowledge in the service of power. Lynn (1963) went so far as to argue professions are vital, not merely for the stability and survival of individual industrial societies, but also to 'maintain world order' (p.653), through their international organisations and identities.

A central feature of the 'stabilising' nature of professions is said to be what is known as 'professionalism'. This, it is claimed, involves a devotion to the collective good, and a minimising of self-interest. That is, notions of commitment to particular standards of work and morality. For example, Halmos (1970) claims that an 'ethic of personal service' characterises those professions such as medicine and social work whose 'principal function is to bring about changes in the psychosocial personality of the client', and that they are 'leaders in the creation of a new moral uniformity, a natural order influencing all industrial societies, whatever their political structure' (Johnson 1972 p.13). Professions are seen, from this perspective, as vanguards of morality as well as stability.

The writers quoted so far all agree that a key function of the professions is that of engendering social stability by moderating and channelling forces pressing for change. This function is considered a positive factor in the development of industrial societies. This sympathetic account of the function of professions has been criticised in various ways. We can consider two main questions: are these accounts accurate – are the professions really stabilising forces? And, if they are, should they be praised or criticised?

Weber's (1964) analysis accepts the 'stability' function of professions, but is critical because he considers the professions to be part of the bureaucratisation of society, which he argues will inevitably lead to individuals becoming subject to increasingly unaccountable authority. C. Wright-Mills (1956) argued that the expansion of the professions was not the expansion of learned and humanitarian forces dedicated to service, stability and democracy, but an explosion of 'experts and technocrats' who would by virtue of their specialisation be narrow and lacking in vision. Abercrombie and Urry (1983) offer a neo-Marxist analysis asserting that the 'service class' (i.e. professional and managerial groups) 'perform the functions of control, reproduction and conceptualisation – necessary functions for capital in relation to labour' (p.122). Such accounts agree that the growth of the professions has been a stabilising force, but has served to influence industrial societies in largely undemocratic ways, ensuring that whatever change does occur serves the interests of dominant power groups.

In contrast to such critiques, others argue that professions are a positive force for change, allowing people from relatively unempowered sections of society to attain a greater share of wealth and privilege through the acquisition of specialised knowledge and skills. Some have argued the professions (or at least some professions) are actually the most potent force for change in society. Abercrombie and Urry (1983) argued that during a recession the threats arising from economic insecurity may serve to radicalise members of the service class. In this respect the experience of the service class during the 1980s is instructive. Both sectors of this class (managers and professionals) have expanded dramatically in the last twenty years. But in the 1980s Conservative governments promoted a managerial ethic which included a barely concealed contempt for professionals. There is some evidence (Edgell and Duke 1991), that the professional sectors of the service class, particularly those working in the areas of health and education, became more radical in their views following cuts in public spending and the extension of managerial power that occurred throughout the 1980s. A cynic could be forgiven for suggesting that professionals only make a fuss and draw attention to the discrimination and deprivation suffered by users of their service when their own position is threatened, and are content to remain silent when their privileges are secure. What we have witnessed (particularly in the health service) is a battle for power between managers and professions, and between the rival professions themselves, usually cloaked in rhetoric about the welfare of patients. A critical view may also suggest that the actual behaviour of professions when under threat reveals how hollow the talk of ethical professionalism is, and that a profession essentially exists to promote the self-interest of its members, rather than to protect consumers.

We now turn to the way in which professional status and power develop and how, as individuals, we may participate in this development. In the following section I may seem to be emphasising the unpalatable aspects of the development of professional status and power. If so, my intention is not to promote cynicism or despair. Rather, my goal is to highlight some of the ways our self-interest might be operating, and in particular to encourage awareness of, and investigation into, the ethical dilemmas which inevitably arise when 'care' is professionalised.

Although Savage (1992) is surely correct to argue organisational and cultural assets are inferior to property as sources of class power, we should not underestimate just how valuable are the organisational and cultural assets bestowed on members of a profession, nor how much power is gained by ownership of these assets. In various ways our immediate experience is determined, constrained and dominated by the operation of organisational and cultural power. This is true of our experience both as professionals and as people forced to rely on professionals for help. A point which brings us to a key question: What sorts of power do professions have and how did they get it?

The acquisition of professional power

The development of professions can be explored from various angles, but I want to focus on what we might call the interpersonal strategy of professionalisation. This aspect has been well documented and described by Johnson (1972).

In any society undergoing industrial development we can observe the growth of occupations with specialised skills. Such differentiation inevitably results in relationships of social and economic dependence forming between those who have the required skills and those who do not. Dependence on the skills of others inevitably results in a lack of discrimination in consumption. Clearly, the more a 'consumer' can be made to feel deficient in skills or knowledge in a particular domain, the less confident they will feel in judging the competence of 'producers' ('consumers' and 'producers' being understood in a very broad sense). The highest levels of uncertainty will occur when a consumer is unable to specify what exactly is required of the producer.

There are two crucial features of the interdependence between producers and consumers: *social distance* and *uncertainty*. Clearly when one party in an interaction has knowledge or skills it wishes to market, and another has needs it wants fulfilled, there is dependence but also distance: the two parties have different interests, goals, motives and functions in the interaction. But this social distance gives rise to uncertainty. What is the nature of the relation? What are the rights and duties of each participant? Who is to specify the terms of the exchange and the format of the interaction? How to assess if responsibilities have been adequately discharged? What are the relative levels of dependence and autonomy between the two parties?

Such uncertainty is especially acute when the consumer's lack of discrimination is at its highest – that is when the consumer does not know how their need can be met. Regarding this uncertainty, inherent in all producer–consumer relationships, Johnson notes: 'Power relationships will determine whether uncertainty is reduced at the expense of producer or consumer' (1972, p.41). The operation of power manifests as increased dependency for one party and a corresponding increased autonomy for the other. In effect power will determine whose definition of the relationship will prevail, and hence whose interests will be given priority. Johnson further notes: 'A significant element in producing variation in the degree of uncertainty and therefore potential for autonomy is the esoteric character of the knowledge applied by the specialist' (1972, p.42). 'Esoteric' is the key word here; esoteric means hidden, obscure, known only to the initiated. Esoteric knowledge is a very potent way in which the uncertainty inherent in the producer–consumer interaction can be reduced in favour of the former. This creates a social distinction characterised by the greater dependency of the consumer and the greater autonomy of the producer. Hence laying claim to esoteric knowledge (and the skills which are claimed to follow from this) offers a powerful means of dominating a producer–consumer exchange, and being able to impose what are to be the conditions of that exchange.

In order to establish control of a domain, or territory, a profession must persuade potential clients that members of the profession possess specialised knowledge and skills in three areas:

1. The capacity to accurately identify a problem.
2. The capacity to understand the cause of the problem.
3. The capacity to solve the problem.

Knowledge and skills in these three areas confer the status of 'expert'. With respect to service occupations, the assertion of capability in these three areas, in terms both of knowledge and skills, must operate through face-to-face contact between providers and consumers. Johnson calls this the 'diagnostic relationship'. The diagnostic relationship rests on the claim that a particular service provider can reliably and accurately identify a problem, understand its cause, and provide a solution. The three features of the diagnostic relationship noted here frequently form the basis of an ideological struggle in which professional groups assert the need for independence and 'professional status' as a necessary condition for fulfilling obligations to consumers. And in fact any profession that, within a particular domain, can persuade potential clients that it alone possesses knowledge in these three areas will be able to exercise considerable autonomy, be free of pressure from competition, and be able to rely on continued dependence and compliance from its consumers.

It is easy to see that possession of esoteric knowledge is a very tempting acquisition. But, as Johnson warns, the imbalance in power between practitioner and client provides opportunities for practitioners to increase social distance, and their own autonomy and control over practice, 'by engaging in a process of "mystification"' (1972: p.43). 'Mystification' refers to a process of obscuring, of bewildering in order to exploit. Mystification attempts to render the ideas and practices of the mystifiers unavailable to assessment and evaluation by outsiders. It facilitates control of the assumed area of competence, helps raise effective demand (which expands the market the professional can exploit) while at the same time preventing potential clients developing effective discriminating powers (i.e., keep them needy but ignorant), and helps secure a monopoly in the particular field by dissuading competitors. Broadly, mystification aims to increase the dependence of the client and the autonomy of the professional. Important elements of mystification include the use of technical language, and what might be described as demanding 'rites of passage', which can strengthen the internal cohesion of the group, and ward off critical examination and competition from those outside the group. Mystification may range from what might be regarded as the relatively innocuous use of professional jargon to various forms of dissimulation, and in some cases to outright fraud. But in whatever guise, mystification is essentially a tool of power and self-interest. As Johnson notes: 'Uncertainty is not, therefore, entirely cognitive in origin but may be deliberately increased to serve manipulative or managerial ends' (ibid., p. 43).

Mystification is closely related to the notion of ideology, which can be defined as the deployment of ideas that obscure and distort reality in the interests of a particular group. If a profession can offer not only merely persuasive grounds for its domination of a territory but also demonstrate usefulness to wider networks of power, particularly political and economic power, then its security will be greatly increased. Any profession that can promote or protect the interests of those with political and economic power, functioning as 'experts in legitimation', will have added another layer of protection to their position.

Although this account applies to the professions in general it is particularly relevant to those working in health and social service areas. As Johnson notes, these occupations have 'particularly acute problems of uncertainty', with the judgement of consumers being largely ineffective. In these situations the seeking of professional help 'necessarily invites intrusion of others into intimate and vulnerable areas of the consumers self- or group-identity'. With respect to these professions the greater social distance and greater helplessness of the client leads to a greater 'exposure to possible exploitation and the need for social control' (Johnson, 1972, pp. 43–4).

COLONISING DISTRESS

What Johnson calls the 'diagnostic relationship' is at the heart of the function and development of the mental health professions, especially those who actually control the diagnostic relation. Examining the operation of the diagnostic relation reveals most clearly the ideological nature of the mental health industry. We will very briefly consider the essential features of the diagnostic relationship in relation to the specific diagnosis of 'schizophrenia', one of the foundation stones of psychiatry.

The diagnostic relationship: the case of 'schizophrenia'

Is 'schizophrenia' a disease? Can 'schizophrenia' be reliably identified? Is the cause, or are the causes, understood? Can the condition be effectively treated? Clearly the answers to these questions focus on the credibility of the diagnostic relationship itself, and on the legitimation of psychiatric power which is based on that relation. However, these matters have been, and remain, highly controversial. Concerning the first aspect of the diagnostic relationship, identifying the problem, there are two questions. Can psychiatrists reliably infer the presence of the construct 'schizophrenia', and is this construct valid? There have been a number of recent reviews of a large body of evidence which cast considerable doubt on the reliability, the construct validity, the predictive validity, and the aetiological specificity of the diagnosis of 'schizophrenia' (for example Bentall *et al.*, 1988; Boyle, 1990). The evidence suggests that the reliability and validity of the construct 'schizophrenia' have yet to be established, hence its use in both clinical and research settings raises serious questions. But what about the second aspect of the diagnostic relationship, concerning cause? (It may be noted that the question, 'What is the cause of schizophrenia?', becomes incoherent if we reject the notion of 'schizophrenia' as a meaningful scientific construct. But we may ask 'Why do some individuals manifest the specific forms of behaviour and experience likely to attract a diagnosis of 'schizophrenia'?') It is important to consider this second feature of the diagnostic relationship as it has implications for the fate of those diagnosed 'schizophrenic' and brings into focus the ideological function of the diagnosis.

There have been various suggested causes of 'schizophrenia', but most psychiatrists have focused on biological factors. Despite the efforts expended in the search for a biological cause, results have been tenuous at best, while the claims have often been optimistic, and at times bordering on fraudulent (Charlton, 1990). But while the search for the assumed biological origins have continued, there has been a gradual accumulation of evidence pointing to the importance of social factors in both the incidence and the course of 'schizophrenia'. In a comprehensive review of this evidence Richard Warner (1985) notes that in particular 'political economy assumes a hitherto underemphasised importance in the production and perpetuation of schizophrenia' (ibid., p. 28). Concerning what may be regarded as typical symptoms of chronic 'schizophrenia', these are more accurately 'attributed to the purposeless lifestyle and second class citizenship of the schizophrenic'(1985, p. 299). And that 'the origins of the schizophrenic's alienation are to be found in the political and economic structure of society – in the division of labour and development of wage work' (ibid., p. 190). Warner is careful to point out that he is not arguing 'that material conditions create schizophrenia in any simple, deterministic way, but rather that they mould the course and outcome of the illness and influence, along with others factors, its incidence'. The point is that the significance of social factors has been dramatically underemphasised in favour of biological theory and research. Given the state of the evidence, it is difficult to see this as other than ideological.

The third aspect of the diagnostic relationship will often be regarded as following logically from the second, although clearly this is not necessarily the case. However, consistent with a biological approach to causation 'schizophrenia' is usually treated with medication. But neuroleptic medication may be much less helpful than often assumed. Crow *et al.* (1986) note that only about 20 per cent of first episode 'schizophrenics' (followed up for two years) respond to drug treatment. It may be admitted that response to medication is unpredictable, but what of the claims that, overall, neuroleptics have dramatically improved outcome? Warner (1985, Chapter 10) presents evidence demonstrating that long-term outcome of 'schizophrenia' has not significantly improved since the introduction of antipsychotic drugs in 1954. It also appears to be the case that despite suppressing symptoms in some patients in the short-term, long-term use of neuroleptics may exacerbate what is assumed to be a basic neurochemical deficit in 'schizophrenia': dopamine receptor supersensitivity (ibid., pp. 218–21). A number of researchers have argued the polymorphic course of the condition is evidence against the conception of 'schizophrenia' as a progressive disease process (for a review of this research see Barham and Haywood, 1990). Recovery from 'schizophrenia' appears to be crucially related to social and economic factors. Warner concludes that we know enough about the origin and perpetuation of 'schizophrenia' to render the condition benign, but 'we may, in essence, have to restructure Western society' to do so (1985, p. 156).

It would appear then that with respect to 'schizophrenia' the diagnostic relationship, which confers power on psychiatrists, is constructed on some highly contentious claims, to put it mildly. It is difficult to see the emphasis which is placed on the concept of 'schizophrenia', and the medically based research and treatment industry such emphasis has generated, as anything other than ideological. Hence we may legitimately ask, whose interests are served by this emphasis? In whose interests are millions of pounds spent on research into drugs and biochemical theories of causation? By promoting the view that 'schizophrenia' is a biological defect we obscure the multifactorial nature of the condition, and in particular we conceal the fact, argued so forcefully by Warner, that we are generating pain and suffering by the way we organise our society. It is in the interests of all those who do well out of industrial societies to support psychiatrists and others working in the field of 'mental health' in perpetuating this view of 'schizophrenia'. All this is part of a process of 'mystification' which serves the interests of power, a means by which those without power are blamed for their condition and given merely token assistance, through medication or therapy.

The diagnostic relationship: the psychotherapy industry

Much the same questions can be raised with regard to psychotherapy in general. What are considered to be problems, the way we identify needs, what experience or states of mind we assume require professional attention, the sorts of explanation we offer, the language we use, and the processes we consider to be helpful, all reflect the basic structure of the diagnostic relationship, which invariably operates primarily in the interests of professionals. It is our definition of the nature of the interaction which prevails.

We find ourselves contributing to a radical disempowering of people, appropriating their capacity to help and support each other, by promoting ourselves as experts in the area of 'mental health'. While, just as with the case of 'schizophrenia' the assumptions of the diagnostic relationship which we employ are largely bogus. Emotional distress of any sort is deemed to be the domain of professionals who have esoteric knowledge and expertise in this field. The professional will seek to locate the problem in the person's history of learning, their belief-system, their family relationships or whatever other model is associated with a particular professional identity. However, the evidence that any of these accounts are true, or that the specific therapeutic procedures based on them are effective, is almost non-existent. But as David Smail has noted: 'We find it virtually impossible to *abandon* the idea of therapy, to contemplate *seriously* the possibility that in fact therapy may *really not work*' (1987, p. 77). And yet therapy 'is of much less help then almost any of us can bear to think' (ibid., p. 78).

The ideological functions and self-interest of psychiatry, psychology and psychotherapy may not be seen as such by practitioners, but the effects are surely obvious. Siphoning off from the community the capacity for understanding and mutual support serves the interests of professionals who benefit from a dependent and disempowered group of 'clients' (the implications of the term do not need spelling out).

An important feature of colonisation is the way it spreads its borders. It is instructive to note the way new diagnoses are invented to incorporate features of human life and experience into the framework of 'pathology'. In an unusual reversal of this trend homosexuality was only removed from the Diagnostic and Statistical Manual in its third edition (1983). Many aspects of human variation are drawn into the orbit of 'pathology', colonised by a professional class eager to extend its borders. R.D. Laing once described this as a 'project of homogenisation': we are all expected to experience and behave in similar ways, and variations are abnormal (not in the statistical sense, but in the sense of pathology). This is clearly a process of extending power and control into as many areas of an individual's life as possible. This process serves the interests of professionals by giving them an increasingly disempowered and heterogenous client group, serving to marginalise difference and potential dissent. If we take this line of enquiry to the point of challenging the ability or the right of any group to legislate on issues of 'mental health' and normality (i.e., to question the terms of the diagnostic relationship) we move into dangerous territory. Colonial powers do not welcome resistance.

Damaging professions?

Ivan Illich (1977) has provided a deeply critical account of the effects of professional health care systems. He outlines three main areas of concern. First, what Illich calls 'clinical iatrogenesis', refers to damage resulting directly from treatment. Second, 'social iatrogenesis', meaning the various forms of damage that result from the 'socio-economic transformations which have been made attractive, possible or necessary' by the development of the professional and institutional structures of the health care system (p. 49). For example, social iatrogenesis arises from the creation of disabling dependence and extravagant expectations, which involves the expropriation of the capacity of individuals and communities to take care of and heal themselves (equivalent to creating a 'client' group which has unlimited effective demand with as little discriminative power as possible). And third, 'cultural iatrogenesis' refers to the damaging consequences of promoting a culture in which suffering, sickness, pain, infirmity, old age and death are enemies against which others (professionals) wage a relentless war on our behalf. In an advanced stage of such a culture alternatives become virtually inconceivable. One way in which this is accomplished is through the control of language: 'Language is taken over by the doctors: the sick person is deprived of meaningful words for his anguish, which is thus further increased by linguistic mystification' (ibid., p. 175). Overall, Illich argues, a professionalised care system 'cannot but enhance even as it obscures the political conditions that render society unhealthy', and will inevitably tend to 'mystify and to expropriate the power of the individual to heal himself and to shape his or her environment' (ibid., p. 16).

Illich is uncompromising in his claims that the professionalisation of medical and psychological care has been deeply damaging to individuals and communities. Although I am inclined to agree with those critics of Illich who argue he has overstated his case, it seems to me that the forms of damage which he sought to elucidate are particularly visible with respect to the mental health industry. It is striking, for example, to see the way various 'experts' (psychiatrists, psychologists, psychotherapists and counsellors) are called in whenever someone undergoes a conspicuous trauma. But we may ask, what has happened to the capacity of communities to care for those in anguish? And if there really is more to the counsellor's trade than care and consideration, why are these 'skills' not disseminated to the population at large?

The problem is of course that a population saturated with various forms of social and cultural iatrogenesis will be convinced that they need the ministrations of professionals, and indeed to suddenly withdraw those ministrations will leave many without any help at all. None the less the habit of deferring to professionals in the field of 'mental health' is a deeply damaging one. Caring for people in distress, even those in psychotic states, is not something that can be appropriated by a professional class without damage to the community as a whole.

It does not follow from this necessarily that there is no role for specialised care (although Illich does draw this conclusion). As far as we know, in every culture, there have been people whose distress and disability are prolonged and profound. The community may well decide these people would be most helped by other members of the community who spend their working lives trying to understand and help those in such difficulties. Clearly this raises important ethical questions concerning principles of distributive justice. I believe a very strong case can be made for the primacy of the principle, *to each according to their need*. But what we have seen in the 'mental health' industry is a shift of resources, skills, and concern away from the more chronic and less glamorous end of the spectrum of difficulties towards the milder forms of disturbance, that are perhaps easier to work with, and felt to be more rewarding. In a recent edition of *Hospital Update* (April 1994), Jeffrey Marks, a consultant psychiatrist, wrote an editorial, the general tone of which is one of outraged indignation that the role of psychiatry should by questioned by what he sees as subordinate groups, in particular nurses and psychologists. He criticises CPNs who have shifted the focus of their work from severe disturbances to those with relatively mild difficulties, under the pretext of 'primary prevention'. As Marks notes, the evidence does not support the claims that such work is effective, and it is surely pertinent to ask whose interests are served by this shift of focus.

Issues of power and domination are of course of much wider scope than we have considered so far. The writings of Michel Foucault have been instrumental in making visible some of the intricacies of what he calls the 'strategies of power', which goes far beyond the familiar Marxist analysis of power resting ultimately with those who control the economy. Foucault saw modern life as a 'dispersed and indefinite field of power relations or strategies of domination', with power manifesting 'in a multiplicity of networks' (1988, Chapter 6). He described what he considered to be a vast 'normalising' project which has extended over centuries, in which various forms of difference have been classified, marginalised and controlled through the proliferation of categories of deviance within the broad domains of criminality and psychopathology. Foucault tried to demonstrate through the historical analysis of various institutions, that more subtle methods of domination and control have largely replaced overt violence. In developed societies various forms of coercion have been exerted towards the production of regimented, obedient, isolated and self-policing subjects. It is not difficult to see how key features of the 'mental health' industry contribute to this process. In Foucault's account the operation of this industry is just one part of a much wider project of domination, control and exploitation. Hence it would be an error to assume that professionalised care in the field of mental health is simply a product of professional self-interest: the 'mental health' industry is shaped by, and serves the purposes of, much wider and much more powerful interests.

To conclude, I would like to emphasise a point implicit throughout this section, true of all forms of colonisation: that colonisation is not merely exploitive it is also formative. The ideas and procedures underlying 'mental health' practice are constitutive of the reality they purport to describe. That is, our accounts of psychological disturbance are not simply mirrors, or even models, or reality. We have noted that the 'mental health' industry in general presents a view of the world that serves to legitimise abuse and exploitation by advancing theories of damage and claims of cure that are primarily personal and internal in nature. However, the application of such views ensures that they are not merely descriptive or explanatory, but in various ways contribute to the production of the various forms of behaviour considered to be the professional's legitimate domain. Psychological theories tend to become instantiated in the phenomena they purport to describe. This is perhaps the most insidious form of colonisation perpetuated by the 'mental health' industry.

DEMOCRATISING DISTRESS

In reviewing the foregoing information it is not my intention to argue that there is no place for paid workers in the field of 'mental health', but rather to emphasise some of the ethical issues inherent in any occupation where there are substantial temptations to mystification. Concerning the general framework of description, classification and explanation, and current treatment procedures, crucial questions arise: how legitimate are they? Whose interests do they serve? To what extent do current understanding and treatment hinder development in other directions?

'Democratising distress' would involve a different way of thinking about and responding to the various forms of suffering currently regarded as the 'territory' of various professionals. By way of contrast it is worth reflecting on the communal approach to psychosis that has often been described by anthropologists in studies of 'traditional' societies. One example is that of the Navaho healing ceremony in which psychosis is regarded as a community disturbance and as such the healing ceremony embraces the whole community. Relatives, friends, and a wider group of participants, all take medicines and undergo the elaborate purifications and rituals of the ceremony in recognition of the community's need to be healed, or made whole. The primary value of the individual's relation to the wider community is thereby re-asserted. In this way psychosis is not personalised or individualised, hence the person undergoing a psychotic crisis is not marginalised, stigmatised or pathologised. This way of responding to psychosis clearly has the advantage of avoiding the secondary symptoms that frequently occur in those labelled 'schizophrenic' in 'developed' societies as a result of the marginal and deprived existence they are forced to live. Elements of a tolerant and communal response to psychosis survive in much of the Third World, and may well be a significant factor in the superior recovery rates that have been noted outside of the 'developed' world (Warner, 1985).

With respect to Europe and the United States Breggin (1993) notes that despite obstacles there have been a number of 'creative alternatives' to the medically dominated treatment of psychosis that are 'by far the least expensive and most effective' (p. 479). He describes a number of these alternatives. I will not address these approaches here, but will instead draw attention to some of the obstacles that are frequently neglected in the search for a more democratic response to human suffering. I believe Breggin is right to point out that 'As long as the psychiatric and medical monopoly controls the delivery of mental health services creative alternatives will be rare' (ibid., p. 479). But I would question his exclusive focus on psychiatrists. Psychiatry is not the only profession in the field of 'mental health' that trades in mystification. All of us who benefit from the sufferings of others are implicated in this question of whose interest are served by the operation of the 'mental health' industry. The question is, of course, not merely a factual one; at its heart it is an ethical question. And answering ethical questions honestly often involves considerable cost. As Sue Holland (1988) has noted: 'It is only by finding a therapeutic practice which will genuinely empower the "patient/client" that we can honestly reject the accusation that we are "poverty pimps", enriching ourselves out of the anguish of others' (p. 135).

Often the obstacles preventing the development of 'creative alternatives' are considered to be the vested interests of psychiatry and the pharmaceutical industry. Breggin's (1993) book detailing the deficiencies of psychiatric treatments and the psychiatry–pharmaceutical industry alliance argues this point forcefully. But this is surely only part of the picture. The operation of power and dominance, and the pursuit of self-interest are not the prerogative of one or two professional groups. All of those who benefit from the suffering of others have a vested interest in promoting particular types of explanation and types of treatment. Promoting certain ideas and practices and attacking others is often only tenuously related to questions of argument and evidence, and appears more clearly associated with ideological struggle. Therapeutic fashions may be promoted for many reasons unrelated to the welfare of the patient. The 'territory' of 'mental health' has been a region exploited for crude financial gain, but also a means for gaining status and prestige, for promoting pet theories, for achieving some sense of dominance, or a way of managing personal conflicts. The challenge of finding democratic alternatives to the current arrangements, riddled as they are with hierarchy, rivalry, mystification and self-interest, is a daunting one, not least because our own assumptions, perceptions and convictions are likely to be as saturated with self-interest as those we would criticise. It is not easy for any of us to extricate ourselves from the intricate web of mystification, dissimulation, wishful thinking, insecurity and self-interest which both ensnares us, and by which we ensnare others.

Not only are self-interest and wishful thinking deeply engrained, so is the tendency (when we are not simply indifferent) to either dominate or defer to others. To talk about 'democratic' alternatives implies both an understanding of democracy, and a capacity to think and act in a democratic fashion. But how easy is that? 'Representative' democracies like the United Kingdom are of course democratic in only a very minimal sense. Our lives are shaped by forces which are extremely antagonistic to democracy, and our capacity to think and act democratically are very severely constrained. The habits of deferring to 'experts', of needing leaders, of accepting injustice and coercion, and submitting to sundry authorities are all very deeply ingrained. We are are not permitted to take control of our own lives, to participate in forming the decisions which will affect us in the workplace and in our communities. Given the poverty of our experience of democracy it is bound to be an extremely difficult process to shift the provision of 'mental health' services in a genuinely democratic direction.

The way in which our responses are informed by assumptions that are often deeply antagonistic to democratic values may be seen by simply reflecting on how we respond to others. Concerning the case studies outlined in the first section, we may note that various professional groups (doctors, psychiatrists, social workers, nurses, psychotherapists, etc.) would diagnose and treat each situation differently. But how legitimate are the competing claims? It is by no means clear just what would be the most accurate account of the problem(s) and its cause(s) in each of these examples. What would be a good 'outcome' – for the patients, for their families, for the professionals, for other interested parties? Whose interests will be paramount? Whose version of the diagnostic relationship will prevail, and why? These questions will usually be settled by considerations of power and interest. Looking back to the outline of the three experiences we may give particular attention to our personal responses. What do we want of Carlton, Clare and Albert, and of the various professionals involved? Do we want to control them? Do we want to feel powerful, knowledgeable or superior? To what extent do our own needs intrude and shape our perceptions of them? As we reflect on the experiences can we get a sense of where our interests and judgements lie? Given the brevity of the sketches, what have we read into the accounts? What alliances and agendas have already taken shape, despite the paucity of information? Have we already categorised and prescribed, judged, exonerated or perhaps condemned? Are we already caught in a web of power, of accusation and justification?

It is important to remember that domination, exploitation and hierarchy are not simply the product of institutions. We create these relations as reflections of what we are. I would suggest that the very desire for professional status and expertise in the field of emotional disturbance is particularly problematic. The struggle for power inevitably creates distinction and separation. The detrimental consequences of this raises pressing ethical questions for all those who earn a living in this field. Alternative approaches may be very difficult to realise. Having lived enmeshed in networks of abusive power all our lives we may well find ourselves unprepared and ill-equipped to respond to another's suffering in non-exploitative and genuinely caring ways.

CONCLUSION

The debt to the work of others will be clear from the references, but I hope I have brought together observations from different fields that help illuminate some of the ethical problems raised by systems of professionalised care. Through this brief exploration I hope enough has been covered to raise questions in the reader's mind about the conflicts of interest implicit in the process of professionalisation (which are particularly acute in the context of 'mental health' care); the ways in which perception and practice may be shaped less by reason and evidence and more by self-interest; the way struggles for dominance and 'territory', and inter-professional rivalries, may damage service users; the way professional self-interest may block the development of more effective, and more helpful forms of care; the way in which the activity of workers in the field of 'mental health' may actually be contributing to a culture that is toxic to psychological well-being. These and related issues present us with the inevitability of making multiple ethical choices with significant consequences both for ourselves and others.

But perhaps the most difficult problems we face are our own capacity for self-deception, and our own inertia. The pressures involved in surviving in what many experience as an increasingly hostile work environment can easily lead to an accentuated sense of personal and professional insecurity, and a blunting of our moral sensibilities. Returning to the metaphor of colonisation we can note the exploitation involved does not only have detrimental consequences for the territories colonised: the colonisers damage themselves. Professional privilege has its costs. Seeing beyond what we may imagine to be our self-interest, to the wider consequences and implications of our actions, may require considerable effort and be profoundly unsettling. We may discover that we are far advanced into a dangerous state of passivity, acquiescence and moral paralysis. But if, individually and collectively, we are ever going to be able to dismantle some of what Foucault calls the 'multiple mechanisms of "incarceration"', – which largely define our personal, social and professional being – then such honest, and potentially disturbing, reflection, is unavoidable.

REFERENCES

Abercrombie, N. and Urry, J. 1983: *Capital, labour and the middle classes*. London: Allen and Unwin.

American Psychiatric Association 1983: *Diagnostic and statistical manual*. 3rd edition. Washington, DC: AMPA.

Barham, P. and Hayward, R. 1990: Schizophrenia as a life process. In Bentall, P. (ed.) *Reconstructing schizophrenia*. London: Routledge, 61–85.

Bentall, R.P., Jackson, H.F., and Pilgrim, D. 1988: Abandoning the concept of 'schizophrenia': some implications of validity arguments for psychological research into psychotic phenomena. *British Journal of Clinical Psychology* 27: 303–24.

Boyle, M. 1990: *Schizophrenia: a scientific delusion?* London: Routledge.

Breggin, P. 1993: *Toxic psychiatry*. London: HarperCollins.

Carr-Saunders, A.M. and Wilson, P.A. 1993: *The professions*. Reprint. London: Frank Cass.

Charlton, B.G. 1990: A critique of biological psychiatry. *Psychological Medicine* 20, 3–6.

Crow, T.J., MacMillan, J.F., Johnson, A.L. and Johnstone, E.C. 1986: The Northwick Park study of first time episodes of schizophrenia: II: a controlled trial of prophylactic neuroleptic treatment. *British Journal of Psychiatry* 148: 120–7.

Durkheim, E. 1957: *Professional ethics and civil morals*. London: MacMillan.

Edgell, S. and Duke, V. 1991: *A measure of Thatcherism: a sociology of Britain*. London: HarperCollins.

Foucault, M. 1979: *Discipline and punish*. London: Penguin.

Foucault, M. 1988: *Politics, philosophy, culture: interviews and other writings, 1977–1984*. Edited by L.D. Kritzman. London: Routledge.

Halmos, P. 1970: *The personal service society*. London: Macmillan.

Holland, S. 1988: Defining and experimenting with prevention. In Ramen, S. and Grannichedda, M.G. (eds.) *Psychiatry in transition: the Italian and British experience*. London: Pluto Press, 125–37.

Illich, I. 1977: *Limits to medicine*. London: Penguin.

Johnson, T.J. 1972: *Professions and power*. London: MacMillan.

Marks, J. 1994: The re-emergence of anti-psychiatry: psychiatry under threat. *Hospital Update* editorial, 187–9.

Marshall, R. 1990: The genetics of schizophrenia. In Bentall, R.P. (ed.) *Reconstructing schizophrenia*. London: Routledge, 89–117.

Savage, M. 1992: *Property, bureaucracy and culture: middle-class formation in contemporary Britain*. London: Routledge.

Smail, D. 1987: *Taking care: an alternative to therapy*. London: J.M.Dent and Sons Ltd.

Warner, R. 1985: *Recovery from schizophrenia: psychiatry and political economy*. 2nd edition. London: Routledge.

Weber, M. 1964: *The theory of social and economic organisation*. London: Collier-Macmillan.

Wright-Mills, C. 1956: *White collar*. New York: OUP.

5

THE ROLE OF THE PSYCHIATRIC NURSE

Ben Davidson

Perhaps we should punctuate the narrative of the text at this stage by making explicit a social contructionist view of psychiatric disorder; it might also be timely to assert that the popular conception of mental illness as a disorder located in the individual is wrong, and that the concepts and techniques of psychiatry and associated disciplines do more harm than good. We now begin to develop an alternative view. Using as a starting point the writings of David Smail and referring to Laing's work as well as professional and personal experience, Ben Davidson argues that the process of genuine 'mental health' care comprises demystification and comfort, and examines some of the benefits and difficulties of this model in relation to clinical practice. The role of the psychiatric nurse and issues of professional identity are considered. Ben emphasises the merits of a reformulation of our role and identity in line with the preceding analysis.

What can be the relevance of the psychiatric nurse to the life of a person who is mentally ill? To do justice to this question, it is necessary to examine what 'mental illness' is, how best to care for those 'suffering from it' and the role psychiatric nurses might usefully play in that care. My starting-point is the position held by David Smail, a senior clinical psychologist and academic, and I will use Smail's work as the basis for examining all of these issues.

David Smail is currently honorary special professor in clinical psychology at Nottingham University and head of clinical psychology services in Nottingham. His reputation as a clinician is widespread but his popularity is by no means universal, particularly as his work since 1973 has embodied scepticism regarding the clinical and theoretical claims of the psychology/psychiatry/psychotherapy industry (the psych industry). Although abnormal behaviour, chaotic experience and states of emotional distress are popularly conceived as disorders located in individuals, Smail rejects any attempt to pathologise people in such states and avoids using ideas from any conceptual system which does so. In this regard, such concepts as 'biochemical imbalance', 'behavioural dysfunction', 'cognitive malfunction', 'faulty learning', 'developmental arrest' and 'family dysfunction' all appear to him to pathologise individuals and thus to mislead, both in terms of theory and clinical practice.

Central to Smail's approach is the belief that we live in a 'dysfunctional' society and emotional, cognitive or behavioural disturbance 'within' an individual (or a family) is essentially a natural result of the intolerable pressures and constraints imposed by that society. These pressures and constraints increasingly impinge on individuals, the lower their position within the hierarchies of wealth and power. Thus, when we observe the emotional, cognitive and behavioural 'symptoms' of the sort of individual, medical ailment that is taken to constitute 'mental illness', we are suffering from a misconception. No matter whether they are classified as neurotic or psychotic, these symptoms are, in Smail's view, more accurately and usefully to be understood as a form of communication wherein the individual is expressing and responding to the havoc wreaked by other individuals or by society at large on her or his embodied experience in the world (Smail, 1984 pp. 92–93 and in this chapter).

Any such extreme expression of intense internal frustration, anger, pain, despair, confusion, misery or fear is unfortunately, according to Smail, likely to be seen as 'illness', for 'being ill' appears to be the only metaphor (or euphemism) available to represent such states. We use similar metaphors in everyday life:

> Recently, when my 4-year-old son was crying, I tried to comfort him, but my comforting was half-hearted. My impatience and irritability undoubtedly showed through and I may well have sounded quite cross with him. He became inconsolably distressed. At the time I concluded (and I caught myself telling him) that he was merely 'tired'. This was easier than acknowledging and validating the real sense of hurt and rejection he felt in response to my behaviour.

In much the same way, according to Smail, the ordinary and inevitable misery and suffering which arise as a more or less direct result of painful and unjust forms of social organisation are represented disingenuously by society as more or less obscure processes of 'illness' requiring professional expertise to diagnose and treat them.

Sometimes I have found that people appear to be reasonably satisfied with this conventional description and treatment of their condition. In many cases, however, individuals seeking (or at least open to) some alternative explanation for their troubles than 'illness', and uneasy about the treatment they expect to receive, have to accept the conventional explanation and treatment anyway, together with its enforcement by assorted agencies and experts.

> At age 4, Craig was sometimes abandoned for days at a time and left to look after two younger sisters. Other times he looked on while his single mother engaged in prostitution in their single room. At age 5 he was taken into care. Despite these and other experiences of severe emotional and physical deprivation, perhaps precisely because these painful experiences were so hard to accept, he retained a desperate optimism and buoyancy through his childhood and adolescence. This optimism was encouraged at the childrens' home where he lived. It was also in conformity with the overwhelming social pressure to accept one's lot and be happy. It did not begin to fade until his twenties. Since the recent death of his mother he has only managed to cling onto some final shreds of this optimism by adopting a set of beliefs which include a view of himself as a Hindu demi-god with superhuman powers to set the world aright and control heaven and earth by magic. When

unable finally to maintain these beliefs he sinks alone into the compounded misery and turmoil of 28 emotionally gruelling years.

Although he desperately wants to understand his experience, his involvement with traditional psychiatric services over two years has not helped. Despite two hospital admissions and intense contact with many psychiatrists and nurses, this contact has served to force him into a reluctant acceptance that his troubles are a biochemical matter (bi-polar affective disorder – manic-depression); that is, they represent something *wrong with him*. He is struggling to free himself from this view with very little support and meanwhile is being treated with psychotropic medication which makes it something of an effort for him even to think.

It is demoralising and uncomfortable to acknowledge and validate the real hurt Craig and countless other clients have suffered. Furthermore, given the ascendancy of a scientific, empirical view of reality wherein subjective experience is generally either devalued or invalidated completely, both clients and those treating them find it hard not to succumb to pressures to accept the conventional wisdom. In these circumstances, it is much easier to call experiential suffering and its results 'illness' and treat them as such.

Smail's ideas, as well as borrowing from some analytic theory, are very much reminiscent of Laing's middle period of work (Laing, 1967) where he reframed psychotic experience and symptom as a form of communication, a pilgrimage and a struggle for freedom and meaning. Smail's work also parallels Laing's in his scepticism regarding the right of society to proclaim itself 'sane'. He calls into question many of the cultural beliefs and values we hold most dear, including the pursuit and idolisation of happiness, the faith we place in science and experts for our salvation and our compulsive view of the self as an object (Smail, 1984, 1988). Laing also contextualised and reframed our conventional ideas regarding 'sanity', for example, he drew attention to 'the condition of alienation, of being asleep, of being unconscious, of being out of one's mind, . . . of . . . normal men [who] have killed perhaps 100,000,000 of their fellow men in the last fifty years' [Laing, 1967; pp. 25–30]. Although one may be inclined to insist that someone whose experience is psychotic appears in some significant way to be 'ill', while the rest of us are not, the most this can really mean is that they are statistically abnormal, for example like a plane no longer flying in formation with the rest of a squadron of planes. Laing urged us not to make the mistake of assuming that society (the rest of the planes still flying 'in formation') is 'on course' and therefore in any particularly superior position (ibid.; pp. 25–30, pp. 55–76). The Holocaust, the Vietnam War, the prevalence of childhood sexual abuse, Western support for and financing of the death squads in Central America, together with countless other examples, show that present-day society as a whole seems also pretty much off course.

As Laing made emphatically clear in his work, however, this is not to say 'that the person who is "out of formation" is more "on course" than the formation' (ibid.: 119) – although, of course, they might be! Likewise, Smail does not believe that a person labelled as 'mentally ill' is, by virtue of their sensitivity to the pressures and constraints that society or life imposes, necessarily more 'sane' than the rest. Neither does he believe that their suffering should be somehow idealised. He simply insists that it is a mistake to see the locus of the problem as within that individual.

Smail argues, furthermore, that, by virtue of the assumptions built into them which pathologise individuals, the various concepts and techniques of 'the psych industry' probably make it more rather than less hard for clients correctly to assess their situation and act accordingly, however innocently these concepts and techniques are used.

> Christine was forced to have sexual intercourse with her father from the age of 4, and subsequently with a group of his paedophile friends. In adolescence her account of her past and her expression of distress were time and again disbelieved by every figure of authority from her mother to doctors and police. Her resulting sense of unreality and dissociation were seen out of context and taken, together with other unextraordinary phenomena, to be 'symptoms' of 'mental illness' (schizophrenia), to be treated chemically. Her belief that she had been sexually abused was taken, subsequently, to be a delusion. And making such claims and expressing distress as she did, was thereafter seen as no more than melodrama and 'attention seeking behaviour', to be discouraged by ignoring or disattending to it, or by sedating her.

Smail suggests that concepts and techniques of behaviour modification, cognitive restructuring, psychoanalysis and chemical control shift both responsibility and blame for their distress onto individuals, worsening their problems by overlaying their misery and suffering with mystification and guilt, as was evidently the case with Christine and Craig.

Now I will summarise what Smail thinks society's response ought to be, and outline my own view of how psychiatric nurses could participate in this response.

THE PROCESS OF 'TAKING CARE'

In place of the techniques of 'the psych industry', Smail suggests the process of 'taking care'. Although he does not say so, I suggest that the psychiatric nurse is particularly well placed to undertake this activity, and that to the extent that any psychiatric nurse does 'take care', she or he becomes relevant in a beneficial way to a person who is 'mentally ill'.

Despite his scepticism, Smail states: 'There will no doubt always be a place for therapy' (1988, p. 142). For Smail, the aims of therapy are demystification and comfort. He defines demystification:

> as establishing what is the case . . . the examination and clearing of the confusions which surround the person's deceived or self-deceiving view of what lies behind [her or his] 'symptoms' [through a process of] negotiat[ing] a view of what the patient's predicament is about which both the patient and therapist can agree.
>
> (Smail, 1984; p. 4)

He continues: 'It seems to me essential for people to enter into, to have the full opportunity to alter and argue with the processes whereby someone else arrives at a formulation of "the problem"'.

Demystification

The process of demystification is a complex one requiring enormous skill and understanding. It is easy to underplay the difficulties faced in keeping one's own prejudices and idiosyncratic views out of this negotiation (Smail, 1978). It is easy also to underestimate the effect on this negotiation of one's being in a position of power over a client. At the risk of oversimplification, however, the spirit of this process may be represented as follows. When we uncover a complete picture of your life history we will realise that it is natural for you to be feeling/thinking/behaving/relating this way. These patterns and states of mind are more than likely 'the reasonable upshot of [your] life history' (Smail, 1984 pp. 12–13) which we can, if you like, explore together. There is a certain humility in adopting and conveying this attitude that, like oneself, the client has a completely acceptable uniqueness. Such humility is essential and all too rare. But perhaps that is understandable. The adoption of this demystifying and normalising attitude often requires a great deal of effort, strength and faith, as significant parts of clients' life histories often appear impenetrably obscure, to them no less than to anyone else. A reductionist view is frequently simpler. Moreover, as already suggested, it is no easy feat to acknowledge and validate the experience of someone who has suffered in a way we prefer not to recognise, particularly if they can hardly bring themselves to acknowledge it. A medical view is frequently less demoralising.

The greater simplicity and reassurance within a reductionist view are extremely powerful motivating factors. Often I meet clients who experience quite bizarre phenomena, such as walls screaming at them, voices instructing them to cut themselves to get rid of the bad blood, their spines crumbling and time bombs primed to go off inside them. Others seems to have been left feeling so precarious and under such threat that they choose not to step outside their homes, sometimes hardly even to move or speak.

> Vernon rarely ventures outside the bedroom of his council flat. He is a handsome man in his early thirties, but he is tortured by an excruciating and overwhelming shyness. Virtually his only human contact is with a community psychiatric nurse who visits him once every week. Vernon insists sometimes that these visits are designed to humiliate him as his key worker is so much more confident and better-looking than he is. At such times Vernon asks his visitor to leave so that he can 'get on with his own life'. Other times he welcomes this contact and talks a little, for example about his hopes of finding a girlfriend. This seems to represent some progress from the situation three years ago when Vernon had no real human contact and was twice arrested and once severely beaten after exposing his erect penis to female neighbours in the street or on their doorsteps.

It seems that some of us, like Vernon, are so overwhelmed by feelings of fear and threat that the ensuing shyness is completely debilitating. In others, this sense of threat manifests itself in fearful hallucinations or delusions and in particular phobias and obsessions. Some people have such fear of making any move at all that they are catatonic. It is difficult to discern where such fear and sense of threat comes from, whether from frightening contact with others, through terrifying experience of society and its enforced norms of thought, experience and behaviour, whether from life itself, or, again, as a result of the treatment received within the psychiatric system. But in any event, the experience and subjective world of clients in such states seem to have been so devastated that I often find it too awful and dismaying to want to explore it. The 'act of faith' I mentioned above seems at such times to be more a plunge into the abyss. And yet I am sure I am not alone in discovering that in response to such an 'act of faith' clients begin to accept their experience so that even the most traumatised begin to unfold as people. This is, of course, not necessarily to cure the individual's 'symptoms'. But it may

> bring them face to face with circumstances in their lives which are distressing, and which they can only ignore at the cost of 'neurotic' [or psychotic] suffering. Often, admittedly, this is to replace one kind of suffering with another, and whether or not this seems a good idea depends on one's values. To me, it seems more constructive, and essentially more hopeful, to recognise that real difficulties, real evils and real pain arise in the world around us through our conduct towards one another than it is to resort, albeit unawares, to self-deceiving strategies which, for example, allow 'illness' to provide the explanation, and indeed the form, of our misery
>
> (Smail, 1984 pp.2–3)

Comfort

Smail's emphasis on comfort as the other main function of therapy makes it clear that a realistic appraisal of clients' predicaments should be followed by empowering and encouraging them 'to do what [they] can to confront those elements of the predicament which admit of some possibility of alteration' (Smail, 1988 p.4). It is an appalling indictment of our society that such basic 'kindness, encouragement and comfort' (ibid. p.142) are in such short supply (and commercial interests are so powerful) that they need to be commodified and sold in the market place by professional 'experts' in the field, or doled out begrudgingly by an overburdened NHS. In ideal circumstances such support and love might be expected and supplied freely and naturally by family and friends for whom we are, surely, but poor substitutes. Nevertheless, 'For many people psychotherapy provides the only source of comfort they are likely to find in what has been, for them at least, a predominantly cruel world' (ibid. p.4). It does appear possible to offer clients something through a relationship with them which serves as comfort and nurturance. In an interview recorded shortly before his death Laing referred to this something as 'co-presence'. He defined this as 'a sort of harmless, inviting presence that doesn't offer threat, isn't felt as threatening, isn't felt as pulling in, isn't felt as doing anything, as just being – but alive, vibrant, actively being' (Tougas *et al.*, 1989). The provision of this sort of comfort is not a product of professional training and is not measurable in terms of some objective criteria of expertise. Neither is it reducible to blind optimism or cheerfulness. Laing defines co-presence further as 'a field effect taking place prior to and behind any words spoken'.

It is more a mark of one's humanity to be able to just be with someone, no matter what state they are in, without needing to act on them in some way, without attempting to change them to suit one's own book, so to speak, and yet still be vibrantly alive to their humanity. But if the distressed and desperate states which are conventionally known as 'mental illness' arise out of our conduct towards one another, then their resolution too must issue from this interface between people, out of a healing common ground that can be established through a therapeutic relationship.

In the context of such a therapeutic relationship, that is, one characterised by this absence of threat, by co-presence and by encouragement and comfort, it seems to me that clients do eventually feel sufficiently safe and courageous to tackle aspects of their experience and life which are amenable to development. Moreover, they often do so without the need for any specialist techniques or esoteric knowledge. What seems often to count for more is the quality of the physical environment (Stokeld, 1990) and the constancy of the nursing care (Strang, 1982). Although there is often little that can be changed and it is frustrating for both the client and oneself to acknowledge that there is neither any way of undoing past experience, nor any cure for the suffering it has brought, one can at least, in such a nurturing, unthreatening physical and psychological environment, work towards a position where the client is seeing things as they really are and accepting their own experience and potential.

THE NURSE'S ROLE?

As nurses, we occupy neither a defined theoretical position with regard to 'mental illness' nor a particularly prestigious or valued position within the hierarchy of 'the psych industry'. This can lead to nurses experiencing a sense of disempowerment, out of which we often rely on a medical framework both for understanding and treating clients, and for our professional and clinical sense of identity. Paradoxically, however, this lowly position and lack of definition in our theoretical approach leave us in a situation where we can more easily accept the adjustment to our thinking and practice that acceptance of Smail's view requires.

Many of the tools for this adjustment are already at hand. For example, Egan's (1990) counselling model which nurses sometimes use encapsulates the range of skills involved in helping someone tell and understand their story. With further training in demystification and empowerment, perhaps with regular involvement in patients' care of groups like Mind and Survivors Speak Out, psychiatric nurses could become more adept in this work. If we do choose to move from the medical view we so often rely on, there is certainly no reason why we should be any less proficient in the dispensation of comfort and in the supply of this unthreatening co-presence than those who have trained as doctors, psychotherapists or other more highly valued professionals. And as 24–hour carers adopting the role both of therapist and friend (Strang, 1982) it may even be that we are more effective. Furthermore, I believe that the adoption of a defined theoretical position and a model of clinical practice as outlined above would probably enhance not only the efficacy of our work, but also our social position by establishing a clear professional role and identity distinct from psychiatry and well beyond the role of hand-servants to the medical profession.

SKILLS AND TRAINING FOR DEMYSTIFICATION AND COMFORT

In order to implement care comprising these elements of demystification and comfort, the skills needed are, of course, considerable. But it is not inconceivable that resources, currently allocated to training nurses somewhat randomly in a hotchpotch of different therapies and a diffusion of antagonistic systems of thought, might be reallocated to training nurses sequentially in:

- awareness of and sensitivity to socio-economic power and interpersonal power issues as they contribute to mental suffering, together with the appropriate skills in demystifying, empowering and facilitating clients in telling their story;
- damage limitation in interaction with clients to prevent the abuses of trust and power;
- working with psychotic people without reliance on medication or other forms of restraint, e.g., employing concepts and skills as used in Kingsley Hall by Laing and Berke in their work with Mary Barnes (Barnes and Berke, 1971) and as still used at The Arbours Crisis Centre[1];
- comfort, encouragement and co-presence, in the context of which, finally, supplementary techniques in dynamic, behavioural or cognitive change may be fully explained and offered to clients *for them* to use if they wish.

If this is done and our identity and role are defined accordingly, I believe that the care we implement will be more effective. But whether or not these changes occur in our profession as a whole, I believe that to the extent that we serve individually to demystify, comfort and empower a person who is 'mentally ill' in the way suggested above, we are both relevant to their life, and also exercise a benign influence on it. Equally, to the extent that our involvement in the life of this person serves to mystify and discomfort them further, we are relevant and, like so many others, do damage. It is imperative that this relevance and benign influence are enhanced.

CONCLUSION

In *The Politics of Experience* Laing wrote (1967 p.110); 'A revolution is currently going on in relation to sanity and madness both inside and outside psychiatry. The clinical view is giving way before a point of view that is both existential and social.' Personally, I have not seen much of it.

In my experience, the general consensus amongst psychiatrists and nurses appears to be that Laing was an interesting and extremely idiosyncratic product of the 1960s psychedelic culture, but best consigned to history and, of course, quite mad. Unfortunately, neither Laing's, nor Smail's, nor anyone else's social and existential perspec-

---

[1] The Arbours Association is a registered charity, set up in 1973 by Morton Schatzman and Joseph Berke, both colleagues of R.D. Laing, three years after the famous Kingsley Hall experiment had finished. The Arbours advertises itself as an organisation founded 'in order to assist people in emotional distress and offer alternatives to traditional mental hospital treatment'. They currently run a Crisis Centre, three long-term residential communities, a consultation service and a psychotherapy training programme. Further information from: The Arbours, 41 Weston Park, London N8 9SY, telephone 0181–340 8125; *see also* Berke's accounts of this work (Berke, 1974, 1981).

tives have taken over from the medical model of madness within psychiatry, nor really even seriously challenged it[2]. Neither does there seem to be much evidence that psychiatric nursing is moving towards an approach resembling the one outlined above, and any attempt to do so would seem to be undermined by our acceptance of the medical model and willingness to encourage the use of medication.

Meanwhile, outside 'the psyche industry', despite attempts to market a rose-tinted version of 'Care in the Community', it is clear from the most cursory examination that neither the political establishment nor society generally have taken up the 1960's call to love and live in harmony with their fellow citizens, especially if they are mad. The clinical view seems altogether more safe and less personally burdensome.

It is clear, therefore, that Laing's optimism regarding this so-called revolution in psychiatry was ill-founded. It is heartening to discover in these circumstances that Smail keeps the lamp burning. It would be even more heartening to discover that there are psychiatric nurses trying to develop this kind of work and interested in forming a professional association based around the ideas above.

REFERENCES

Barnes, M. and Berke, J. 1971: *Mary Barnes: two accounts of a journey through madness.* London: Free Association Books.

Berke, J. 1981: *I haven't had to go mad in here.* Harmondsworth: Penguin.

Egan, G. 1990: *The skilled helper: a systematic approach to effective helping.* 4th edn. California: Brooks Cole Publishing.

Laing, R.D. 1967: *The politics of experience.* New York: Ballantine.

Laing, R.D. and Esterson, A. 1964: *Sanity, madness and the family.* Harmondsworth: Penguin.

Segal, H. 1957: *An introduction to the work of Melanie Klein.* London: Heinemann.

Smail, D. 1978: *Psychotherapy: a personal approach.* London: Dent.

Smail, D. 1984: *Illusion and reality: the meaning of anxiety.* London: Dent.

Smail, D. 1988: *Taking care: an alternative to therapy.* London: Dent.

Stokeld, A. 1990: Building on metaphors. *International Journal of Therapeutic Communities* 2(4), 233–6.

Strang, J. 1982: Psychotherapy by nurses: some special characteristics. *Journal of Advanced Nursing* 7, 167–71.

Tougas, K., Shandel, T. and Feldmar, A. 1989: *Did you used to be R. D. Laing?* Channel Four, London and Third Mind Productions Inc., Vancouver (TV documentary transcript).

[2] Ironically, at the same time as Laing's views appear to be more or less universally discarded within psychiatry (if they were ever given credence) many psychiatrists do what they can to covertly hijack and sanitise Laing's social and existential insights in a way that makes them almost support a reductionist view, as for example, with recent work on High Expressed Emotion in the families of schizophrenics, in which nurses and other practitioners now undertake specialist training. This work seems to me to issue directly from Laing's and Esterson's insights e.g. 'Sanity, Madness and the Family' (Laing and Esterson, 1964).

6

ANTI-PSYCHIATRY: THE ETHICAL AND PRACTICAL ALTERNATIVES TO TRADITIONAL TREATMENT

Joseph H. Berke

There is, of course, a context to the principles outlined in the previous chapter. For a century now within Western, industrialised society, there have been voices insisting that experience labelled 'mad' is meaningful, and *breakdown* of an individual's normal social functioning may better be seen as a *breakthrough*. Here Joseph Berke extends the critique of professional status and conventional psychiatric wisdom. He concentrates here on the anti-spiritual implications of traditional approaches, and he considers alternatives. He develops the theme that there is a way of working which validates clients' experience rather than turning it into an 'illness'. The context is discussed in which it becomes possible to work in this way, referring to the experience of other cultures where the religious and healing potential of dream states is validated. Linking this with mystical experience, Joseph elaborates his own story of setting up a community for those in crisis where people have not had to go mad to be there.

'Anti-psychiatry' essentially means a strong opposition to the theories and practices of traditional Western European psychiatry. By this I refer to the medical model of mental illness and the physical methods, usually drugs, electroshock and institution-alisation, that comprise psychiatric treatment. The term was coined in the 1960s by R.D. Laing and David Cooper.

I discovered 'anti-psychiatry' as a medical student in New York during the early 1960s. I had to spend several months on the psychiatric ward of a large city hospital. During this time I was taught to distinguish different categories of disease, from the neurotic to psychotic to psychopathic, as well as their prognoses. Since the ward was psychodynamically orientated, neurotic patients received psychotherapy. But those diagnosed as psychotic received drugs or electroshock. We were told that one third of them got better, one third got worse, and one third stayed the same, no matter what you did for them or to them. Moreover, we were assured that the rambling speech of 'schizophrenics' was a sign of their damaged thought processes and was inherently unintelligible.

Imagine my shock when I discovered that I could easily talk with many of the 'schizophrenics' and that these people often made perfect sense to me. I thought I was crazy too. Two teachers helped me sort out my confusion and upset. One was John Thompson, an unusual and original man, 'an existential psychoanalyst', who used to sit silently with his disturbed, catatonic patients, week after week, month after month, until they were ready to converse with him. He explained that these people were not sick, rather very frightened, and that their symptoms were a self-protective shell, to keep the world from destroying them, or to keep them from magically destroying the world.

My other mentor was R.D. Laing. I came across his book, *The Divided Self* (1990a) by accident in a medical bookshop, and was attracted by the interesting title. I quickly discovered that this young Scottish psychoanalyst, who was unknown in the States at the time, held views that were remarkably similar to Thompson, 'that schizophrenic behaviour is a special strategy that a person invents to live in an unlivable situation'. Moreover, Laing meticulously related 'mad' behaviour and experience to the social context in which it occurred, thereby making it intelligible, even obvious.

I liked Laing's social critique. His perspective covered the way individuals were treated in small interpersonal settings, like the family; and large settings, like schools or hospitals; and finally society at large. In addition, his analyses covered a much wider range of phenomena than traditional psychiatry, for he not only discussed interpersonal events, that is, behavioural transactions, but inter-subjective events, how people influence each other's experience.[1] Laing's work seemed especially relevant to America in the 1960s, a period of intense social ferment – civil rights, the Vietnam war and flower power. The latter refers to the attempt by youngsters to replace hate with love and guns with hugs. Really, the whole culture was in turmoil.

A seminal film was Ken Kesey's, *One Flew over the Cuckoo's Nest*. The action concerned a group of patients who tried to escape from a repressive, soul-destroying mental hospital, representing America of the 1950s. The plot was, of course, a phantasy, the internal world of the writer, a psyche trying to break the shackles of childhood. But the film also depicted actuality. I was personally asked to help people who were sent to mental hospital for singing in the street, or dressing unusually, or for demonstrating against atomic bombs. And the public hospitals to which they were sent often held between 20,000 and 30,000 souls, in highly oppressive conditions, with treatments that were often degrading and dangerous. These included excessive medication, electrical and chemical convulsions, endless incarceration, and, if none of these worked, psychosurgery, a direct physical assault on the brain. Here we can clearly see how alleged issues of 'psychopathology' mask a more basic agenda: institutional authority, social deviance and political control.

Concomitantly, a wide variety of scholars found they could query the way society worked, indeed the very foundations of social policy, by examining the ways mental patients were diagnosed and treated. The psychoanalyst Dr Thomas Szasz, called the whole concept of mental illness 'a myth'. And in a dozen or more books he showed

---

[1] Laing explored the issue of subjectivity and inter-subjectivity in a number of books, most notably *The Divided Self* and *The Politics of Experience*, Penguin Books, 1990.

how this myth justified institutional sadism. Similarly, the sociologist Irving Goffman pointed out that social deviancy and 'mental illness' were identical. For him diagnosis equalled labelling, the transformation of 'bad' to 'mad'.

Significantly, the anthropologist Gregory Bateson studied patterns of communication in the family. He proposed the 'double bind theory of schizophrenia', which concludes that an individual exposed to an array of contradictory communications, may go mad. For example, a little girl is eagerly awaiting the return of her mother from work. The mother comes home and the little girl runs to her shrieking, 'Mommy, Mommy.' In response the mother stops, scowls and tenses. The little girl, a bit confused, sees this and stops. The mother replies, 'What's the matter, don't you love mommy?' Her daughter is confused but starts towards her again. But the mother does the same. Usually the little girl can't articulate what is happening, and often withdraws. But if she could comment on the transaction, her mother might reply, 'Don't be rude, I did no such thing, I only wanted a hug.' Later in life, when exposed to a similar pattern of communications with a parent or close friend, Bateson noted that the girl might enter a catatonic state, or a suicidal depression.

As a medical student and young doctor I was fascinated by these issues, all of them a central focus in the work of Laing. So in 1965, I decided to go to London to work with Laing and his colleagues, David Cooper and Aaron Esterson. I wanted to learn more about strange states of mind. I thought men and women should be treated humanely and with respect regardless of their condition. Moreover, I believed one could transform their life-situation by validating their experience, rather than turning them into mental 'in-valids.' (I refer to the basic meaning of 'invalid' – sick, incapacitated and worthless.) At the time Laing had just established Kingsley Hall. This was meant to be a special place, a therapeutic milieu without staff or patients. It was to be a community of men and women 'obstinately trying to recover the wholeness of being human through the relationship between them'.

For Laing, breakdown carried with it the possibility of breakthrough. The fundamental idea was that mental and social breakdown was an opportunity for growth and development. Laing himself thought that psychosis, a term he used to denote a state of being, was akin to a mental and spiritual voyage. He thought that an individual could pass through a psychosis, and become stronger in himself, if he were given the necessary support and encouragement.

The healing potential of regression, as Laing knew, was a feature of many spiritual traditions. The ancient Greeks used the term 'incubation'. At the temples of Aesculapius or Demeter physically or mentally damaged people were invited to spend days in a special cave, awaiting a healing dream. When it came, their symptoms were relieved. In our day and age, I think the most common form of regression is 'a cold'. The mild fever and pains provide the good excuse to refrain from work and stay in bed. Conscience permitting, after a few days one usually returns to the world feeling refreshed.

These ideas fascinated me. Therefore, I was very pleased to be invited to join the Kingsley Hall community, and within a few weeks, to be asked by Laing to establish a close relationship with Mary Barnes. Mary was a 45-year-old nurse who had a long history of mental breakdown. She had been in and out of hospital many times and had all the usual treatments; drugs, ECT, rigid institutional 'care'. But she had the idea that what she really needed was to be allowed to regress, to literally become a fetus, and then grow up again. As her wish coincided with Laing's theory, Mary was soon a prestigious, although difficult resident of the community.

Little did I know what I was getting into, or how I would be affected. The basic story has been told in the book we wrote together: *Mary Barnes: Two Accounts of a Journey Through Madness*. It describes how I fed her with a baby bottle, cleaned her and played sharks and alligators, while always having to withstand the ravages of 'IT' as she called her dark rages. The book also relates how Mary became a very talented painter and writer. Perhaps more importantly, it demonstrates how her self-perception, as well as others' perception of her, changed from mental patient to human being.

Subsequently, Mary published an account of her life after leaving Kingsley Hall entitled, *Something Sacred*. She concludes with this poem:

Softly we touch,
   here, and there,
as the current
of our life, flows
   on its way.

How lightly we step on the
                  Sand
How soon comes the
                  Tide.

Kingsley Hall closed in 1970. The owners refused to renew the lease on the building. But the reality was more complicated. Laing had gotten involved in other ideas and projects, and so had I. Was Kingsley Hall a success or a failure? A former resident remarked, 'Those who live here see "Kingsley Hall" each in his own way . . . simply [put], Kingsley Hall is a place, where some may encounter selves long forgotten or distorted.'

After 1970, the therapists who had been involved with Kingsley Hall split into two groups. Laing's original organisation, The Philadelphia Association, emphasised existential therapy as part of a wide educational and support programme. A new organisation called 'Arbours' was started by myself, Dr Morton Schatzman, our wives and others. We thought of the temporary dwelling places, in Hebrew, 'Sukkot', where the Israelites lived in the wilderness after the exodus from Egypt. The English equivalent is Arbours, places of shade and shelter. The name also sounds like 'harbour', a place of safe anchorage for ships during storms. We felt people in distress needed a similar haven or sanctuary, one with a more consistent degree of support than Kingsley Hall had provided.

Let me quote from a statement in one of our first brochures as it presents some of our motivating beliefs:

We feel it is more helpful and humane to give persons who have been or could become mental patients a chance not to be seen as mentally ill, called mentally ill, or treated as mentally ill. There are practical reasons for this approach. The label 'mental patient' remains a severe social stigma. It may limit work, travel and educational opportunities. Other people – friends, relatives or strangers – behave differently towards those they perceive as 'mentally ill'. They are often intimidating, rejecting or patronising. Furthermore the term 'mental illness' can be confusing and unhelpful for the people to whom it is applied. The 'mentally ill person' tends to take on others' unsympathetic attitudes and abdicate responsibility for his life to outside authorities or institutions, all to his detriment. He or she may become type-cast and see no possibility for himself other than to embark on a long term career as a mental patient.

We are aware that certain experiences and behaviour may be unusual. However, what is regarded as odd or bothersome in some social circles may not be seen that way in others. Many people who might otherwise be trapped within an ill identity need the opportunity and encouragement to come to terms with their problems. We intend that the Arbours should be a place where people may encounter selves long distorted and forgotten, where they can regain and contain their experiences, and achieve a sense of integrity and autonomy.

The first Arbours community was in the home of Morton Schatzman and his wife, Vivien Millett. For several years they and their children shared their house with several people who might otherwise have been in mental hospital. About the same time, we rented a house in London and established a community which has continued until this very day. Now the Arbours has three houses, each with 7–10 residents who share comfortable accommodation in North London. In these households residents know and sympathise with each other's emotional and social problems. Two psychotherapists co-ordinate the activities of each household and offer personal and practical support. Psychotherapists-in-training also live in and contribute to the life of the communities.

No one is cast in the role of mental patient. Residents are responsible for shopping, cooking, cleaning and managing communal affairs. And they go to great lengths to look after each other. I recall a young man who lived in our South London household. He had become very agitated, so much so that the community found it hard to cope with him. So Morty Schatzman suggested that he moved to his house. Still the man found it hard to calm down. Instead he decided to live in my old three-door taxi which was parked outside the house. We obliged by arranging for his therapist to see him daily in the rear of the taxi, for a pint of milk to be delivered to the taxi each day and for him to be able to take a loaf of bread at the local bakery. The arrangement seemed to be working and the man began to calm. Regretfully the story does not have a happy ending. Although known and generally tolerated in the neighbourhood, this person was picked up by a policeman who did not know about his circumstances. When he refused to talk and appeared peculiar, he was taken to a mental hospital, forcibly detained and was not allowed to return to us. Sadly, this episode precipitated his career as a mental patient for a long time.

Others have been more fortunate. Many men and women with severe psychiatric histories have managed to return to their homes or establish themselves in separate living quarters after residing in our households for periods of a few months to a few years.

During these first years we tried to accommodate a wide variety of people who sought refuge with us. But we often found this to be a difficult task, either because of their own immediate needs which conflicted with the long process of joining a community, or because they needed a degree of consistent support which the communities could not give. After long discussions we decided to establish a staffed community where individuals, couples or families who were acutely upset could obtain immediate and intensive support, with or without residential accommodation.

Our first effort to get a house for the project was scuppered by alarmed neighbours. This was in November 1972 when we learned a direct and painful lesson about the extent of the public's fears of 'mental illness'. At the time a friendly vicar told us that we could use a disused church hall to establish a new community, to be the forerunner of our Crisis Centre. We were overjoyed. But before we could move in, the vicar insisted that the project was given the OK by a neighbourhood community association, a group which had not met for many years. We did not realise this would be a problem, and, after informing local residents, organised a meeting to explain our project. To our astonishment no less than 70 angry locals showed up for the meeting. One rage-filled tradesman was especially vociferous and seemed to articulate collective concerns. He shouted that the women and children of the neighbourhood would not be safe to walk the streets if Arbours had use of the hall. Mental patients, actually he used the word 'deranged', were extremely dangerous. He was convinced that violence, rape, maybe murder would be perpetrated by the members of the proposed community. At the least, immorality and chaos would be let loose onto a quiet North London neighbourhood and his family would be stricken. To the sounds of heavy applause, his speech carried the vote. The project was turned down. The streets remained 'safe' and we all came down with bad colds.

This might have been the end of the matter. But some months later a close colleague took on a new patient in psychotherapy. She lived a few blocks from the hall and was having an affair with a local tradesman. But he had become very jealous and had taken to sitting all night in front of her house with a loaded shotgun, convinced that she was two-timing him. The woman was terrified, both for herself and her boyfriend. Fortunately no one came to any harm. But, the jealous lover and the angry local who carried the meeting were one and the same person. By a stroke of luck we were able to see clearly how private passions can go public. The man suffered from well-founded fears, of himself, of his own immorality, violence and rapacious impulses, which for him, if let loose, or even acknowledged, constituted insanity. He dealt with this dilemma by projecting his fear and impulses onto others, the unknown people, the 'nutters' whom the Arbours proposed to bring into the neighbourhood. Without the coincidence of his girl friend seeing an Arbours therapist, we might never have been able to make sense of the meeting where our project was turned down, nor known for sure, why the locals were so frightened of us.

In fact, these scenarios go on all the time and make it difficult for any community-based mental health projects to get off the ground. Therefore, when we establish new communities we make sure never to announce ourselves in advance. But we also make sure that our gardens, front and back, are well tended and the residents get on speaking terms with the neighbours. This policy has paid dividends on several occasions, including the time when we were forced to seek planning permission for one of our long-stay communities. The council sent letters to nearby residents. Soon afterwards the household was confronted by a highly anxious next door neighbour, a mother of six, who came to tell people that some group called Arbours was threatening to set up shop here and flood the area with mental patients. No one would be safe. After inviting her in, the residents of the community gave her a cup of tea and calmly explained that they were Arbours. 'Oh, you are nice. I feel so much better.' Subsequently she wrote a letter to the council praising the community and saying how much she supported it. Planning permission came soon afterwards.

With all this is mind, we eventually rented a small house in North London to establish the Arbours Crisis Centre, which opened in January 1973. Two therapists lived in the house, it was their home. They became known as the resident therapists. This arrangement has continued and worked well right through to the present.

People whom we help come as guests, not patients. This simple shift in roles makes a tremendous difference in the relationships that unfold. 'Guests', are less likely to play 'being crazy' or replay the role of 'mental patient'.

The first house had room for three guests. Subsequently, we were able to purchase a much bigger house in North London. The Crisis Centre moved there in 1980. It has room for three resident therapists and six guests, including a family suite. To the best of my knowledge it is the only facility I know that can take in an entire family, including children and, if necessary, the family pet, on short notice.[2] The Crisis Centre uses a team approach. The therapy side of the Arbours' team consists of a resident therapist (the RT), an experienced psychotherapist known as the team leader (the TL) and an Arbours trainee or other professional studying at the Centre.

The first intervention is on the phone. Sometimes this will suffice. If not, an appointment will be made with a team to meet at the Centre, or occasionally, at the caller's home. The team may decide to do a focused short-term intervention using only a few consultations, really brief psychotherapy. But if the situation is more serious it may invite the caller or other family member to be a guest.

Inevitably, people who do come for a stay are deeply disturbed. They may be frankly psychotic, or suicidally depressed, or as happens more frequently in the past decade, they may be anorexic and self-mutilating. Our aim is not to stop bizarre or disruptive experience or behaviour, but to contain it and make sense of it. These goals are interconnected. The guests need help because they are no longer able to keep in themselves, and to themselves, wildly distressing thoughts, feelings and wishes. We make things bearable again by tolerating the pain and discomfort in ourselves. In other words, the essential point of being a therapist has to do with being able to suffer on behalf of another without losing one's own integrity. It's not easy. In this regard we don't rely on medication to keep others' feelings at a distance. Quite the opposite. We try to be very sensitive to the emotional currents swirling around the Centre. Technically I am referring to countertransference exchanges.

Once I came to the Centre for a meeting. No one was about, but I heard loud noises coming from the kitchen. When I walked into the room, I was assailed by the sight of 'Ingrid,' a very large woman, holding a knife to her wrist. Upon seeing me she started to scream, 'Joe, I'm going to do it, yes I will, I'm going to kill myself, no-one can stop me.' The RTs who were present seemed immobile. They had their hands out is if to stop her, but they were almost catatonic for fear she would cut her wrists, if they made a move. My reaction was total panic. But curiously, within a few moments, I noticed that I had started to feel sad, even tearful. So I said, 'Ingrid, I can't stop you from killing yourself, but when I think of you doing so, I feel very sad, for I will miss you.' Ingrid's immediate response was to put down the knife and exclaim, 'Oh Joe, you know I was only joking.' Then she walked away. In retrospect we realised that Ingrid

---

[2] Arbours Crisis Centre, 41 Weston Park, London N8 9SY; telephone 0181–340 8125; fax 0181–342 8849.

was very sad about other guests who were leaving. But she couldn't tolerate feelings of sadness or depression. The self she wanted to kill was her depressed self. But once she had induced it in me, she felt free of this burden in herself, and no longer needed to use the knife.

On another occasion, the Centre was being terrorised by a guest who used to go up to people and put his hands around their throat. One day he did this to Andrea Sabbadini, a team leader. Instead of screaming or yelling at him to stop, Andrea replied, 'You know, I am frightened when you do that, but I think you really want to make contact with me, but are frightened to do so.' The man put down his hands and began to cry. Incidents like this are very dramatic and not very frequent. Mostly both therapists and guests have a daily struggle to make sense of their experiences.

The Centre includes three separate but inter-related and inter-relating systems. These are the milieu, the group and the team. The milieu is the Centre in its role as an overall therapeutic environment. The examples I have just given illustrate the task of the milieu to contain and defuse very disturbing outbursts.[3]

The group consists of all the residents, therapists and guests, and meets four times a week. Essentially these house meetings are an opportunity for people to express their experiences and gain feedback from others about themselves. Also the 'house culture' tends to be passed on during these meetings. Often guests who have been at the Centre for a while teach newcomers what to expect. For example, one man who himself had been completely inarticulate about his feelings, took the lead in explaining to a new guest that the reason she had come to the Centre was, 'to learn to know what you feel'.

The third therapeutic system is the team. The team includes the guest and his or her RT, TL and student. This is quite a unique arrangement. The professional literature is full of articles about therapeutic groups which include several patients and one or two therapists. But the Arbours team consists of several therapists and one guest. This approach enables us to work intensively and relatively quickly with very chaotic individuals, and to bring about significant changes in their lives without relying on biochemical or other forms of physical restraint. Nothing is more uplifting both for the RTs and TLs than to see someone who had been dismissed as a 'hopeless case' regain hope and vitality. The outcome of our work is that three-quarters of all guests return home after a stay at the Centre. About 15 per cent go to an Arbours long-stay community or other hostel. And about 5 per cent require hospitalisation.

In conjunction with the work of the Communities and Crisis Centre we saw the need for two further services, a training programme in analytical psychotherapy and social psychiatry, which now has fifty trainees, and a psychotherapy service. The latter provides training cases for our students and low-cost therapy for clients who cannot afford full fees.[4]

The first anthology on the work of the Arbours called, *Sanctuary: The Arbours Experience of Alternative Community Care* was published in 1995. The book includes

---

[3] For further and extensive discussion of the different ways the Centre works with guests, see my papers: The Conjoint Therapy of Severely Disturbed Individuals within a Therapeutic Milieu, *International Journal of Therapeutic Communities*, **11**, (4), Winter 1990, 237–48; and Psychotic Interventions at the Arbours Crisis Centre, *British Journal of Psychotherapy*, **10**, (3), Spring 1994, 372–82.

[4] For information about Arbours facilities and activities contact: The Arbours, 6 Church Lane, London N8 7BU, 0181–340 7646.

reflections by Arbours therapists, trainees and clients, the residents and guests. Collectively we have tried to provide a detailed description of the individual, group and institutional dynamics that provide the foundation of the Arbours' practical and theoretical accomplishments.

But does the Arbours really succeed in helping people who are severely disturbed, chaotic and self-destructive? Does 'therapy', that is, listening to another with a 'third ear', with an attentive mind, really work? The answer is yes. Yet, this is also a strange question. If we do not cure, we try to do no harm. We hope that people who come to us for help may find the selves they have lost, and the soul they never knew existed. Perhaps given time, given luck, they may hear the beat of their hearts and be able to elucidate the rhythm. Probably this is the goal of most therapists who have worked under the heading of 'anti-psychiatry'. But are we still anti-psychiatrists? Well, yes and no. Laing himself disavowed the term many years ago. He didn't like the fact that it had been hijacked for political purposes.

There have been and still are centres and therapists in many countries which do justice to the basic principles of humane, self-enhancing interventions. In Italy Franco Basaglia saw his life's work culminate in the passage of Law 180, which created the basis for a whole new approach to mental health. In America Loren Mosher has pioneered non-institutionalised and non-institutionalising interventions at Soteria House in California, and more recently, Crossing Place, in Washington, DC. A disciple of Laing, David Goldblatt, has continued his work at Burch House in New England. And the Philadelphia Association continues to sponsor communities and training in London.

But the problem of dehumanising treatments remain. One need only consider the massive use and abuse of psychotropic medications, the resurgence of ECT, the absence of adequate funding, and the relative unsophistication of mental health services in most areas, to ponder how much more can still be accomplished.

And if this were not enough, we have to deal with the pervasive bureaucracy which envelopes every therapeutic intervention. The 1993 government White Paper on mental health was supposedly designed to enable people to get help for mental problems. In practice, the opposite is the case. The new rules and regulations mean that clients have to pass through a further layer of administrators, who often seem to be charged with the task of obstructing support, rather than facilitating it.

Let me not be unjust. I meet and continue to work with social workers who act promptly and efficiently. Yet, we find that people in acute distress almost never are able to get grants to come to Arbours facilities, even though they are theoretically eligible for them. And others, with long-standing difficulties, may have to wait an inordinate amount of time before help is made available. Then, even when funding is agreed, the contracts are so complicated that it is a wonder anyone could comply with them. The net effect is that the monies on offer pay for more and more administration and less and less direct clinical help.

If this weren't bad enough, the various bureaucracies involved in client care try to dictate how we should practise. Directives concern the size of the rooms, the number of therapists, the width of doors, and so on. Mostly this arises because the Arbours is so unique that the Crisis Centre and Communities get lumped with the category of old people's homes. The regulators then regulate accordingly. Administrative procedures supersede clinical judgement. There is little room for taking risks and to live, rather than to batten down the hatches and behave. The result is that we, as therapists, as human beings trying to assist other human beings, become more concerned with re-covering, than recovery, more preoccupied with playing safe, than with enabling those people who wish to do so, to descend into their darkness and emerge renewed.

In the face of all these pressures, can Arbours therapists remember their vision and retain their integrity? Or will the Arbours become a somewhat offbeat, but basically conventional purveyor of therapy? And the same question assails all students and colleagues with a comparable outlook: can we practise what we preach, become mainstream, or will we be marginalised by the forces of medical tradition, bureau-cracy, politically correctness and the pervasive influence of neurobiology?

In the 1960s Laing bequeathed a vision which had become obscured by the 1980s. He fought battles and gained ground which need to be refought and regained during the 1990s. So in this sense the Arbours, myself, kindred spirits, are very anti-psychia-tric, indeed. The task remains to comprehend the knots that bind the heart and soul, and to bring the 'treat', or joy, back into treatment. Then people can ascend from the abyss of self-torment and rediscover the inherent satisfaction of making bonds with each other and to life itself.

REFERENCES

Barnes, M. 1989: *Something sacred: conversations, writings, paintings*. London: Free Association Books.

Barnes, M. and Berke, J.H. 1991: *Mary Barnes: the accounts of a journey through madness*. London: Free Association Books.

Berke, J.H. 1990: The conjoint therapy of severely disturbed individuals within a therapeutic milieu. *International Journal of Therapeutic Communities* 11(4), Winter, 237–48.

Berke, J.H. 1994: Psychotic interventions at the Arbours Crisis Centre. *British Journal of Psychotherapy* 10(3), Spring, 372–82.

Berke, J.H., Masoliver, C. and Ryan, T. 1995: *Sanctuary: the Arbours experience of alternative community care*. London: Process Press.

Laing, R.D. 1990a: *The divided self*. Harmondsworth: Penguin.

Laing, R.D. 1990b: *The politics of experience*. Harmondsworth: Penguin.

7

CREATING FROM CHAOS

Eibhlín Inglesby

'Only out of chaos may there be born a dancing star', argued Nietzsche. Such an event may be manifest in the sort of breakthrough where an individual's psychic reality shatters the convention of a false self, also, by implication, the breakthrough, in the sense of moral triumph, of their spirit. Part two of the book will offer accounts of clients' and clinicians' experience where turmoil, uncertainty and chaos could be used as an opportunity for change and growth. Here Eibhlín Inglesby explores in more general terms this *process* of growth and development, symbolised as a spiritual journey or pilgrimage. She discusses the use of creative symbolism and religious imagery as an aid to facilitating such growth, emphasising the religious perspective rather than any one manifestation of it. She then focuses on two specific religious frameworks and urges us to remain alive to the hazards of imposing beliefs on those already vulnerable, also to take frameworks such as these seriously as a means to facilitate the creative use of crisis to effect growth.

INTRODUCTION

Madness is, to our Western view, unintelligible. Persons entering into madness are somehow lost to us. Mad persons are, almost by definition, those whom we do not recognise. To admit this fact is not only to acknowledge the low civil status (and the historical and contemporary abuse) alloted to those we call mentally ill, but to admit also, as any honest carer must, that there are times when the mad appear to go beyond the boundaries of our understanding and to recognise them as persons is to stretch to the limits our credulity.

None the less, 'moral conduct' is surely meaningless without a concept of person-hood, and surely impossible if we have no perception of 'the person' affected by our conduct. When this perception of a person is lost or veiled, we enter an amoral, and often in our conduct towards that person, immoral sphere.

How do we redeem the situation for both the mentally ill and for ourselves?[1] If we accept that we need to 'hang onto' the 'person' in order to act morally, we must find

---

[1] It must be understood that only in doing justice to others do we do justice also to ourselves. Moral action is necessarily relational; a two-way process.

ways of understanding personhood in madness. I would suggest that symbolic imagery, the worlds of religious language, myth and artistic creation, can help us 'find' the persons we feared 'lost' beyond our understanding and do them the justice of behaving with moral integrity towards them.

I recommend the use of such spiritual or symbolic perspectives to interpret madness because I believe that they can work where others fail. By 'work' I mean provide a 'lens' for viewing the person within their mental chaos and thus offer a basis for just action and relationship with respect to them. In other words I wish to provide a moral framework. I believe that such imagery and interpretation have the potential to render meaningful, both to the carer and also to the sufferer, the dark and hostile world that madness so often inhabits. If it succeeds in doing this, then mental illness might be seen by both as a journey with light at the end of the tunnel, a pilgrimage rather than lost time. The agony, isolation, and chaos which are so often experienced may result in creating new life. This may not be a life free from all 'symptoms' of 'madness', but it will be one that has meaning and integrity for the individual concerned. It seems to me that as carers we could have no greater moral goal.

The theme of this chapter, then, is that the healing of ourselves and others, using this sort of lens, is the moral imperative of our work, perhaps of our lives. I shall elaborate this by discussing the ways in which the story that the mentally ill person tells may be the focus of healing. This will entail analysing the principles behind the conventional and the alternative ways in which that story may be interpreted. I shall then demonstrate the significance of alternative methods of interpretation in relation to a pair of case studies. Finally, I shall discuss some symbolic images which may be useful contributions to the healing process, namely, hell, redemption, pilgrimage, the yurodivy from Russian folklore and the Buddhist middle way. The yurodivy may, through participation in the pilgrimage, guide the pilgrims, so that they return from the extreme edges of both an inner and outer world that is split, redeemed people.

GLOSSARY OF TERMS

One of the problems of introducing a spiritual dimension to care is dealing with the presuppositions associated with spiritual and religious language and imagery. I have therefore defined the specific ways in which I have used terms that may have a variety of interpretations.

Spiritual/religious

The word 'spiritual' is more acceptable to a multicultural, post-Christian society to define the meaning we give to our lives. The word 'religious' is usually associated with organised ritualistic activity and belief in a particular set of ideas regarding our purpose in the cosmos, as a manifestation of that search for meaning. While I do not wish to enter a debate about the value or truth of any particular religious framework, I would wish to attribute a positive value to the word 'religious' because I believe that traditional religious wisdom can contribute much to our understanding of the spiritual dimension of our life and its meaning. However, I do acknowledge that sometimes what is *called* religious truth may be extremely unhelpful.

The distinction I make between the terms 'religious' and 'spiritual' may be particularly helpful in a caring situation where orthodox religious activity such as formal worship may be either unwanted or inappropriate, but where spiritual questions concerning meaning, purpose, identity and relationship remain central to the process of healing.

Redemption

I do *not* wish to use the word 'redemption' in its specifically Christian context as associated with Christ's death and the meaning Christians attribute to it, but, rather, more generally, as a term that implies that (new) life can be created from that which had seemed irrevocably lost.

Mental illness/madness

We are all familiar with the problems of the interpretation of madness as mental 'illness'. It is, none the less, the common usage within our society and so I have used the terms 'madness' and 'mental illness' interchangeably to widen the categories of each. By using a spiritual interpretation of madness I am not seeking to deny either that there may also be organic components to madness, or the possible benefits of medical interventions such as drug therapy. Whilst not all medicine has had to offer has been therapeutic, one has to view a complex situation in a way that does it justice. A spiritual interpretation runs alongside other interpretations as one way among many of trying to understand madness.

Evil

In philosophical discussion the 'problem of evil' refers both to wrong-doing and to the unexplained suffering which pervades the world. Many religious traditions have posited an objective force of evil (such as the devil), which is responsible for the suffering and devastation wreaked around us. My own interpretation of evil is that it is an objective reality only in so far as there are people injuring each other and bringing suffering into our world.

Those who suffer in madness may do so for no *apparent* reason. Conversely, they may have been the obvious victims of abuse. In both cases they could be said to participate, in some sense, in the 'problem of evil'. This is in no way to assert that the mad themselves are evil, although their action, like the action of all of us, might sometimes be so.

Most of the symbolism in this chapter comes from the Judaic/Christian traditions. This is purely because of my own familiarity with them. I am particularly aware of the potential of the eastern religions to offer meaningful symbols and their absence here is a reflection of my lack of knowledge rather than a deliberate choice to elevate one tradition over another.

SPIRITUAL EXPERIENCE, MADNESS AND TRUTH

Conventional views

In order to show how a *spiritual* interpretation of madness may present a clearer moral framework it is necessary to examine how these concepts have been linked historically: religion and madness have an age-old connection. In a world where all interpretation had a religious perspective, madness was seen as the inspiration of either God or the devil and tolerated accordingly. Much political use was made of these types of inter-pretation , e.g., Joan of Arc. A contemporary, popular view of madness, stemming from this medieval, religious world view and the Victorian outlook, which emphasised moral inferiority, is that the mad are possessed by spiritual inadequacy of some sort. A second contemporary view, the conventional wisdom which represents a more secular outlook, suggests that madness, particularly in the form of subjective, religious interpretation of experience, is simply the product of an outmoded world view or meaningless disturbance, possibly reducible to organic change and cognitive malfunc-tion. Maybe, as argued elsewhere in this text, such views have as much in common with the political dynamics of the Joan of Arc story as they have with genuine religion or science. In any event, the negative effect of both such perspectives has invariably been to isolate people experiencing things this way and confirm their madness to the 'sane' world. Coulter (1993) quotes the response of such a person. 'When I talk to God, I am praying. When God talks to me, I am a schizophrenic' (p. 87).

Despite the inroads made by concepts of holism in health care, subjective, religious interpretations of experience are generally still associated with one of the above views. Anyone claiming direct experience of spiritual reality is likely to be seen either as blighted by some kind of bad spirit, or as holding an outmoded world view and making an irrational interpretation of their experience. In these circumstances there appears neither any authentic relationship between the person experiencing things this way and reality, nor the possibility that any sort of moral development may be taking place. I suggest, however, that while such experiences may represent the disturbed and the outmoded and arational,[2] the disturbed and the outmoded and arational may have as much access to the truth as the modern world has to offer. If psychiatry has learnt anything in the last hundred years, we might hope it is that in every realm, the foundations of what we take to be reality can shift; thus we should not deny the experience of others, even if that experience remains unintelligible.

Alternative metaphors

Contemporary society rationalises both God and madness, and may redefine both as pathology. Nevertheless, the belief in spiritual possession is not redundant (Perry, 1987). It may be that madness has, at its core, the potential to recreate images and ideas into symbolic forms, just as art forms can convey experience more fully. Whether or not these forms are 'religious' in any orthodox sense, I view this as a religious or spiritual potential. The crux comes with whether this potential leads to healing.

I do not wish to attribute the status of objective truth to such symbolic forms of

---

[2] I have used the word *arational* here instead of *irrational* because it denotes that which is outside of the sphere of the rational, rather than that which merely falls short of the rules of logic.

experience and expression. Nor, however, do I agree with Kristeva (1989) that religious interpretation of experience is only imaginary, when she says:

> aesthetic and particularly literary creation, and also *religious discourse in its imaginary, fictional essence,* set forth a device whose prosodic economy, interaction of characters, and implicit symbolism constitute a very faithful semiological representation of the subject's battle with symbolic collapse. [Such] representation[s] possess . . . imaginary effectiveness that comes closer to catharsis than to elaboration; it is a therapeutic device used in all societies throughout the ages.
>
> (p.24: emphasis mine)

Thus it may be prudent to stand neutrally with respect to epistemological difficulties regarding 'subjective' and 'objective' truth. I prefer to emphasise, like Kristeva above, the *pragmatic* value of spiritual forms of expression and interpretation of crisis to the sufferer. For the purposes of this discussion, therefore, I will take the truth to mean that which heals, and reiterate that the healing of ourselves and others may be the moral imperative of our lives.

CASE STUDIES

Patrick McGrath grew up in the grounds of Broadmoor Hospital where his father was the last medical superintendent. He relates:

> Once at dusk, when I was crossing the yard inside the hospital with my father, a terrible scream came from one of the high windows of block six (the secure unit), a scream charged with utmost misery. Startled, I looked up at my father. 'Poor John', he murmured and by his tone I understood that *he* understood why poor John had screamed and the fact that he understood it robbed the scream of its terror for me.
>
> (McGrath, 1989, p.159)

For McGrath, to understand changed everything. Someone who has a shared understanding of her 'madness' may not be able or willing to alter her situation, but here I shall demonstrate how her life may nevertheless be rendered meaningful and dignified again.

Cath (A)

Cath's real name is Catriona but she has become used to being called Cath by her husband and family even though she thinks of herself as Catriona. She grew up in a Scottish Catholic family in Glasgow. Her father died when she was seven and her mother worked relentlessly to care for Cath and her younger brother. Cath describes her relationship with her mother as alternately 'close' and 'claustrophobic'. Passing school examinations with ease she studied history at university and then became a hospital social worker. In her late twenties she married Paul, a junior solicitor, and continued in her job for another two years until having her first child. After eight years of caring for her three children, Cath came to her GP, saying that she had been feeling suicidal for months. She described her behaviour as 'loathsome', constantly shouting at her children, crying all the time, feeling that her body was 'out of control'. Her GP prescribed a course of antidepressants and suggested some counselling. Cath agreed to both treatments and described her counselling in the following way:

> I saw the counsellor for several months. At each session I would weep uncontrollably. I could not understand where all the grief was coming from. I had come to have two very contrary views of myself. One was feeling that I did not exist – when I looked in the mirror, the dull-eyed blank reflection did not seem to be 'me'. But I also perceived myself as a miserable pathetic woman and had a terrible sense of self-loathing. I did not want to exist. My husband was kind and sympathetic. He treated me as someone with an 'illness'. But I see things differently now. I feel that I have always been defined by other people – my mother, my husband, my colleagues – in such a way as to stop me being myself. I was being remade in order to keep the family going – a sort of pivot or linchpin. If I broke out, they would have to redefine themselves and they were not able to do that. I thought that I was the weak, pathetic one, but now I see that I was bearing all the strain. I am a Christian and believe in redemption but I had never understood it properly until now. This experience, although very painful, taught me that I could not tolerate the 'living death' that my life had become. By reclaiming myself I can find a new way of being. Christ chose the role of the scapegoat, but it was being forced upon me. My choice had been taken away. I now may choose that role for the sake of the family but it will be I, Catriona, who decides and defines my own roles.

Cath's husband said that he did not really understand Cath's interpretation of things but he supposed that it was her way of getting better. He felt that the antidepressants had made a lot of difference and he hoped that things would soon return to normal.

Cath (B)

Cath's real name is Catriona but she had refused to be called anything except Cath over the six months prior to her hospitalisation. She was admitted as an emergency to an acute psychiatric unit, suffering from severe paranoid delusions. She believed that her husband was trying to kill her and had drawn a kitchen knife threatening to 'stop him'. Her parents met with similar rebuffs. Eventually her 16-year-old daughter, Beverley, managed to persuade her to put the knife down. The GP and the police had been called and Cath consented to being admitted to hospital on condition that her daughter came to 'protect' her. On her arrival the staff recorded Cath's behaviour as withdrawn and suspicious. She would sometimes talk through Beverley or huddle in a corner with her hands over her ears. When the family tried to take Beverley home Cath became very distressed and screamed that 'he' would rape her if she (Beverley) left. When asked who 'he' was, she replied, 'God'. A compromise was reached when she was persuaded to take some sedation by Beverley and the family then departed. Over the next few weeks Cath remained very suspicious and withdrawn.

Cath's family history appeared unremarkable. Her parents ran a shop in the north of England and their three daughters had been able scholars. Cath's mother felt that her other daughters had done well for themselves. One was a teacher and the other a nurse who had married a doctor. According to Cath's mother, 'Cath was not so good at sticking at things. She fell pregnant at eighteen and had to give up her nurse training. She might not have stuck at it anyway.' Cath married the baby's father

(Jeff) and the marriage appeared to be successful. Two more children were subsequently born.

Neither her parents nor Jeff could understand Cath's outburst. Her mother said that she had always been 'difficult to fathom' and Jeff thought that she had been quieter than usual. Beverley had noticed that her mother often came to sit near her but had supposed that this was just making the most of their time together before she (Beverley) left home to go to college.

Gradually Cath began to confide in one of the younger nurses but her account remained obscure. She claimed that her mother had always wanted to kill her and that her father had never intervened. She said that her mother and Jeff had tried to kill her by getting her pregnant but that 'Bev and I tricked them. They can't get me when she is there.' When asked why they should wish to kill her she refused to answer but would laugh. Her reasons for staying with Jeff in the circumstances were 'because of Bev. But they'll kill me when she leaves home.' In answer to the question of her change of name she would often make cryptic comments: 'It's the name they use to kill me'; or 'the name will kill me and save them the bother'; or 'the name means Catholic, guilty ones. God told me to use it.' Cath was diagnosed as suffering from schizophrenia and began a course of medication.

Both Cath (A) and Cath (B) are fictional characters. This is in no way to deny the truth of their experience.

Intelligibility and validity

There are a variety of ways of defining the difference between the experience of Cath (A) and Cath (B). The classical formula has been the neurotic/psychotic division, which is in some respects a mere sliding scale of the severity of symptoms. Arieti and Bemporad (1980) prefer a distinction based on the sufferer's experience of their interior world: 'psychosis indicates not only actual . . . severity, but it also connotes that an *unrealistic* way of appreciating the self and the world is accepted and tends to be accepted by the sufferer as a normal way of living' (p. 59: emphasis mine). Whilst realising the epistemological problems of accurately defining the nature of reality, they wish to focus on the psychotic's acceptance of their world:

> In practical terms we can say that no matter what transformation the psychotic patient has undergone, that transformation becomes his way of relating to himself and to others and of interpreting the world . . . The distortion of character neuroses . . . are susceptible to at least partial adaptation to the demands of society, whereas in psychosis such adaptation is impossible or very difficult.
>
> (ibid.)

The crucial concept here is not severity but intelligibility. Cath (A) has found a bridge between her experience and the exterior world that enables her to live with integrity in both worlds. For her this link comes in the form of spiritual symbolism that has rendered her experience intelligible to herself and made it communicable to the outside world. Her interpretation of her experience may still not be accepted as legitimate, but there is, at least, the possibility of dialogue. Cath (B)'s account is also rich in symbolism, but the doors to a shared encounter with her experience appear, as yet, to be firmly closed.

The difference in the experience of these two women is as much to do with redemption as it is with organic disorder. Redemption occurs when a situation, hitherto unintelligible, becomes an experience that can be shared, and where appropriate moral stances can be taken.

In the following pages I shall show how understanding a person in their madness may change everything. To be understood is to be redeemed.

HELL AND REDEMPTION

Metaphor as a bridge

To care for another human being suffering 'mental illness' is in some way to share their experience. Validating such experience is not necessarily to say that it is 'good' or 'right' or 'true', but to testify that the experience exists and deserves to be treated as significant. To be a witness in this way is the basis of moral action because it shows another respect for their person. It is to show that they are considered to be of worth.

This is not always easy to do, however. The painful confusion we all feel in the face of mental illness is a startling form of much everyday misunderstanding. It parallels our inability as a society to construct a shared language around our differing interpretations and conceptualisations of the world. This is not to say that these differences in our outlooks, between viewing the world from the perspectives of, say, emotion and reason, morality and amorality, religion and the secular world, are wrong. Perhaps, though, such dichotomies in our understanding are too absolute and special work is required so that they can be bridged.

Metaphor is a bridge that can link these worlds. It is an important and valid way, sometimes perhaps the only way to give someone lost to our ordinary view this sense that they are understood and respected. Religious/spiritual language as metaphor (rather than as doctrine)[3] has traditionally sought to render intelligible just these experiences that the scientific, rational, 'sane' world tends to deny, attempting to bridge the gap in understanding and offer sustenance to the person suffering. Thus:

> the death of Christ offers imaginary support to the non representable catastrophic anguish distinctive of melancholy persons . . . A suspension of meaning, a darkness without hope, a recession of perspective including that of life . . . the recollection of traumatic partings, [which] thrust us into a state of withdrawal. 'Father why have you deserted me?' Moreover serious depression . . . represents a true hell for modern individuals, convinced as they are that they must and can realise all their desires of objects and values. The Christly dereliction presents that hell with an imaginary elaboration, it provides the subject with an echo of its unbearable moments when . . . the meaning of life was lost.
>
> (Kristeva, 1989 pp. 132–3)

---

[3] The difficulty in the doctrinal use of religious language in this context is that the issues involved may be seen as 'clear-cut and evident' in an almost scientific sense and thus leave little room for the ambiguity necessary for healing to occur.

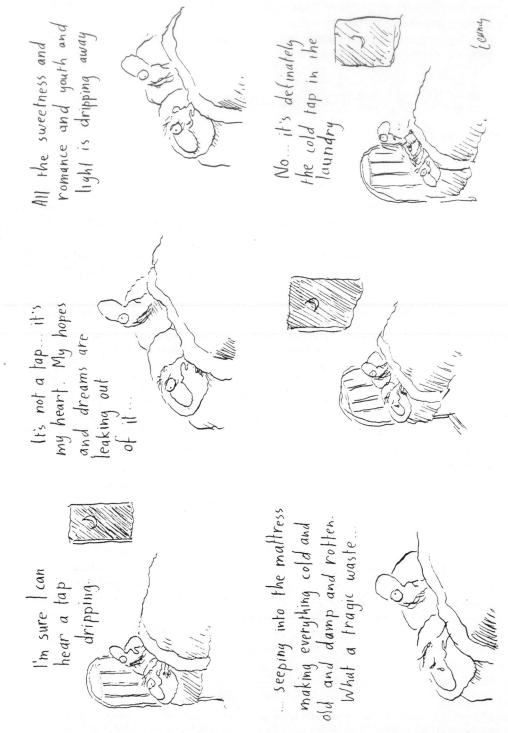

Figure 7.1 (Leunig, 1990)

Metaphor allows for creative expression on one side and creative interpretation on the other. The speaker communicates her meaning without denying the listener an opportunity to invent an interpretation. As it is in art so it may be in life.

(Barker, 1992 p.9.)

In relation to the metaphor of Christ's death, Kristeva points out that Christian symbolism does not leave Christ in the tomb but, with the resurrection, offers a hope of salvation – even within this earthly life. The hope offered may not be as concrete as the traditional Christian doctrine of life after death; it may be, as Kristeva points out, that the catharsis of identification, which can begin a healing process, is itself a form of resurrection. Laing endorsed the possibility of such resurrection: 'Madness need not be all breakdown. It may also be breakthrough. It is potentially liberation and renewal as well as enslavement and existential death.' (1990 p.110).

The author William Styron is one of the many who have suffered from severe depression and been able to clarify their experience with an imagery of descent into hell. Styron's descent into hell had been preceded by a history of self-abuse, such that it might be considered he opened the door to hell himself by his behaviour. His alcoholism and subsequent 'madness', however, were a complex evil, probably precipitated by his relationships with significant others in his life, his mother's early death and by his lack of ability to cope with these relationships None the less, the opening of the door to hell for Styron, whether an evil inflicted by his own hand or by 'circumstance' may have been a redemptive necessity. Hell is perhaps a confrontation with ourselves that many of us need to face before self-acceptance is possible.

Styron was fortunate enough to rise as from Dante's inferno into the light. Mary Barnes, who was a participant in the Kingsley Hall experiment set up by R.D. Laing (see Chapter 6), described her experience in a similar way:

The feeling of shame and guilt that brings us to a dead stillness, makes all giving and receiving of love impossible, is a barrier to all creativity, causes us to feel as ghosts and bury our souls and bodies in a 'living death' and is a very great sickness . . . To be helped, to make the break, to go through madness, is salvation.

(Boyars and Orrill, 1973, 223)

Implicit in the imagery of death and resurrection above is also the richly symbolic concept of journeying. The spiritual quest is often described as a journey and translated into physical journeys in traditional pilgrimages. Its importance in this context is that it may give madness a sense of direction and thus of purpose. Much of the ethos of modern health care is of a 'return to a former state' – a rehabilitation of some sort. It was this concept which grieved Laing so greatly for he believed that we profoundly damage the mad by our attempts to drag them back to the world which we call sane. If one does find oneself in hell, it is probably, as Dante said, that one has lost one's path or been taken along the wrong path. In either case healing seems unlikely if one is merely being taken back to the point of one's descent. Moreover, the descent may have been necessary in order to find a path out to the light.

The mad are not necessarily those who are afraid of the darkness. Those who witness their descent may also quake with fear on the precipice. Madness is often a dark, chaotic and painful experience which poses a moral quandary for both sufferer and carer. The questions we need to address as moral agents are, 'How may I help this person face their personal hell?'; 'How may I best relate to this person and their madness in order to act with justice and integrity towards them?'; 'Do I stand back and watch or do I brave the journey of understanding too; join them in their pilgrimage?'

Psychotic episodes are invariably chaotic. Such chaos could, however, in itself, be a symbol of hope in madness, for although in its original sense the word 'chaos' meant a 'void', it has now come to mean 'turmoil' and 'confusion', and within these there is constant movement. As Nietzsche (1892) said, 'Only out of chaos may there be born a dancing star'. If one can keep moving, continue to journey through the darkness, even if accompanied only by such metaphors as I have explored above, there remains the hope of light at the end, the possibility that Creation has begun. The journey itself may be the beginning of the creative process. It is only when one stands still in the dark with no hand to hold that annihilation becomes a reality and fear takes hold. Both sufferer and carer have then entered a moral void.

Redemption throught participation

Iulia de Beausobre, a Russian *émigré*, describes a figure from Russian folklore who existed in order to make such 'foolhardy' journeys with others. The 'yurodivy' or 'born fool' could be male or female, itinerant or mendicant. The 'yurodivy'

> prefers for the most part to live on the people, and in return for his meal and night's lodging will give them a piece of his mind, seldom mincing his words. Though he has no formal schooling at all, he is always ready to express his views upon the world of matter and the world of the spirit . . . from a practical point of view the yurodivy serves no useful purpose. He achieves nothing . . . The aim of the yurodivy is to participate in evil through suffering . . . Where evil is most intense, there too must be the greatest good. To us (Russians) this is not a hypothesis, it is axiomatic . . . He participates in all the badness and degradation and believes that in doing so he helps in the great drama of redemption.
>
> (1954 p.33)

This figure becomes more understandable in the context of another aspect of Russian tradition. De Beausobre speaks of the traditional Russian view of the social world which is seen as split, not horizontally (as in England with the upper classes on the top and the lower classes below) but vertically. On one side of the vertical line is all that is good and on the other side is all that is evil. People and actions of all classes fall onto both sides of the line dependent upon virtue and not status. She saw the English system of 'doing good' as that of 'dropping handouts' both material and spiritual down into the lower echelons in order that those below, if they have enough moral fibre, may drag themselves up. The Russian notion, however, is this:

> He who pities another must leave his place among the good on the sunny side of the gap, must go out and find where the other *is* – in the darkness, on the side of evil – and be ready to stay with him there; if he returns at all, it is with the other at his own pace. This looks an unpractical attitude . . . but [it] rests on the conviction that evil can be overcome only through knowledge, the knowledge of evil, and it seems to the Russians that man can *know* a thing, as man, *only through participation*.
>
> (1954 pp.30–1: emphasis mine)

De Beausobre's concern was to render intelligible, redeem for herself and for others, both oppressed and oppressors, the very real evil of torture. Thus her use of the words 'good' and 'evil' have a quite tangible meaning. It may be misleading to apply these terms directly to our current context, however, and so I shall substitute the terms 'healing' and 'damaging' for 'good' and 'evil'. The participants in the Kingsley Hall experiment, which is apt to be seen as a crazy (i.e. foolhardy) stunt, bear the marks of the yurodivy. A venture to set up a therapeutic community for the mad, and for those who had decided to accompany them on their journeys, took considerable courage and conviction. When all the labels were removed and there were no 'doctors' and no 'patients', the core of human relationship was exposed and the damage suffered by each was laid bare. The yurodivy is not at liberty to return to the side of healing unless he returns with his fellow sufferer. The stakes at Kingsley Hall were very high. The stance taken by the participants may well have been 'foolhardy', but it was above all a moral stance. It was seen as the most likely way for the true nature of the participants' suffering to be revealed and for healing to occur.

There is much religious imagery which echoes this theme: Buddhism has the notion of the 'bodhisattva', a saint-like figure who postpones the enlightenment that he has already achieved, and remains in the world in order to help others toward enlightenment. The Christian notion of the incarnation of God in Christ and the many incarnations of Vishnu in Hinduism point to a similar meaning – that which is complete and whole participates in that which is in need of being made whole as an act of solidarity, generosity and love. As humans, not only the well-being of our fellows but our very wholeness is said to be dependent upon our ability to participate in the journeys of others.

In *The myth of mental illness*, however, the radical theorist Szasz states, in his critique of the Christian metaphors I have endorsed above: 'Christian ethics is the ethics of partners in misery' (Szasz, 1961, 197). This definition is meant as a condemnation of the oppression that Szasz believes traditional Christian society has inflicted upon people – making them into 'mad' people. He continues elsewhere:

> This is the grand strategy of discrimination, invalidation and scapegoating. Man searches for, creates and imputes differences, the better to alienate the Other. By casting out the Other, Just Man aggrandizes himself and vents his anger in a manner approved by his fellows.

(1971, p.292)

Szasz's perspective on religious and societal structures is penetrating and valid. There are, however, two sides to the coin he describes. To be seen as a partner in misery may be a redemptive and not an oppressive activity. Moreover, it is arguable that the life of Christ itself bore witness to the scapegoating that Szasz abhors. A spiritual interpretation of Christ's life sees it as an endeavour to highlight the reality of humanity's (sinful) alienation of self and others by becoming the scapegoat voluntarily. His message was always one of accompanying the Other, not of invalidating him, no matter what his social or mental status. Christ as scapegoat is the symbol of the Other at his most marginalised. His life and death remain meaningful and important not as masochistic surrendering, but by the fact that it is possible for meaning and solidarity to exist at the margins. The symbol of Christ as scapegoat can be seen to show that meaning can be redeemed even amidst the most terrible suffering.

In his account of the 'ten day voyage' of Jesse Watkins, Laing describes Watkins' 'journey into madness', which took the form of entering into a different time and space in order to face the ultimate questions of life. Watkins faced this task with fear and trembling and was helped by linking his experience with the agony and isolation of Christ.

> I remember going through that night struggling . . . curiosity or willingness to open myself up to experiencing this, and the panic and the insufficiency of spirit which would enable me to experience it. And during that time I went through . . . the Stations of the Cross, although I've never been what you might call a really religious sort of person
>
> (quoted in Laing, 1990, pp. 130–1)

In some sense Christ's suffering made Watkins' suffering meaningful, but this was only possible through participation. Such participation may mean the individual's authentic involvement in the experience of their own chaos as well as the solidarity of participation of others.[4]

But at the same time as flying high with religious images of self-giving and with the spiritual experience of particular celebrated cases, one must anchor one's efforts in a tangible reality. It was always recognised by the Russian people that the role of the yurodivy was a relatively unique one as a result of the harsh demands it made upon a person. How can we translate the power of such imagery into practical forms of care? How can we be moral agents through participation? One of the most obvious attempts at the task of the companion in suffering has come from the realms of psychotherapy. Fromm-Reichmann is described as seeking to 'be there' in the following way: 'She would for instance sit in a patient's urine with them to show that there was no difference between them. Or a patient would give her his faeces as a gift and she would take them' (Boyars and Orrill, 1973, p. 132). This description was given as an example of a therapist who was able to enter into her patient's world without verging into madness herself. It struck me forcibly because of a situation I once found myself in.

As a general nurse, in charge of a small residential unit of elderly people, I had in my care a woman in her late eighties who, though physically mobile, had a number of non-specific 'mental disorders'. She certainly exhibited gross anxiety and severe memory impairment, both common features of dementia, but she also appeared to have an underlying personality disorder and was highly manipulative. She created havoc amongst the other residents, and both staff and residents found her extremely difficult to like.

On one occasion I assisted her to the toilet and asked her to remain there whilst I answered another bell. I returned within two or three minutes to find her standing outside the toilet. Both she and the floor were covered in faeces. She proceeded to wipe her soiled hands all over my uniform. My response verged on complete loss of control. Managing to summon an assistant carer, I retreated for a few minutes to calm down before returning to the situation, outwardly composed but inwardly seething with anger.

I had looked after many elderly people prior to this and had been soiled many

---

[4] Watkins' case is actually very interesting, for not only was he actively participating in his own suffering, but participating in Christ's by way of contemplating the Stations. It may be that this act of solidarity with Christ, as well as Christ's with him, had therapeutic and redemptive power.

times in the process. None of this bothered me – it was part of life. I knew that the woman had probably forgotten that I was coming back and was panic-stricken. But in that situation with her I could feel no motivating compassion. I had no image with which to penetrate the unintelligible realms of her mind and actions and therefore could not treat her as a subject, a person of moral worth. I did not make the descent into hell with her because I lost sight of her humanity. It was only her metaphorical demons which showed themselves to me.

It was not until I read the passage about Fromm-Reichmann that a different perspective appeared, a bridge which enabled me to relate to her isolation and unhappiness. Dealing with that woman had been like a battlefield. We each spoke from our own side of no-man's-land. The situation was futile. It was impossible for that lonely old woman to share anything except her excreta because in a metaphorical sense that was all that her life consisted of. For my part I could do nothing but reject her in her filthy state. I do not think that I should have joined her in it either, but for me to have accepted her state and not been horrified by it might have redeemed the event for *both* of us. This may have been a way of creating from chaos, of descending into the hell of someone else's life, if I had had the courage not to teeter on the precipice.

As Szasz said of the mad, 'If they are not people, then what are they?' (1971, p. 289). If we leave them on the margins, as people without definition, then we also margin-alise ourselves. But to see those who are on the fringe of our experience as within our moral sphere remains a gargantuan task. There is more keeping us away from the precipice than lack of moral fibre:

> One of the fundamental reasons why so many doctors become cynical and disillu-sioned is precisely because, when the abstract idealism has worn thin, they are uncertain about the value of the actual lives of the patients they are treating. This is not because they are callous or personally inhuman: it is because they live in a society that is incapable of knowing what a human life is worth.
>
> (Berger and Mohr, 1981, pp. 165–6)

Yet we are either all people, or none of us are. It is not only the mad who need to see their experience as meaningful and of moral worth, but we, their carers also.

Redemption and the middle way

As a complement to de Beausobre's ideas it is helpful to consider another image of the divisions within which we structure our lives. Like many people who have worked in Africa, Michael Wilson, a medical doctor and theologian, grew to love and respect many aspects of a world view radically different from his own. He describes the polarities of truth which represent a harmony of opposites in Christian worship and theology but emphasises our Western mistake of relying too much on the 'left brain' – that is, our legacy of Enlightenment rationalism. He feels that, whilst not negating the good aspects of rationalism, we need to redress the balance in favour of the 'right brain' picture of the two-thirds world.[5] In Wilson's list (*see* Figure 7.2) the reason/

---

[5] Wilson uses this phrase as an alternative to the rather elitist first and third world labels. The two-thirds world covers two-thirds of the globe.

INDIVIDUALITY←	→MEMBERSHIP
CASUALTY CARE←	→GROWING COMMUNITY
HOLY PLACE←	→EVERYDAY PLACE
PROFESSIONAL←	→LAITY
(accreditisation, specialisation)	(amateur)
OBJECTIVE←	→SUBJECTIVE
(arm's length)	(mutuality, share, participation)
SERVICE←	→FRIENDSHIP
THERAPY←	→GROWTH
(disease, sin)	(suffer)
THE FALL←	→THE FULFILMENT
(look back)	(look forward)
LOVE←	→JUSTICE
(private faith)	(public issues)
MIND←	→MATTER
(vision, idealism, theory)	(practice, reality, action)
LEFT BRAIN←	→RIGHT BRAIN
(Western, verbal)	(two-thirds world, artistic, ritual)

Source: Wilson, 1988, p.219.

FIGURE 7.2 Wilson's 'Polarities of Truth'

emotion, science/art division already mentioned and the need for a shift of emphasis to set up an equilibrium – a Buddhist 'middle way' – is implicit.[6] Wilson believes that the 'West' has defined life and experience in terms of the 'private' and the 'professional' with the result that power is possessed by a few, truth is the monopoly of those with power and we characteristically suffer problems of alienation from our world and our experience. In contrast, the cultures of the two-thirds world have retained a community-based view of life and thus placed technology and rationalism as peripheral rather than central to experience. Both of these polarities have helpful and unhelpful aspects. Wilson seeks to harmonise the two in order to create a healthier and more just world.

Lidz describes one aspect of the reality Wilson is mapping:

> Some people become artists and create worlds of their own, but most of them know that these worlds are not reality. The schizophrenic is apt to retreat into a world in which he can solve things purely on his own. And he will not refer this world back to the real one at any point.
>
> (Boyars and Orrill, 1973, p.144)

Although one may wish to challenge Lidz's notion that some definitive 'real world' exists, his point is nevertheless important. Barham in his excellent book 'Schizophrenia and Human Value' uses Alistair McIntyre's concept of man as a story telling animal to clarify this idea: Barham (1984; p.89) writes: 'We are never more (and sometimes less) than the co-authors of our own narratives. Only in fantasy do we

---

[6] This Buddhist analogy is mine and not Wilson's.

live any story we please'. Using Wilson's schema it is possible to see the person with psychotic illness at the extreme end of the right-hand side, so far over that she can no longer reach back to the middle. Whereas the state of mental and physical wholeness we are aiming to achieve in ourselves and others, 'health' in any spiritual sense, must be a broad margin around Wilson's middle line.

There is undoubtedly much illness on the extreme left-hand side of Wilson's division too: individualism, indifference, materialism, and alienation. Living exclusively on either side is unwholesome. But generally we view these latter characteristics as normal. Whilst recognising psychopathy as deviant behaviour we do not perceive that it may be an extreme extention of these *left* brain characteristics. We might usefully employ Laing's imagery here, and see the left brain as denoting the outer world and the right brain as the inner world. 'The outer world divorced from any illumination from the inner is a state of darkness. We are in an age of darkness. The state of outer darkness is a state of sin, i.e. alienation or estrangement from the inner light' (Laing, 1990, pp.116–17). We need to stretch our hands across the 'oceanic abyss' (the chaos?) from both sides of the polarised world Wilson has depicted. It is not just a matter of the left pulling the right back into sanity but the reverse also.

Wilson's division must not be confused with de Beausobre's good/evil split which is of different categories. Good/healing remains close to Wilson's midline and evil/ suffering at each extreme edge. One may see how the yurodivy may exist on each side of Wilson's line and thus the psychotic has a chance of being an active part of redemption and not merely a passive recipient.

Redemption and creativity

The title of de Beausobre's book (*Creative Suffering*) is important. Suffering can only be redeemed if it is allowed to be creative.[7] We have only recently recognised the link between mental illness and creativity in such people as van Gogh, Kierkegaard, Nietzsche, and Woolf. Most people who suffer do not produce such works,[8] but the creations of some do testify to the struggle to understand and to be understood. Their efforts to understand may have brought them to mental darkness and their need to be understood may have created their works. The fact that most were not valued in their own lifetimes may have precipitated their demise into irredeemed psychosis or suicide. They were perhaps yurodivys who were not able to return from their experience of suffering because no one would take their hands. The significance of these artistic lives in the current context is to show that creativity and chaos are inextricably linked. Berger sees this as a universal truth:

> When you look up at the balcony of the sky from Barra, another answer comes to one of the oldest questions – a different answer to the one given in the Age of the Enlightenment. With things changing every hour, and forever repeating themselves like the tide, you understand that Creation for all its beauty, was born of suffering.

(1992, pp.223–4)

---

[7] Perhaps it would be helpful if we thought also of moral action as a creative art rather than as the 'science' of ethics.

[8] This may be due to lack of opportunity rather than lack of ability.

As creativity is born of suffering, so suffering may only be redeemed by creativity. Creative redemption may, in a few cases, involve the reception of works of art, but for most people it will be as a result of their carers' willingness to understand them, rather than seeing them simply as Other, no matter how bizarre they seem. This is a creative process for both parties. When the Other is understood she is then free, if she so wishes, to return to the mid-point of healing and bring others back with her.

Such participation is, however, a complex event for it means accepting the experience of others as meaningful to *them*, and as an aspect of reality, while understanding that alone it may not represent that which is healing:

> Of course the perception of a schizophrenic may be different from anything you or I can have, so closely in touch is he with things we have to block off. These special perceptions may have more to do with things that myth deals with – a deeper understanding of human motivation often.

> (Lidz, quoted in Boyars and Orrill, 1973 p.141)

Szasz's (1961) definition of 'myth' differs from the word's connotation in this passage by Lidz in an important way. His description of mental illness as a myth emphasises its falseness. His was a damning interpretation. Lidz's rendering is of 'myth' used in its biblical sense, another way of expressing truth.

The story of our lives is our own myth. We cannot simply have scientific understanding or simply artistic understanding, for as we have seen these lead to the illnesses of Western rationality or of 'living every story we please' (psychosis). A myth is that which joins both of these understandings and gives them meaning and human value. Myth may be what is lost and lacking in our world, which seems not to 'know what a human life is worth' and its lack may be what makes moral action with respect to the mentally ill so difficult.

CONCLUSION

It has been my aim here to demonstrate the importance of retaining the image of the 'person' in their madness. Professional carers of the mentally ill face, daily, the very hard task of relating with integrity to those whose experience, and expression of that experience, may appear vastly different from their own. Such carers may be required to cross over the abyss that appears to separate the mad from everyone else. To cross this abyss is not to enter into madness but to stand where the mad person is and see the world from their viewpoint. I do not underestimate the difficult nature of my prescription. It may not be a matter of 'doing' certain things but of 'being' in a new way.

We are the result of our own stories, no less than the mad are of theirs. I do not believe that we should leave our stories behind when we cross the abyss (for maybe this would be to become mad too), but in taking our stories with us and in allowing them to be open to the very different story of another, we are then exercising our moral duty appropriately: It is to show respect for the person; to treat their experience as equally valid to one's own; and to acknowledge that the symbolic account being offered has meaning for us too. I hope that in elaborating some such symbolism I have offered another way of understanding madness.

I described Cath (A) and (B) as studies in the concept of meaning because it seems to me that we have a moral obligation to view mental illness as meaningful experience. It would be over-simplistic to view Cath (A)'s experience as less severe or important than Cath (B)'s. The difference in their experience is probably better defined by our ability to bear witness to it. It was possible for Cath (A) to share her journey with another (her counsellor), who in a sense gave her a point of reference with which to situate her experience. The counsellor becomes the one who links the polarities of experience that Wilson describes. Cath (A) did, however, always maintain a link with the 'rational' world whereas Cath (B) appears not to have done. The ability to maintain this link should not be underestimated. Many people like Cath (A) commit suicide precisely because of the burden of having a 'foot in each camp'. The view from 'both sides' may be too much for many to contemplate and this may be one of the reasons why those who care for the mentally ill are very wary of crossing over traditional boundaries of explanation and participation. Our moral responsibility to those in our care may, however, ask this of us. None of us is ever completely healthy. We all sway too far over to the left and right of Wilson's divide at various times in our lives. Our moral responsibility to our selves and to others is to maintain some sort of balance. Cath (A)'s counsellor was able to help her integrate what had previously been a divisive and destructive experience that she was being overwhelmed by. Instead of stradling the divide precariously, she can now stand Janus-like in the centre and view both directions simultaneously.

Caring for Cath (B) presents different challenges. The fact that her experience is less recognisable than Cath (A)'s may make it less distressing to care for her, as identification is so much more difficult. But as a greater step away from one's own experience needs to be made in order to make sense of her world, there may be other risks which have to be taken. The yurodivy metaphor seems most apt in this situation. The carer will recognise the damage sustained (the evil) and like the yurodivy she will need somehow to participate in it. She will need to participate in the symbolic world that Cath (B) has created, in order to make sense of the suffering she so intensely feels. It is not exactly a matter of translating the symbolic story back into a more rational language but of understanding the truth that each story may yield. In Cath (A)'s case this may mean exploring the Christian metaphor with her; in Cath (B)'s situation it may necessitate an investigation of the 'God language' that she uses and what 'being killed' means to her. If we can help restore a sense of meaning to these women's lives, we will have fulfilled our moral obligation to them; we will have behaved with integrity as one person to another.

If mental illness is understood as myth, that is as an attempt to understand and to be understood, then the chaos of many may, at last, have potential for creativity and value. Cath (A) prepares to create a new life for herself because she can share her story, arguing her moral worth to the world. Cath (B), however, must wait, isolated within her own story, until some soul is brave enough to cross over to her side and reinterpret the world *with* her (but not for her). Redemption comes through our moral participation: it can never be a distant academic exercise. Only through this redemption will Cath (B) no longer feel that she is being killed at the margins of our world.

REFERENCES

Arieti, S. and **Bemporad, J.** 1980: *Severe and mild Depression: the therapeutic approach*. London: Tavistock Publications.

Barker, P.J. 1992: *Severe depression: a practioner's guide*. London: Chapman and Hall.

Berger, J. 1992: *Keeping a rendezvous*. London: Granta Publications.

Berger, J. and **Mohr, J.** 1981: *A fortunate man*. London: Readers' and Writers' Press.

Boyars, R. and **Orrill, R.** 1973: *Laing and anti-psychiatry*. London: Penguin.

Coulter, K. 1993: *The sociology of religious madness*. Unpublished MA dissertation. Department of Religious Studies, University of Newcastle upon Tyne.

De Beausobre, I. 1954: *Creative suffering*. London: Dacre Press.

Kristeva, J. 1989: *Black sun: depression and melancholia*. New York: Columbia University Press.

Laing, R.D. 1990: *The politics of experience and the bird of paradise*. London: Penguin.

Leunig, M. 1990: *Ramming the Shears*. Australia: Penguin.

McGrath, P. 1989: A childhood in Broadmoor Hospital. In *Granta 29, New World*. London: Granta.

Nietzsche, F. 1892: *Thus spoke Zarathustra*. trans. R.J. Hollingdale (1961), Harmondsworth: Penguin.

Perry, M. 1987: *Deliverance*. London: SPCK.

Styron, W. 1991: Dark night of the soul. In *The Independent on Sunday Review*. 24 February, 3–6.

Szasz, T. 1961: *The myth of mental illness*. New York: Harper and Row.

Szasz, T. 1971: *The manufacture of madness*. London: Routledge and Kegan Paul.

Wilson, M. 1988: *A coat of many Colours*. London: Epworth Press.

8

PSYCHIATRIC NURSING AND THE MYTH OF ALTRUISM

Joy Bray

Psychiatric nursing is moving, in theory at least, closer to a position where a central aspect of the nurse's role is to offer the sort of healing relationship outlined. Offering help, that is, so that people can experience their distress and then see it both as the reasonable upshot of their life history and an opportunity for growth. Perhaps, as argued, within the psychie-industry nurses occupy the ideal position to adopt this role. Here Joy Bray discusses the theoretical background to this move. She examines whether it is in fact taking place and then suggests another way in which self-interest operates within psychiatric nursing to interrupt progress. Drawing on themes developed in previous chapters in relation to pathologising the Other, Joy holds up a mirror to explore the 'illness' of being a mental health professional. She insists that proper attention be given to our own mental health needs if we are to work effectively. In particular Joy addresses the need for therapeutic supervision and staff support groups. She acknowledges how unlikely it is that these needs will be adequately met in the current social and economic climate.

INTRODUCTION

There is a cherished idea within nursing, infrequently challenged, that the nurse and the patient have a close, collaborative relationship within which the person in need finds solace and relief from an overwhelming experience of psychic pain. The question that is seldom addressed is whether it is the nurse or the patient seeking the solace and relief, or both.

In the following chapter I address this question by exploring a number of related issues: first I examine the ideology relating to nurse–patient relationships. Then I ask what patients want from their relationships with nurses and whether they get it. Third I pose similar questions of nurses in their relationships with patients. What might they hope to get and what do they get from the experience? And then, crucially, given the apparent frustration of both patients and nurses in their aims, finally I offer an analysis of the problems we face, and a view of the potential for improvement.

The central ethical dilemma with which I am concerned relates to our status as mental health carers. We are viewed, and we may see ourselves, as in less need, as mentally healthier, as saner than those we enter into relationships with to offer them care. Is this right?

Setting the scene: the 'collaborative' relationship

The close relationship between nurse and patient is usually considered the essential component of psychiatric nursing. Peplau (1994) acknowledges the significance and expected therapeutic benefit of the nurse's interactions with patients, stating 'It is the responses of nurses to patients within nurse patient relationships, which provide the stimuli for constructive changes that psychiatric patients need to make in their thinking and in their behaviour' (p.5). This emphasis on the centrality of the relationship within good nursing practice as a method of helping the patient is characteristic of Peplau's writings. Many other leading nurse theorists agree with her views, presuming almost without question that this sort of close relationship is firmly entrenched within nursing practice.

Even if this presumption is questionable (Dartington, 1993) there are structures within psychiatric nursing practice that underpin the close nurse–patient relationship, notably 'nursing process' and 'primary nursing'. Nursing process, the fourfold schema of assessment, planning, implementation and evaluation, was first presented in the UK in 1975, following work in America (de la Cuesta, 1983). Ideas within the nursing process have become subsumed into primary nursing (Pearson, 1988) with its emphasis on accountability, and these two theories together are now being developed as the organisational structure for delivering care, underpinned by the statutory concept of the 'named nurse'. These structures all emphasise the need for nurse and patient to spend time together writing care plans, carrying out structured pieces of work, partaking in counselling sessions, evaluating outcomes, and so on. The emphasis throughout is on closeness, on time together.

Cementing these theoretical and structural trends towards nurse–patient collaboration, the Government's long anticipated report on mental health nursing recommends that care plans be developed with individuals based on their wishes and needs, not the convenience of the service (Department of Health, 1994). The report also emphasises that mental health services should be arranged so as to ensure that nurses spend the majority of the time responding to the needs of service users (Butterworth and Faugier, 1994). The implication is clear: nurses will need to spend time with patients to discover their wishes and needs, and in order to respond to these.

If we accept that the essence of psychiatric nursing is indeed a close, collaborative relationship between nurse and patient, two points need to be addressed. First, do patients want or get a close involvement with their nurse? If so what do they value within it? Second, what type of closeness might nurses either want or get from their involvement with patients? And why?

WHAT DO USERS OF THE SERVICE WANT AND GET?

Rogers *et al.* (1993) in their survey of users' views of psychiatric services found that a preferred model of practice involved personal contact and understanding, being listened and responded to empathically. Users viewed the appropriate response to their distress as working, or talking through their problems with someone ready to listen, within a supportive and caring environment. Similarly, McIntyre *et al.* (1989) asked, 'What do psychiatric inpatients really want?' The patients rated most highly getting out of the hospital environment! They also rated as helpful talking to a nurse. Carson and Sharma (1994) concurred with this, finding also that nurses, when considering what was therapeutic for patients, rated most highly 'talking to nurses'. Looking into the value ascribed by patients to different forms of treatment, Pollock (1989) found that having already achieved their main objective, leaving hospital, community-based patients continued to value very highly nurse involvement. Such patients identified 'the interest and concern' shown by their community psychiatric nurses as 'very considerably' helpful. These studies all thus reflected the felt importance of nurses' talking to patients, both for nurses and for their patients, both in hospital and in the community.

It may be worthwhile at this stage to examine the characteristics of the nurse–patient relationship historically. The research findings reproduced here will shed some light on whether in the past service users have in fact got what they all seem to agree they want and need. Two studies observing what happened between nurse and patient were completed at the same time as the nursing process was introduced in the UK. Cormack (1976) observed psychiatric nurses working on an in-patient unit and found a discrepancy between what recent literature had suggested the nurse ought to be doing and what was actually happening. Cormack found that the nurses' interactions were on average of very short duration, typically thirty seconds to four minutes. Three-quarters of such interactions were terminated by the nurse. This suggests very poor conditions for close, empathetic work. And it was not just staff nurses whose contact with patients was limited. Cormack's observations of charge nurses suggested that their managerial role precluded them from: 'indulging in the prolonged patient contact which would be necessary for the performance of the prescribed role' (p. 87). One suggestion was that the charge nurses were using their role as a way of avoiding patient contact.

Towell (1975) was studying similar phenomena in England from a sociological perspective. His findings closely replicated Cormack's: an avoidance of prolonged patient contact by all grades of nurses. There was some evidence, however, that uninitiated (most frequently student) nurses did become 'involved' with patients. Ironically, this involvement was felt as a *threat* to staff norms. The involved member of staff was considered deviant and a variety of strategies were put into operation to reduce what would characteristically be termed *over-involvement*. An example of such a strategy was open discussion of the relationship in a staff meeting where strong group pressure could be applied. If such control processes were unsuccessful, a breach was likely in the staff group and the involved nurse was herself perceived as 'having a problem'. Naturally enough, having had this difficult experience, the 'deviant' nurse was likely to enter into subsequent relationships with patients at a more superficial level, seeking to avoid a repeat experience of being labelled deviant, then ostracised.

If we accept that these findings were true of psychiatric institutions generally, then, evidently, two decades ago nurses were being discouraged from spending time with their patients. More recent studies suggest there has been little improvement. Haugen Bunch (1985) studied aspects of nurses' communication with schizophrenic patients in a psychiatric ward in America. The findings have a familiar feel. The nurses engaged in passive nursing strategies when the ward was quiet, such as short episodes of social talking with patients. When the ward was busy the nurses engaged in strategies such as 'business talking', medicating and 'scheduling' patients. There was virtually no evidence of meaningful, therapeutic relationships.

Handy (in Carson *et al.*, 1995) too, has noted the lack of time spent with their patients by all but the most junior of nurses. She describes one of the methods used to deal with nurses deviating from the professionally accepted norm: senior staff suggest that the involved nurse is herself mentally ill.

Over the past few years there has been a series of observational studies carried out by either non-nurses or nurses now practising as psychoanalysts (Sinanoglou, 1987; Donati, 1989). Their method (psychodynamic observation) represents an attempt to gain access to the unconscious life and functioning of the institution and its participants (mostly patients and nurses). Sinanoglou's account is poignant:

> My initial impression of the atmosphere was one of intense anxiety, unknown fear, despair and chaos. The staff seemed harassed, overworked and with no time to breathe, let alone waste . . . The faces of the patients were ghostlike, with an empty dead expression desperately looking towards the door which symbolised life.
>
> (p.28)

All these authors' presentations of their perceptions reflect the lifelessness felt, the predominance of apathy over enthusiasm and the defeat of any attempt to create a positive culture. Why might it be that the goal of collaboration between nurses and their patients seems so rarely, if ever, attained? It is surely short-sighted to suggest that nurses be held individually to blame for this situation. However, it might be instructive to explore what nurses want and get from their involvement with patients.

WHAT DO NURSES WANT AND GET?

The myth of altruism

Josie

Josie was a 28-year-old nurse, the only child of professional parents who were absorbed in their careers and had left her between the ages of 1 and 11 with a succession of nannies, none of whom stayed for longer than two years. At age 11 she was sent to boarding school. After qualifying as an RMN she joined a rehabilitation unit for patients with enduring mental health problems. She developed very rewarding relationships with the patients to whom she was primary nurse, most of whom had histories either of childhood neglect or abuse. Josie had difficulty in establishing close peer relationships and frequently felt that her most worthwhile relationships were the ones she had developed with her patients. Other staff were impressed with her work and noted patient improvement. During a session of clinical supervision, Josie was asked to consider whether and how she might be meeting her own needs as well as her patients' in bringing a stable relationship to them. Unfortunately this interpretation was made insensitively, with destructive results. One week later Josie became ill and subsequently left nursing. The patients were all delegated to other care workers.

Helping others is not an altruistic act. Dartington (1993) suggested that people are drawn into the caring professions out of a need to make something right, to heal one's own emotional wounds and the damaged figures of one's imagination. This is not necessarily a bad thing. It makes good psychic and economic sense to heal oneself whilst promoting healing in others. Moreover, as Skynner (1989) emphasised, mental health professionals are the only people willing and able to sustain their very difficult task of caring for others' mental illness *perhaps precisely because* they are getting something from it psychologically, something which they have been unable to obtain in the normal course of their life. Skynner suggests that a mutual satisfaction of needs is quite reasonable. Indeed, the same needs may be satisfied in both worker and patient, though the worker has a responsibility to ensure that the exchange is not totally symmetrical.

The need for support

In order to ensure an asymmetry whereby the patient's needs are looked after by the worker in at least equal measure to her own, it is crucial that the worker's needs are given some space outside of her time with her patient where they can be acknowledged. As a supervisor it becomes clear just how crucial this space is when one considers the ill advised clinical decisions that can be averted by helping nurses to address their own unresolved turmoil and unmet needs.

Susan

A very competent and caring charge nurse brought to clinical supervision a case that was bothering her: 'This woman is manipulating the team. I want to consider how to set really firm boundaries on her.' When asked to describe the problem behaviours she found it difficult to quantify any. Eventually she said: 'I know she's supposed to be depressed but I hate the way she ignores her children when they visit.' It eventually became obvious to us both that what she was feeling was out of proportion to the situation. Then she spoke about her own childhood where her mother had suffered recurrent bouts of depression, during which she had largely ignored her children. The charge nurse had of course found this extraordinarily painful. She had never spoken about it though, as she knew that 'Mum was ill and couldn't help it'. Instead, her unvoiced feelings about her own experience, her difficulty in this area, had become invested in the patient.

The transference onto a patient of feelings that one has towards a significant figure in one's own life, as in the case above, is quite natural. It is one aspect of a process known as 'counter-transference'. A mother ignoring her children was, understandably, a sore spot for Susan. Significantly though, the reason for the decision Susan was inclined to make in relation to this patient could easily have gone unnoticed, had there not been the space to explore what was happening. More worrying still, the angry, possibly punitive aspect of Susan's plan to 'set really firm boundaries' on the patient is very likely to have remained unacknowledged without a safe relationship where such dynamics could be explored. Without a way of acknowledging this aspect of her feelings towards the patient, this anger may in turn have been attributed to the patient herself, in a process known as projection. If the patient 'resisted' being treated in the way planned, she would no doubt have been said to be *angrily* 'acting out' as a result of her inability to accept and work with the 'appropriate boundaries' Susan had attempted to enforce. Susan's limitations would have become the limitations of the therapy and the resulting impasse may in turn have been characterised as a product of the patient's pathology. This ethically dubious picture must be familiar to many nurses, if allowed the time to reflect on it.

The individual and institutional reasons why relationships with patients so often take this sort of turn are issues I shall return to. For now, I want to develop the idea that nurses have needs in their relationships with patients, and that this can be both acceptable and constructive. I shall now contrast the potential hazards to a therapeutic relationship if it is given insufficient support, with the potential benefits to both nurse and patient if the relationship is properly tended.

Therapists can grow too

Clearly, a lot can go wrong when there is no space to disentangle one's own emotional experiences from one's patients', and at very least the therapist must be ready to be open about the feelings and experiences she has had in the therapeutic setting if she is to confront the problems that she is struggling with in her work. But when the nurse is willing to acknowledge that she is there for herself, not just the patient, there is immense therapeutic potential in the work situation for both patient and nurse, which has ramifications for the nurse in her life way beyond her work situation. For Susan in the above example the self-exploration she undertook, encouraged and supported by her supervisor, was not just an embarrassing difficulty to face as part of her job; it was a growth experience that affected her whole sense of self and her life. Indeed, Peplau (1988) advocated that the very purpose of therapy is for the patient and therapist to grow together. Certainly there is no clear difference in principle between exploring the blind spots in our self-awareness and helping our patients to work on theirs.

In the light of such arguments, any mental health care would best begin with an exploration by the worker of the self, an appraising of motives and a willingness to face parts of oneself normally kept hidden. Indeed, psychiatric nurse education, in parallel to Peplau's writings, has, since the 1982 Mental Health Nursing Syllabus, consistently endorsed this view, with 'self-awareness' or 'group dynamics' sessions prescribed as an integral part of training. Rioch suggests that quite a powerful and potentially life-changing experience of growth and development should be encouraged: 'If students do not know that they are potentially . . . murderers, crooks and cowards, they cannot deal therapeutically with these potentialities in their clients' (Hawkins and Shohet, 1989; p.5). However, something seems to be failing. The work previously reviewed suggests that psychiatric nurses are not working consistently in close relationships with patients. Perhaps the depth of self-awareness encouraged in training is inadequate and inconsistent? And again, could it be that there simply is not the structure or time in busy clinical settings for staff to continue this work of reflection and individual growth and development, post-training?

AN ANALYSIS OF THE PROBLEM

Why then is it so difficult for nurses to get on with the work of disentangling their emotional material from their patients, to their mutual benefit? Why do nurses view having vulnerabilities and needs as failure? And why do the structures and cultures of the organisations in which they work seem invariably to inhibit the sharing of such vulnerabilities?

Psychic complexity

The need to control

Lawton (1982; p.266) developed a framework to help understand the processes described below.

1. Helping others is not an altruistic, selfless act, rather it serves the needs of the helper.
2. The need to control stems from the social worker's childhood and points to the fact that there is a family-specific type of 'professional' personality contributing to the maintenance of the system.
3. The agency serves as a fertile field for the expression of the worker's needs because its structure and process broadly resemble the worker's family of origin where the needs were formed in the first place.
4. The agency serves as a theatre in which social workers, especially those who remain longer than a year or two, are able to relive important aspects of their childhoods. This psycho-historical relationship strongly influences why people choose the work in the first place, and the nature of the institution in which the job is carried out.

He demonstrated how there was a need, shared by the social workers who were subjects of his study, to be in control.[1] This need originated from their childhood. Lawton maintained that there is a fairly specific type of 'professional carer' personality, which contributes to the maintenance of a system wherein relationships of control predominate. He described the type of child-rearing encountered by children who go on to work in this field as that of psychic control, where the parents communicated a number of very strong expectations about how their children were to conduct themselves, usually in unspoken ways. The idea of deviating from these expectations seldom occurred to these workers when they were children. They were controlled without ever realising it, awareness of this and the resulting features of their character coming only in adolescence or adulthood. Many had felt close to their parents and were not considered especially rebellious as children.

The nursing staff of a small, specialised unit have a good reputation for care of acutely distressed patients. They work hard to deliver 'good' nursing care. However, the 'good' nursing care that is planned is seldom delivered. The staff complain

---

[1] The feelings described by Lawton (1982) as belonging to social workers, could parallel the feelings experienced by others in the helping professions. Although mental health nurses are not social workers, Aldridge (1994) argued that the two professions do now closely reflect each other. She emphasised how in 'new nursing', as she termed it, like social work, the major component is working with the individual in a close, collaborative relationship. With the movement of nurses into the community and the heightening of their accountability for patient care, their job now resembles even more closely that of a social worker.

that 'they' (by this they mean unspecified management figures) are preventing them from carrying out 'good' nursing care. This perception is never challenged, the nursing staff never confront the management team about the fantasised lack of autonomy. Their self-confidence is limited, compounded by a nagging sense of failure, of never quite reaching the ideal of being a 'good' nurse.

Evidently the issue of control may move from the family to the place of work, where the 'controlling' management blocks both the creativity and fulfilment of staff, or even of a whole staff team. There is hostility felt towards the parent/management who never quite cares enough. This can not be expressed openly, however, because the result may be to lose whatever care there is. So it is absorbed, masochistically. This suffering, and the ability to endure it, may make a nurse feel special, one reason perhaps why we take a perverse but grandiose pleasure in being able to survive the institution. How often do nurses hear 'I couldn't do your job'?

We have experienced psychic control in our childhoods and we may imagine we are still suffering it, as above. We are also likely to exercise similar control in our relationships with patients. Lawton's suggestion is that we are bound to see the patient as childlike and dependent in order to live out our dependence and vulnerability through him. We identify with the patient as 'troubled child', we attempt vicariously to care for ourselves, as child, within the patient and we therefore 'enjoy' our patient's dependency. Instead of setting conditions where the patient (the person ostensibly more in need of help) can achieve independence, it seems that in general we unconsciously foster her dependency. The patient in our care helps us to feel good about ourselves, for we are repairing something important that has gone wrong; it is as if helping her to work with her problems *is* helping ourselves. The control we exercise is in the more or less subtle manipulation of the role into which we place and in which we attempt to keep her.

There is a further aspect to the masochism described earler. We may not only enjoy the continuation of our being controlled, we may also enjoy experiencing an almost inevitable frustration of our own attempts to control.[2]

> A patient with a long-term psychotic illness was discharged after an admission of six weeks. He was very stable and was returning to a job and a supportive family. In handover the charge nurse said: 'Things look good at the moment but you wait; he'll be back within a couple of months.' The charge nurse was unable to let control go, was unable to allow the patient to be anything but dependent and was unable to feel good about what the patient had achieved. Through presumably either envy, masochism, a need to maintain the *status quo* in their respective roles, or all three, he could only feel good about the patient's prospective failure and the failure of his own attempts to heal.

The need to deny

Henry Lawton's (1982) paper's main theme was the ambiguous nature of altruism in mental health carers. He hoped unrealistically that it would be well received. On

---

[2] The frustration is almost inevitable, since we have two mutually exclusive needs in this situation: to experience a vicarious healing through our sense of the patient's improvement, also to experience a continued sense that they remain the patient, the vulnerable one, not us.

studying his group of social workers Lawton had found not the altruistically motivated workforce he expected, but a group of very needy people. The amount of need seemed to mirror, if it did not overtake, that of their clients. This view was intolerable, it seems, to the workforce in question.

Skynner (1989) provided a picture of the health professional's family that explains to some extent this phenomenon. While agreeing with Lawton's basic premise regarding the 'psychic control' described above, he offered a different emphasis. He suggested that in a typical 'deprived' family, which maintains some sort of cycle of deprivation and control in the psyches of its children, the deprivation itself is not the main problem. Rather, it is the denial of such. As I shall now describe, such denial functions as a form of protection to avoid the intolerable pain of loss or neglect that would otherwise be felt.

For our social worker or RMN, the cycle of control, deprivation and denial originates at some point in their family. Their parents, themselves deprived, would have been unable to face and control the pain of this and so would have split off and repressed the feelings of need within themselves. They would have just had to stay in control and cope. As Lawton depicts, they would then have projected the feeling and perceived the need not as their own but as if it were within their children. Instead of being able to perceive their own deprivation and therefore do something about it, they decide to give their children what they did not have themselves. The motive may have been good but the mechanism is flawed. The parents have not seen their children with their own individual and unique needs, but rather saw themselves and their needs within their children.

On reflection, many parents can identify with this mechanism. When you think about the needs you perceive in your children, they may bear a remarkable resemblance to your own unmet childhood needs. But the result is that children in these circumstances do not have their own needs met. Rather, they have their parents' needs met in them. They get emotional warmth, for example, in circumstances where as a child the parent might have needed it, not when *they* do; or when the parent is currently feeling lonely, not when *they* are. The parents remain deprived and the children ultimately grow up deprived too. The convolutions of the cycle continue as the children perceive and identify with the role subtly foisted on them. This is known as projective identification. At some level the child will know that their role is to make their parent feel better, and may as a result try to nurture the parent. But the only way the child can nurture the parent without actually confronting the denial and thereby exposing the parent to distress, is by enhancing the parent's self-esteem by treating him/her as the 'good' parent s/he pretends to be but is not. In this way they are joining in the collusive denial and perpetuating the cycle. What remains unacknowledged is the rage felt by the child (and the parent) at the deprivation suffered. This may be expressed in devious ways such as by disappointing the parent's expectations. By failing, they make the parent fail too. In turn the parent may undermine successes their children have.

This pattern can be related to nurse–patient relationships:

Steve

Steve was primary nurse to a patient who was well known to the service and had a history of alcohol abuse. He had been admitted following an overdose of tranquillisers and alcohol. Steve worked closely with him, concentrating on working through his feelings about his marriage break-up, considering this the exacerbating factor for the overdose. The patient was readmitted within a week of discharge, having taken another overdose. On readmission the patient told the admitting nurse that he felt confused and desperate as he was beginning to relive the feelings he had as a sexually abused child and was terrified he may in some way abuse his son. This readiness to tackle such painful issues may have been framed as a breakthrough. Instead, Steve refused to become his primary nurse again as he felt bereft of the empathy that he had previously felt. He had given everything and the patient had let him down. It was surely no coincidence that Steve's parents had divorced when he was 6 years old and he was currently experiencing profound difficulties in his relationship with his partner, which he was not discussing with anyone, feeling that he should just somehow cope. In working closely with this patient, Steve had clearly been seeing his own vulnerabilities in the patient's situation and missed a large area of the patient's own distress. He had not managed to heal the wounds he perceived in his patient, as that patient had bigger problems to tackle first. Neither had he therefore worked through his own deprivation and turmoil, as he saw it *in* the patient. All he could feel was let down by the patient's remaining ill after his caring input, and depressed, and all he seemed able to do as a result was punish and deprive the patient by rejecting him.

In nursing we feel so much more empathy if we can understand a person's pain as something that we have experienced and can identify with. In these circumstances the mechanism of projection described above is more benign. We perceive a patient's need because it has been our own. Hawkins and Shohet (1989) give the example of an unsympathetic GP who was avoided by all patients until his grandson had leukaemia and 'slowly, through his own hurt and anger, he was able to touch his patients again.' (p.153). By relating our own experience to our patients' we can achieve empathy. However, it may be that we are more likely to be taking care of our own denied distress by projecting it onto the patient and looking after it there, as in Steve's case, whatever the nature of *their* pain and distress: The patient is a passive figure in this equation, whose needs are not perceived individually, who is rather a receptacle for the professional's denied distress, whether such identification helps them or not.

This denial of need elaborated by Skynner relates to a suggestion made by Carson *et al.* (1995) that staff in the NHS feel guilty when considering their own needs. Nurses view having needs as a failure on their part and suspect that any serious admission of need will mean that they lose credible professional standing in the eyes of their colleagues and superiors. There is an almost exact fit with the picture described by Skynner, a denial of need, ensuring feelings of guilt, inadequacy and despair develop when this need starts to surface at a conscious level, as for example in Steve's situation above. Such feelings were perhaps also behind Josie's compulsion, described above, to exit the situation as soon as aspects of her experience were named.

So far I have considered the question 'why do nurses not get what they want from their involvement with patients, or even manage to collaborate properly with them?' in terms of complexities within the psyche of the individual nurse. I have implied that, at some level, the nurse desires to recapitulate former relationship(s) through contact with patients, but is hindered by her emotional material. But a question still remains unanswered: why is any *authentic* form of such contact so rarely, if ever, attained?

After all, the aim of therapy, we should recall, is for patient and therapist to grow together. And we have understood the mechanism of denial and the need to be in control in the context of the family dynamics experienced in childhood by individual nurses, i.e. as areas where such nurses may be ripe for growth. There is no obvious reason, therefore, why nurses should not be ready to leave behind the emotional conditioning they have received, and learn, along with their patients, new ways of being.

Perhaps it is now time to consider the nature of the organisation in which the individual works. How does it happen that mental health workers frequently find themselves working in institutions which are as depriving and unrecognising of their own needs as their parents were, equally controlling and apparently dedicated to maintaining such cycles of control, deprivation and denial in their staff?

Organisational complexity

Hiller (in Carson *et al.*, 1995) suggested that the culture in which nursing takes place is one that seeks to inhibit the development of close professional and supportive ties among nurses, leaving a residue of mistrust, hopelessness and alienation, such that vulnerabilities of any kind are unlikely to be shared.

Lawton (1983) described the public service agencies that he worked in and observed, as sharing certain characteristics.

1. Being resistant to change.
2. Showing a high turnover in senior administration.
3. Being unsupportive to their case workers.
4. Being secretive and restrictive in their communications.
5. Controlling in an infantilising way.
6. Being rigidly bureaucratic, valuing conformity and disliking criticism or opposition.
7. Using their social workers rather than respecting them as persons.

He observed that these organisations demanded loyalty without encouraging adequate training. They generated rage in the workforce but also forced them to suppress it. Lawton summarised the position as follows: 'The agency is like a paradoxical bad/good mother, implacable in her power and appearing implacably dedicated to hampering the effectiveness of her workers/children at every turn' (p.289). The parents want to be seen as excellent but are actually making rather a mess of bringing up the children. Although Lawton suggested that workers who remain longer than a year or two might be able to relive important aspects of their childhood, he became increasingly uncertain that his agency was actually helping people. He began to realise that the agency, comprising both those working in it and those served by it, was an interrelated system, neither good nor bad, but human, functioning on a social level in a way that replicated the primitive intra-psychic mechanisms of defence such as control, denial and projection described above. Skynner (1989) concurred that agencies working with clients trapped in a cycle of deprivation, often manifested a parallel cycle in their staff and organisational culture.

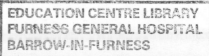

Both Lawton and Skynner suggested that within the arena of mental health care as a whole a division exists where public (i.e. state-funded) agencies are worse in this respect. Lawton (1982) distinguished two types of worker. First, there are those that cling to the institution because they fear change and loss of support, they repeat patterns and use energy in maintaining the *status quo*. Second, there are more confident workers who become dissatisfied at the lack of change and move elsewhere. This mirrors the findings of Menzies-Lyth (1959) with student general nurses, the more mature and confident of whom were more likely to become dissatisfied and terminate their training early. This is a bleak picture indeed, where our most deprived institutions are thus left with the most deprived and unconfident residual workforce.

Private institutions are apparently different, workers there having higher self-esteem. Exceptions to this rule can be found in the UK, where institutions may be state-funded but have access, for various reasons, to more of a lion's share of resources, e.g. the Cassel Hospital and the Maudsley Hospital, both of them clinical and teaching areas with excellent reputations. However, in all areas there are institutional as well as individual difficulties in removing the mechanism of denial described above, as its removal allows the experience of pain.

The complex economic and political frameworks supporting the maintenance of the sort of patterns of relationship described within an institution are vital to understand this situation. Some of them have been addressed in earlier chapters. The question to be asked now, however, is what to do about the situation within the context of the health service and social services in the 1990s.

Even if individual nurses are ready to understand their motivation in becoming RMNs, give up their need for control of their patients and cease operating mechanisms of denial, are there structures in place, at an institutional and wider level, to support them and enable truely collaborative relationships with their clients to develop?

THE POSSIBILITY OF CHANGE

Holden (1991) and Skynner (1989) have prescribed the implementation of supervisory structures offering education, insight and support within a framework of psycho-analytical thinking. Zagier Roberts recognised the importance of interventions focused in this way:

> It is therefore of the greatest importance for helping professionals to have some insight into their reasons for choosing the particular kind of work or setting in which they find themselves and awareness of their specific blind spots, their valency for certain kinds of defences and their vulnerability to particular kinds of projective identification.
>
> (1994, p.116)

Skynner (1989) suggests an actual structure which can be implemented, the result of which would be a sympathetic awareness in the professional of his deprivation and its denial, of his needs and his defences, and of his inability always to be the generous parent in relation to patients or the grateful child in relation to management. If the very real pain of this realisation can be accepted, then the professional carer will be able to experience his own need and want to satisfy it. This change will in turn evoke appropriate responses in others and the carer will be able to take the emotional food offered, integrate it and begin a maturing process whereby he will in turn also be able to give more authentically to others. 'The vicious cycle of deprivation becomes a virtuous cycle of mutual nurture' (Skynner, 1989, p.167). When working with the deprived health worker, Skynner suggested that the worker's self-esteem be carefully protected with a period of supportive teaching, highlighting skills and strengths, before any insight into dynamics can be considered. He suggested three types of groupwork, each related to a certain level of deprivation and denial. Peplau (1989) has made similar proposals, as depicted below where I have integrated her ideas into Skynner's suggested levels:

Level One

This would be for the least confident professionals, where the group leader would focus on case discussion. This would increase self-esteem as individual attention is given. It would also increase an understanding of the skills being used and needed.

The case discussion would take place within a supportive environment where blame is not apportioned for any difficulties being experienced by the nursing team, rather, an attempt to understand what has happened is encouraged.

Peplau justifies this on a very basic level by saying that as nursing actions have consequences for patients, nurses have a responsibility to study what goes on in the nurse–patient relationship. One method is via case discussion. By this study the nurse is afforded choices about interventions rather than delivering routinised responses.

Level Two

The intermediate level would again focus on case discussion, but the professional's counter-transference would be used also, *as a way of gaining more information about the case*. Here the counter-transference feelings are acknowledged and are attributed to the patient; work is then discussed from within that framework.

Level Three

This is a more sophisticated level where the group is run close to a model of therapy and would focus on the individual's motive in choosing nursing as a career. Case discussion would of course remain relevant, but it would be placed within the content of the individual's defensive system or psychopathology, where the counter-transference is attributable to the worker and his/her own needs.

Peplau (1989) describes the 'supervisory conference', where the focus is on the nurse's interactions with patients, but 'Eventually the supervisor may wish to concentrate on patterns of behaviour between the staff nurse and the supervisor' (p. 165). Issues of transference are then acknowledged. Crucially, she adds, if the nurse indicates a disturbance of relationship that goes beyond the remit of supervision, she should be referred for therapy.

The suggestion is to give staff the time and support to think, reflect and learn about themselves, where they can be given permission and encouraged to acknowledge and express their own needs and conflict within a supportive environment in order to achieve greater self-awareness.

The above might seem a hopeful prospect. However, two issues need addressing. First, how will nurses feel about acknowledging their needs openly, needs which may well be severe enough to need help from the mental health services within which they are currently working? Second, the three suggested levels of intervention are not new in nursing. Other writers, notably Dartington (1994) and Franks *et al.* (1994) all suggest that work be carried out based on an awareness and acknowledgement of psychody-namic thinking and defensive structures. Lawton (1983) agreed that the types of system suggested by Skynner can be implemented but asks the vital question 'But will they?'.

How will nurses feel about acknowledging their needs?

Perhaps a good indicator of how we accept need in the profession would be to look at the way nurses who have expressed mental health needs are treated. The answer is, with great fear and ostracism. The need to keep the evidence of mental breakdown 'in the family' is so strong that a special psychiatric unit has been created to deal with health service staff (Day, 1995), preventing patients from seeing evidence of nurses, social workers and other mental health professionals having the full extent of pro-blems that they themselves suffer. There may of course be good reasons for the unit's development. Perhaps only away from other patients can health service staff be allowed the full exhibition of their 'madness'. But it seems, nevertheless, an example of our collusion in the idealisation of ourselves, whereby our mystique and alleged mental health remain unchallenged. It seems that we have to turn our backs on the possibility of patients being able to perceive us (and by implication themselves) as whole people and possibly learning to relate to such. Even when our mental health is such that we can no longer cope without support, it seems we remain locked within our family of origin and our defensive structures, terrified of any authentic, close relationship, acknowledging mutual need. The reality is that nurses are drained, used up and discarded, perhaps so much so that the thought of taking away our defences is intolerable.

Nursing staff feel guilty about acknowledging need and fear a loss of credibility. (Carson *et al.*, 1995). Radsma (1994) concurs with this in a literature review that strongly suggests caring behaviours between nurses are lacking. There is fragmenta-tion, abuse and divisiveness amongst nurses, which she suggests is indicative of a lack of professional self-esteem. The underlying theme of this review seems to be that nurses work from a position where the idealisation of our own group has become a way of life and inevitably results in the denigration of another (e.g. patients, other nurses). This is borne out in nursing theory: 'if caring is to be sustained, those who care must be strong, courageous and capable of inner love, peace, joy – both in relation to themselves and others' (Watson, 1990, cited in Radsma, 1994, p. 448).

In circumstances where respected nursing theorists are making such statements, one begins to lose any hope at all, as the nurse is subjected to an almost painful idealisation. The myth of the strong, loving nurse compounds the myth of altruism. We are not loving and caring at all times. If we pretend to this image it is likely that we will exhaust ourselves and be left unable to carry out any caring task, even care for ourselves.

At the moment the only credible way to explore needs and defences is to become a specialist, preferably working in a unit based on psychotherapeutic principals, where of course one must have therapy to do the job. This is a professionally acceptable way of getting help. As for less 'specialised' work situations, however, Davey (1992) put the case succinctly: 'If and when emotionally damaged people need to create a life in which their own vulnerabilities are never challenged there is in many respects, no better place than working on a psychiatric ward' (p.7).

Barker (1994) publicised a movement begun in the America generating the idea of the prosumer, a link between the professional and the consumer, where people with mental health problems can develop a professional service role and professionals can acknowledge their use of mental health services. The sad rider is that such acknowledgement may be difficult in the wake of the Clothier Report, one of the recommendations of which almost lends itself to a form of witch-hunting: no one with a major personality disorder, including those who have attempted suicide, should be employed in nursing (Friend, 1994). The acknowledgement of mental illness is already a problem, as preliminary research at a London hospital demonstrates in its finding that mental health workers do not seek help early enough for mental health problems (ibid.). It seems likely that nurses will continue to find it difficult to acknowledge mental health needs.

To make matters worse, the NHS has moved from being perceived as a caring employer to something approximating the social service agency described by Lawton. It is now seen as an uncaring, brutal and at times devious employer. Obholzer (1993) views the health system as one which was at the time that Menzies-Lyth wrote, admittedly, defence-ridden, committed to maintaining a denial of the stress, anger and other feelings associated with the work it undertook. Yet it was functioning. It has, however, clearly now moved into a more sinister, paranoid, split position, resulting in a much more menacing and dysfunctional 'us and them' stand. The good and bad are split. *We*, the good workers, against *them*, the bad managers; *we*, the sane staff, against *them*, the mad patients. This is the schizoid aspect of Klein's 'paranoid–schizoid position'; the suspicion of *their* motives (management's desire to dominate; patients' desire to manipulate) and fear of what *they* are planning (attacks on us) is an example of its paranoid aspect.

Nursing takes place in a psychologically complex and often painful relationship with another person. Nurses have learnt how to prevent that hurt by seldom taking part in the relationship to any deep level and by operating the defence mechanisms described. It seems we are resistant to changing this state of affairs. Although one might presume that any nurse would welcome an interest in their individual development via clinical supervision, Castledine (1994) suggests that this is not so. Because of the increase in numbers of general managers and decrease in nurse managers, many nurses may see supervision primarily as a method of control, of spying on their work. I would concur with this suggestion, having been involved with the development of clinical supervision over several areas. Nurses either do not attend or have problems maintaining any consistency. There are, I am sure, multiple reasons for this, all valid, relating to pressure of work, shift patterns and so on, but I suspect that underlying all such reasons are psychic mechanisms of denial, splitting and paranoia described above. Not that these are exclusive to nursing. Clulow (in Obholzer and Zagier

Roberts, 1994) writes about the ambivalence expressed by probation officers towards a supervisory experience. In all such professions there is at some level no doubt an inability to take freely given emotional support and care. This is part of the cycle of deprivation already described. There are areas where clinical supervision is a way of life and where there is no question of whether nurses should attend. Usually these are small, high profile units where staff feel valued and, as Skynner suggests, where they are the least deprived because they have moved themselves into working in such an agency. These are in contrast to the 'have nots', the emotionally deprived individuals working with emotionally deprived individuals. There seems an impasse in the latter situation which it may be hard to break, even with the provision of properly trained personnel who can work with this deprivation.

Holden (1991) suggested that in these circumstances nurses should stick with their primary *practical* tasks in nursing their patients, as a way of mitigating against emotional stress. However, the primary task seems now to be the survival of the Trust (Obholzer 1993). Where does this leave the nurse and the patient? It seems even more unlikely in this climate that nurses will feel able to express real individual needs or collaborate with patients in authentic relationships, or even just practical, work-related ones. Rather, they will feel safe maintaining their self-idealisation as a professional group, resulting in a continuing need to view the patient as the only needy person.

Will adequate support frameworks be created?

It seems that an arena is needed where nurses are allowed to feel and are encouraged to talk, where self-understanding can be generated. Franks *et al.* (1994) suggest a way forward is to establish support groups for student nurses where problems can be addressed intellectually, and presumably engaged with emotionally, in the context of ongoing peer-group relationships. The expectation is that the groups would be based on psychoanalytic principles and psychoanalytic theories of nursing. The individual would be initiated into them during training and would continue with them, once having finished training. Skynner's (1989) three levels of groupwork, allied with Peplau's Supervisory Conference (1989) could be instigated.

The structure of clinical supervision is currently being investigated (UKCC, 1994) with a view to adopting a particular, suitable model. I fear that the implementation of any model may naïvely be seen as an immediate, cure-all answer to all the problems described above, whilst the underlying pathology simmers away. Perhaps this makes it all the more urgent now, while the UKCCs offer consultation, for mental health nurses to state what they want from clinical supervision and what model they want developed, remembering that one of the reasons for advocating clinical supervision is to enable us to work in a close relationship with our patients. I would argue that in these circumstances there is no model, other than the psychoanalytical, adequate to the task.

I am not advocating a totally psychoanalytical service provision, rather, that an ecletic model is adopted, where there is an understanding of unconsious processes, which in turn generates the ability to carry out sustained work with patients utilising other models of therapy. It may be necessary to move towards a more pragmatic idea of nursing, where no intervention is devalued for its simplicity or brevity, neither is any upheld as the only worthwhile therapy because it takes a long time and deals with the 'underlying cause'.

The past decades have seen an emergence of psychodynamic nursing, fuelled in part, I suspect, by individual nurses' needing to know about themselves. The intention may be good, but I have seen wards where this is implemented in such a way that the patient then gets a rather raw deal: regular formalised sessions with little contact between, and worse. This rather goes against what the users of the service have said they want, someone to listen to (not interpret) them and time out of the hospital enviroment. Such developments cannot be seen as progressive when there are practical techniques emerging for use with quite intractable problems. For example, Westacott (1995) reviews methods which may enable an individual to gain some control over auditory hallucinations, one of which is social talking. Recall that patients also rated highly going for walks in the grounds, an activity which has a reassuring normality about it. Peplau has also suggested that patients need to be encouraged to keep active and to stay in shape physically (Smoyak, 1994). There seems a comfortable fit between these activities and what Laing suggested is the ability to 'just be with someone, no matter what state they are in, without needing to act on them in some way, without attempting to change them to suit one's own book, so to speak' (Davidson, 1992, p. 203). The remaining and persistent problem is that, without an adequate support framework, a deprived individual, that is the nurse, may find it almost impossible to offer this presence.

CONCLUSION

Although Menzies-Lyth's work has been acknowledged in nursing for thirty years now, the processing of anxiety and other feelings within institutions has changed very little. Ramon (1992) suggested that feelings both of anxiety and guilt (as well, presumably, as despair, vulnerability and need) are normal reactions to an abnormal situation for a mental health professional. It would be difficult not to agree with her. For sanity's sake, our own and our patients, we need a resolution to the current situation. Understanding our situation, such as I have offered in this text, may help. It will be a beginning when you have a glimmer of understanding that you are not alone and that perhaps your feelings of inadequacy, confusion and failure represent no fault in you, but arise out of family structures and social defence systems (Aldridge, 1994). Alongside this, paradoxically, there is a need for the denial to be allowed to continue. But there should also be some gentle encouragement for insight, enough insight at least to recognise that the collaborative relationships with our patients that we are finding so hard to implement are hard for a reason: we resist them, rightly, to protect our emotional well-being.

To some, the above counsel may appear embarassingly naïve. But we can only begin to address the lack of collaboration and relationship between professional and patient with an acceptance or at the least an exploration by mental health professionals of their own psychopathology. It is crucial that this at least becomes a focus for honest discussion amongst staff members and between staff and users of services, whilst retaining the necessary imbalance mentioned by Skynner (1989). This would be helped by an understanding of the psychodynamics of the institutions within which we work and the families in which we have grown, so that blame is not attributed either to them or to us; rather, an attitude of acceptance and understanding is fostered. This may be impossible in the current climate. In which case, perhaps, there should be a return to task-centred nursing, the tasks based around what patients value. Would it be so bad to resurrect what Bradshaw (1995) terms the classic framework of nursing? This may result in nurses' doing a richer variety of things with patients, working with them. I believe that not all nurses will be distressed to relinquish their quasi-therapeutic role. Who, in any case, asked the patients if that was what they wanted? In any event, there must certainly be an acknowledgement of the emotional labour that each nurse is carrying and acceptance that they may only be able to labour in this way for a few patients at any time. Nurses, who I believe are usually caring, genuine people, and who for all the reasons stated in this chapter, are finding nursing an almost impossible task, are unlikely to acknowledge such burden and needs without genuine permission and encouragement.

How long can we continue to conceive of our needs as subsumed within the patient? It is living a lie and makes our work and our lives impossibly hard. As Peplau (1991) has argued, until we access our own needs and vulnerabilities, nursing is a facade:

> A nurse cannot pay attention to cues in the situation when her own needs are uppermost and require attention in the situation. Her observations are, unwittingly, focussed upon the way her unrecognized needs are met by a patient . . . Until the actual needs of the nurse are met or identified so that she is aware of what they are and how they function as barriers to the patient's goals, she does not have control such as is required for carrying out all of the 'shoulds' and 'musts' indicated in nursing literature.

> (quoted in Farkas-Cameron, 1995, p. 32)

REFERENCES

Aldridge, M. 1994: Unlimited liability? Emotional labour in nursing and social work. *Journal of Advanced Nursing* **20**, 722–8.

Balint, M. and **Balint, E.** 1961: *Psychotherapeutic techniques in medicine.* London: Tavistock Publications.

Barker, P. 1994: Inspired to alternatives. *Nursing Times* 3 Aug **90**(31), 59–60.

Bradshaw, A. 1995: What are nurses doing to patients? A review of theories of nursing past and present. *Journal of Clinical Nursing* **90**(45).

Carson, J., Fagin, L. and **Ritter, S.** 1995: *Stress and coping in mental health nursing.* London: Chapman and Hall.

Carson, J. and **Sharma, T.** 1994: In-patient psychiatric care – what helps? Staff and patient perspectives. *Journal of Mental Health* **3**, 99–104.

Castledine, G. 1994: What is clinical supervision? *British Journal of Nursing* (**3**)21, 1135.

Clulow, C. 1994: Balancing care and control: the supervisory relationship as a focus for promoting organisational health. In Obholzer, A. and Zagier Roberts, V. (eds) *The unconscious at work.* London: Routledge, 179–86.

Cormack, D. 1976: *Psychiatric nursing observed.* London: Royal College of Nursing.

Cuesta de la, C. 1983: The nursing process: from development to implementation. *Journal of Advanced Nursing* **8**, 365–71.

Dartington, A. 1994: Where angels fear to tread: idealism, despondency and inhibition in thought in hospital nursing. *Winnicott Studies* 7 Spring.

Davey, B. 1992: One user's view of psychiatric nursing. Unpublished paper presented at conference 'Working Together' Cambridge.

Davidson, B. 1992: What can be the relevance of the psychiatric nurse to the life of a person who is mentally ill? *Journal of Clinical Nursing* 1, 199–205.

Day, M. 1995: Health workers to be treated privately as 'Lifeline' closes. *Nursing Times* 18 Jan 91(3), 18.

Department of Health 1994: *Working in partnership: a collaborative approach.* London: HMSO.

Donati, F. 1989: A psychodynamic observer in a chronic psychiatric ward. *British Journal of Psychotherapy* 5(3), 317–329.

Farkas-Cameron, M. 1995: Clinical supervision in psychiatric nursing. *Journal of Psychosocial Nursing* 33(2), 31–7.

Franks, V., Watts, M. and **Fabricius, J.** 1994: Interpersonal learning in groups: an investigation. *Journal of Advanced Nursing* 20, 1162–9.

Friend, B. 1994: Asylum seekers. *Nursing Times* 6 April **90**(14), 18.

Haugen Bunch, E. 1985: Therapeutic communication: is it possible for psychiatric nurses to engage in this on an acute psychiatric ward? In Altschul, A. (ed.) *Psychiatric nursing.* Edinburgh: Churchill Livingstone.

Hawkins, P. and **Shohet, R.** 1989: *Supervision in the helping professions.* Milton Keynes: Open University Press.

Hinshelwood, R.D. 1994: *Clinical klein.* London, Free Association Books

Holden, R. 1991: An analysis of caring: attributions, contributions and resolutions. *Journal of Advanced Nursing* 16, 893–8.

Lawton, H. 1982: The myth of altruism: a psychohistory of public agency social work. *The Journal of Psychohistory* 9(3), Winter, 265–308.

Lawton, H. 1983: Comments on the 'myth of altruism'. *The Journal of Psychohistory,* **10**(3), Winter, 399–401.

McIntyre, K., Farrell, M. and **David, A.** 1989: What do psychiatric in-patients really want? *British Medical Journal* **298**, 159–60.

McIver, S. 1991: *Obtaining the views of users of mental health services.* London: Kings Fund Centre.

Menzies-Lyth, I. 1959: The functioning of social systems as a defence against anxiety. In *Containing anxiety in institutions.* London: Free Association Books.

Obholzer, A. 1993: Institutional forces. *Therapetic Communities* 14(4), 275–83.

Obholzer, A. and **Zagier Roberts, V.** (eds) 1994: *The unconscious at work.* London: Routledge.

Pearson, A. (ed.) 1988: *Primary nursing.* London: Croom Helm.

Peplau, H.E. 1988: *Interpersonal relations in nursing.* Basingstoke: Macmillan.

Peplau, H.E. 1989: *Hildegard E Peplau: selected works.* (eds) Werner O'Toole, A. and Rouslin Welt S., New York: Springer.

Peplau, H.E. 1991: *Interpersonal relations in nursing: a conceptual frame of reference for psychodynamic nursing.* New York: Springer.

Peplau, H.E. 1994: Psychiatric mental health nursing: challenge and change. *Journal of Psychiatric and Mental Health Nursing,* **1**(1), 3–7.

Pollock, L. 1989: *Community psychiatric nursing: myth and reality.* Harrow: Scutari Press.

Radsma, J. 1994: Caring and nursing: a dilemma. *Journal of Advanced Nursing* 20, 444–9.

Ramon, S. (ed.) 1992: *Psychiatric hospital closure.* London: Chapman and Hall.

Sinanoglou, I. 1987: Basic anxieties affecting psychiatric staff and their attitudes to psychotic patients. *Psychoanalytic Psychotherapy* 3(1), 27–37.

Skynner, R. 1989: *Institutes and how to survive them.* London: Routledge.

Smoyak, H.S. 1994: Hildegard E. Peplau awarded honrary doctorate. *Journal of Psychosocial Nursing* 32(11).

Towell, D. 1975: *Understanding psychiatric nursing*. London: Royal College of Nursing.

UKCC Register 1994: *Clinical supervision for nursing and health visiting practice*. No. 15 Autumn, London: UKCC.

Westacott, M. 1995: Strategies for managing auditory hallucinations. *Nursing Times* 18 Jan, **91**(3), 35–7.

Zagier Roberts, V. 1994: The self-assigned impossible task. In Obholzer, A. and Zagier Roberts, V. (eds) *The unconscious at work*. London: Routledge.

9

DISSENT

Ben Davidson

For any practitioner subscribing to the views endorsed so far, the journey is likely to be a solitary and difficult one (unless, that is, they are fortunate enough to land up in a working environment similarly endorsing these views – but as already emphasised, environments like this are rare). Such a practitioner will encounter many incidents of practice which is at best irrelevant for the person supposed to be being healed, at worst downright damaging. What are the options open to someone in this position? Ben Davidson argues that there may come a point for any of us when we are compelled on moral grounds to break the terms of our contract with an employer and blow the whistle. The experience of speaking up for patients when it involves going into conflict with one's managers or colleagues is inevitably painful. Ben attempts to convey a true picture of the personal cost of whistle blowing. He also discusses whether it is truly possible to act as patient advocate when our interests (e.g. having a stress-free life, even keeping our job) are at stake. He delineates at both a societal and a personal level the place of dissent. Ben sketches, finally, a recent history of public servants' attempts to effect change by going public when their conscience dictated there was no other way forward, and looks ahead to part 2 where clinicians offer their accounts of work they have undertaken which may well have brought them into conflict with the establishment.

Sandra

Well, I was a student nurse when this happened. Apart from one nursing assistant on the ward and me, all the rest of the staff were men and it was just an incredibly macho atmosphere. I think I did try to pick them up on things a couple of times, like the way they'd tell patients to fuck off if they interrupted a conversation in the staff room. They just laughed at me. I ended up not bothering to say anything, just sort of sitting back and letting them get on with it and thinking I've only got a few more months here. I was very powerless.

There were four other staff, all men. A young black patient had been incontinent of urine. His trousers were absolutely saturated. He was refusing to get changed. The staff had tried to drag him to the bedroom. He was fighting. The qualified nurse said, 'I know what will do it'. He disappeared off to the clinic room and came back, I think it was with a 50ml syringe, it was certainly a large syringe, filled with water. And proceeded to threaten the patient with the syringe . . . pretending it was medication.

I didn't *want* to blow the whistle. I'd hoped for local action to be taken. Then somehow things were taken out of my hands. The loneliness of that position is the worst thing.

It must be said, in contrast to the spirit of Joseph Berke's writing in Chapter 6, that going into conflict with the group, whether the group is a powerful political force or a small number of colleagues or friends, is not always experienced as a spirited, right-eous crusade. It can also be a grim, traumatic struggle. Throughout this chapter I shall be referring to my own and others' experience to explore some of the different dimensions of dissent as they affect mental health workers. In the first part, I shall discuss themes related to dissent as a social phenomenon, both in abstract terms and also using case material. In the second part, I explore the implications of this discus-sion for our supposed role as patient advocate, drawing on personal experience and suggesting aspects of our situation that might get in the way of genuine advocacy. And finally, in conclusion, I shall discuss some means of dissent and sketch a recent history of whistleblowing in the public services in Britain as particular cases in point. The main purpose here is to explore the experience of being in that grey area between two moral imperatives: loyalty to the group and the duty to follow the call of one's conscience.

GOING AGAINST THE GRAIN

In this chapter I shall refer to interviews with the student nurse quoted above, I shall call her Sandra. Sandra and I were both members of a set of ten students. We were one of the last sets to undergo a 2½ year modular RMN certificate course at the school of nursing in a London psychiatric hospital before the introduction of the more academic Project 2000 diploma training there in 1992. Our school was one of the last in Britain to hold out for the old system of nurse training. Its courses all emphasised experiential learning via groupwork. Didactic teaching and academic development for its own sake were not highly prioritised. The school held out for this form of learning until its existence was in jeopardy.

I have put Sandra into some context. I want to ground the experience she shares in a specific place and time. This, together with my using her story at all, is to bring alive some of the abstract and universal themes I shall be discussing related to dissent. More, however, I want to make the most important point about dissent first. Sandra was encouraged in dissenting by the ethos and the structure of the course at her school of nursing, and by the character and value-set of her peer-group and tutors.

Support from Sandra's group

Sandra was not the only dissenter in her group. Among its other members were two black women not prepared to let the racial discrimination ingrained in the hospital's systems and procedures pass unobserved. There was a recently bankrupt estate agent, newly separated from his wife and child yet powerfully optimistic about his ability to change the course of psychiatric nursing. There was a homeless parent living with partner and child in a squat, shortly to be evicted, holding out for their right to an alternative lifestyle. There were four Scots with a fierce sense of cultural identity. Although there were several who were unready to give themselves fully to the experience of who they were and their madness, amongst the mental health disorders of those more comfortable with their experience, mutually and proudly disclosed as early as the third week of the course, were bulimia, personality disorder, two drug-induced psychoses, anxiety disorders and chronic shyness. There was a lot of honesty. There were also a lot of fights, about many things. There were three psychology graduates, two philosophers, a would-be doctor dropped out from medical school training, a trainee psychotherapist and a number of avowed behaviourists. There were several people experimenting with their sexuality, those willing to scrutinise the flaws in their relationships, those not prepared to even look at theirs (at the start, anyway). And there were those hoping, unrealistically, to have a quiet life. A ship of fools? A hothouse for ferment and growth? There was a lot of trust.

Sandra

You all had so much to say. At first I was intimidated. Then I realised a lot of it was bullshit, I had to learn to speak out and point that out to you, just to keep my sanity. Being in a situation where I trusted people to be able to say things has helped me realise its actually OK to speak my own mind. Its given me confidence in speaking out.

The weekly experiential closed group we attended as part of our training changed its character as time passed. Many times it served as a forum in which our relationships could be explored. Occasionally material from outside was introduced, such as when some members of the group attempted to live communally together with explosive results that spilled back into the group. Other times the weekly group served as a focus for us to develop an identity and fight the school on matters that affected our training. We took the fact that space was given in which all this could be done as encouragement to find a voice for our experience and make our voices heard. The school's validation of our identity in this way and its emphasis on self-teaching and experiential learning coalesced with the individual characters and interpersonal dynamics of the ten of us to create a powerful group. We all ended making a noise one way or another.

Sandra

I say offensive things, but I appreciate the group; I couldn't have done it, or at least got through the shit I'm talking about now, without you, particularly Julia; and I wouldn't be who I am now without that experience. It helped me grow up.

Moral fibre?

There are various qualities manifest in someone's standing alone for what they believe is right and risking being an outcast in the face of a hostile group. Courage, confidence, self-esteem, compassion too, are all examples. Yet these are not aspects of someone's character so much as qualities of their conduct, and their conduct can be seen to arise out of certain conditions, including both their current circumstances and their past experience.

People can develop a skill in acting confidently, or acquire over time the habit of conducting themselves courageously if circumstances work in their favour, in which case their skill or habit may come to be seen as if it were a personal quality, an aspect of their character. Perhaps we collude with the trick language plays on us here in denoting with words such as 'courage' or 'confidence' some sort of emotional particle that one stores, or a mental object of some kind, in one's psyche. It suits our predilection for fixing things as if they were permanent, unchanging entities, even when they are dynamic and evolving forms of life. Nevertheless, although a person's behaviour or their conduct can be described as courageous (*she stood alone courageously*), the person cannot be described this. 'Courage' and 'confidence' are abstractions, mere linguistic conventions to convey something a lot more complex. Which is not to say that courage and confidence do not exist. 'Our experiences like [feeling courageous, confident] etc. are . . . properly expressed in language as normally used [e.g. '*I felt a lot of confidence*'], as long as we do not . . . imagine that the word[s used] must refer to *some thing* (Wittgenstein, 1958, p. 56, emphasis mine).

Skills in particular (e.g. courageous) forms of conduct, habits, of acting certain ways patterns of emotional response can better be seen as resources that one has acquired and can draw on. Such skilled or habitual activity inevitably results from the situations a person has been in and their experiences. Self-esteem, a habitually good estimation of self, may come into being out of a consistent feeling of being (or having been) esteemed; the habit of acting confidently, trusting in oneself, may come about through the consistent sense of being (or having been) trusted. I may have had these experiences (of encouragement, trust etc.) from significant others such as parents or siblings and have internalised them so they are always with me. Or I may have a very current sense of others' standing by me, from colleagues or friends as it seems Sandra felt. But either way, this sense of support that gives one the necessary resources to draw on is crucial to an individual's dissenting.

Dissent occurs then on the basis of certain conditions, including the dissenting individual's sense of support and affirmation from the internal and external worlds they inhabit. The image of someone important standing with one can sustain an individual's acting alone in the face of hostility for what they believe is right. I maintain that it is this sense of having someone standing beside one, a sense of solidarity, that sustains one in successfully facing adversity. It is not a question of moral fibre. Dissent 'does not originate within some kind of moral space located inside . . . which [one] can choose to activate or suppress; [behaviour, moral or immoral,] has to be accounted for by the influences which operate on [one]' (Smail, 1993, p.38). Although this is not to say that solidarity and support are always sufficient conditions for dissent to arise. Other societal and cultural influences are also at work.

The scariness of conflict with power

Sandra
I really didn't want to tell tales, though; I got my tutor to promise confidentiality before I told him.

To some people dissent has a negative connotation. As Longman's dictionary defines it, to dissent is to 'refuse to conform to . . . orthodoxy', 'to hold a declared contrary position'. Dissent seems as if it could be related in this context to being contrary. It sounds like it could be about setting oneself apart, stubbornness, contrariness. It also seems from these definitions that dissent is more a conscious than an unconscious activity. It relates to 'positive opposition', a 'declared contrary opinion'. Putting these elements together it sounds as if dissent could almost relate to a sanctimonious attitude, perhaps like when someone takes the moral high ground.

Sometimes the negative valuation of dissent escalates to dangerous extremes. Where dissent is really looked down upon there may exist a culture of conformity and obedience such that anything may be accepted if it is sanctioned by the majority or the powerful. Disagreement with, or dissent from, the 'orthodoxy of the established church' is not undertaken lightly, or at all, in many fascist cultures[1]. During this century there have been many clear and extreme examples of this social phenomenon. For example, the Nationalist Socialist creed in the culture of Nazi Germany, Stalinist Communism in the former Soviet Union, and the many right-wing regimes in South America, to name just a few. Political dissent in cultures such as these is actually seen as bad and can be punishable by death. In such a culture people know to keep their heads down.

Indeed, in Nazi Germany, *non*-dissent and conformity were *positively* valued to such an extent that in the war-crime trials at Nuremberg in 1946, one Nazi after another used the defence for their actions that they had been ordered to carry them out by their superiors. It was as if obedience and unquestioning conformity with the group were seen as superior moral qualities in themselves, and quite sufficient to justify any actions taken in their service. Even Adolf Eichmann used this defence:

the architect of Auschwitz, the introducer of conveyor belts into crematoria, the greatest customer in the world for the gas called Cyklon-B . . . simply a soldier, . . . taking orders from higher-ups, like soldiers around the world [as if] . . . he had invented his own trite defence, though a whole nation of ninety some-odd million had made the same defence before him.

(Vonnegut, 1968, p. 106)

There is a substantial body of psychology literature and experimental research on individual behaviour in relation to social influence and group norms. One particular experiment worthy of note is by Stanley Milgram (1974). Following the Second World War and questions about responsibility for the atrocities that took place during the Holocaust, Milgram constructed experiments to investigate the extent to which individual autonomy in making moral judgements may be compromised by obedience to authority. This was controversial as essentially it was addressing the moral question how much could the 90 million citizens of Germany, or at least those who knew genocide was being committed on the Jews but did nothing, be forgiven for allowing and apparently being complicit in the Holocaust? These would have included not only politicians and the military, of course, but also the townsfolk around the death-camps and the employees of the railway and other companies who manufactured and delivered the equipment used there, as well as their relatives.

Milgram's experiment tested unknowing subjects' willingness to administer painful and dangerous electric shocks to people, on the pretext that they were involved in a legitimate, socially sanctioned group activity, an experiment being carried out under the highly respected auspices of a Yale University science department. The subjects

---

[1] *The 'church'* in Longman's definition, against whose doctrines one may fear to disagree, may be seen in the wider sense, that is as a church of creed, a church of opinions including political views.

had answered newspaper advertisements recruiting paid participants in a 'study of memory'. The subjects believed the experiment was to see if the administration of electric shocks would somehow be correctional, improving recall (of pairs of words) in the person being given the shocks.

The electric shocks to be administered were graded from 15 to 450 volts and the different levers on a panel of the machine supposedly generating them were labelled variously from 'Slight Shock' up to 'Danger: Severe Shock'. The man being given the shocks (an actor referred to by Milgram as the 'victim') was behind a partiton wall so that the real subjects of the experiment could not see him. Needless to say, the apparatus, the personnel and the laboratory were designed to appear very realistic. Indeed, the subjects themselves were given a 45-volt shock from the machine before the supposed memory testing began, to show it was for real.

The actor playing the part of the scientist in charge (the experimenter) instructed subjects to increase the strength of shocks administered as the 'victim' made each error in recall. Although no shocks were actually administered, the 'victim' began to protest loudly as the shock level was increased. He shouted and cursed as they increased further. When the subjects applied what they believed was a 300-volt shock, they heard the 'victim' begin to kick the wall. At a subsequent increase in strength of the electric shock, and thereafter, the 'victim' stopped making any noise at all. The 'experimenter', in the same room as the subject, told the subject to obey his instructions and continue administering shocks, using one of a number of standardised verbal injunctions and commands.

The staggering result was that every one of the subjects continued to follow the instructions to apply electric shocks beyond the point where the 'victim' was kicking the wall and shouting in protest. Two-thirds of the subjects continued to obey the commands to apply electric shocks right to the end of the scale – past the point where the person behind the wall had fallen silent. A remark attributed to Edmund Burke is significant in this respect: 'For the triumph of evil it is necessary only that good men do nothing.' The conclusion drawn was that Nazis and other German civilians were not evil in some sense of being wholly callous, murderous monsters. The very notion of evil is more subtle than that. Milgram's findings concurred with Hannah Arendt's (1963) study of Eichmann in which she emphasised the *banality* of the part Eichmann and others like him played, seeing themselves as small and relatively powerless cogs in a big machine and divorcing themselves from the real nature and effect of their individual actions. 'This is not an easy conclusion to accept because it suggests that each of us might be capable of such evil and that [the Holocaust] was an event less wildly alien from the normal human condition than we might like to think.' (Atkinson, Atkinson and Hilgard, 1981, p. 573).

Sandra

At that stage I wasn't the sort of person that would have made a fuss. It was only the first year of our training, I really wasn't very sure of myself, still felt a bit, very new to nursing. . . . And to be honest I didn't intend to make a fuss about that one incident. But I went into supervision and was telling my tutor I was having quite a lot of difficulty coping there and he started pressurising me to find out what was going on. I told him about this one incident and he just changed. It didn't feel any more like he was supporting me. He was going against my wishes. It was like he was suddenly on some sort of crusade to right all the wrongs on the ward. In the group I felt quite proud to be a part of that reputation, making a noise, being outspoken; but on my own it wasn't me.

The romance of heroism

The *Concise Oxford Dictionary* definition says that dissent is simply to 'think differently' or 'express disagreement'. This sounds more neutral than the definition quoted earlier, perhaps with even a slight romantic tinge. Speaking out against the establishment has a quite positive valuation in our culture. Perhaps the reader finds the tutor wanting to right all the wrongs on the ward mentioned by Sandra above an attractive image, particularly after the foregoing account of Milgram's experimental results and the bleak picture they paint of human nature. The hero, the cultural vandal, the outlaw, are often positive icons. A whole genre of films over several decades reflects this, *Rebel Without a Cause, One Flew Over the Cuckoo's Nest, Cool Hand Luke,* for example, all of which reinforce a positive image of the lone hero taking on some impossibly powerful orthodoxy or institution or status quo. In nearly all his movies, both the early 'spaghetti Westerns' and also the later cop movies, Clint Eastwood plays anti-heroes of this sort. A particularly clear example is in *The Outlaw Josie Wales* where he plays the lead role as an uniquely authentic character, alone, suffering the painful memory of his children and wife's murder by Government (Yankee) troops and vigilantes, unprepared to compromise or surrender, uncompromisingly honest about his experience and thus somehow a warrior, truly courageous and insightful, having to live because of this the life of an exile along with an ever-increasing band of other social outcasts, with whom he finally sets up a community. *One Flew Over the Cuckoo's Nest* (Kesey, 1973) is another example, where Jack Nicholson as R.P. MacMurphy takes on Nurse Ratched and the controlling institution she symbolises in a battle to restore sanity and life to an asylum and its inmates, only to succumb finally to the institution's control in the form of a lobotomy. But not before he has managed to reawaken primitive forces of creativity and life, represented in the newly healed person of the American Indian Chief Bromden.

In the West, dissent by Russian dissidents in the latter decades of the Cold War was popularly seen in a similarly positive light. Indeed, in some quarters, it was seen from an even more romantic perspective, perhaps as some sort of crusade against evil, *the evil empire* as President Reagan called the USSR.

Pursuing again the idea of dissent as an attractive and positively valued activity, Henry David Thoreau wrote a political essay in the late nineteenth century entitled 'On the duty of civil disobedience'. A well-respected essayist and novelist, Thoreau has been seen by some as a kind of prototype beatnik/hippy/traveller, born 100 years too early. At one stage he built his own retreat hut in the middle of some woods and lived in it for a year, meditating, writing and cooking food he caught in the woods. 'On the duty of civil disobedience' argues that society and its values are morally flawed, and when coming up against these flaws one should use *any means necessary* to put things right. This may mean going against not only social custom and taboo, but also the law (see also the writings of Malcolm X). In some circumstances 'civil disobedience' is thus not only a right but a duty. From this more reasoned perspective, too, dissent is to be viewed in a very positive light.

Sandra was no crusader and held with none of these sort of views.

I was afraid of the staff on the ward, I didn't want to get anyone in trouble and in the end the whistle was blown despite me, not because of me.

A resolution

But can things be quite so clear-cut? From the above it sounds as if one decides to be either for or against, and that is the end of the matter: one either hides one's head in the sand or takes on the world. When it came to the dilemma between loyalty to the group or blowing the whistle Sandra was inclined to hide her head in the sand but someone else forced her into taking on the world!

However things may at first glance seem, I maintain it is not as simple as this. Not even in Clint Eastwood movies. A gut feeling of uneasiness with something going on may change at a certain point for some into the conscious knowledge that one is going to have to put oneself out on a limb, to make a stand against it. But maybe for others who do it, dissenting is not a conscious process or a type of decision-making on the basis of moral principles at all. It stays, perhaps, on the level of a gut feeling of uneasiness and is more an activity than a conscious taking of stands. In terms of Sandra's thinking and the stand she took, she would much have preferred to have what was happening dealt with 'at a local level' without recourse to disciplinary procedures and the possibility of someone losing their job, certainly without her having to put her head above the parapet. Indeed, if she made a decision at all, the decision she took was *not* to blow the whistle or 'dissent'. She is quite clear on this.

And yet in another way, in terms of activity, also quite clearly, she did dissent. She felt something was wrong and spoke out about it, even if only to her tutor. Although it is clear she intended not to blow the whistle formally, there *was* intentionality, Sandra intended at some level to dissent from what was going on. In these circumstances perhaps dissent could be said to come to the individual as a sort of instinctual response, as when Sandra told her tutor what had happened all the time at some level knowing that he may well not be able to keep confidentiality. Thus, at the same time as being a declared, positive opposition to something, perhaps dissent can also take a more subversive form, remaining relatively quiet, remaining perhaps even an *unconscious* process in response to facing a duty to perform tasks that one feels in one's guts to be wrong.

Sandra
I hated having to make that formal statement and attending the disciplinary hearings as a witness. But something must have been ready to give. It only took so much prompting from [my supervisor] back at the school of nursing. At some level I guess I must have known he couldn't guarantee it, confidentiality, he couldn't have just colluded with *anything* I said and ignored it, just because I didn't want to get someone in trouble.

An interesting illustration of this is from the 1950s when American soldiers in their bunkers in the Arizona desert, in charge of controls that would fire nuclear missiles at the USSR, were called upon, during a simulated exercise, to press the launch button. They did not know it was a simulation though and 40 per cent of them are said to have refused to obey the orders. They subsequently regretted their mutinous conduct; they had no record of conscientious objection – they were at a level of seniority where they could be entrusted with this task. They were nevertheless unable to bring themselves to carry it out.

ADVOCACY COMPROMISED

The foregoing discussion raises a number of interesting questions in relation to psychiatric nurses' self-styled role as patient advocate. Namely, when our peace of mind is at stake, when our popularity and acceptance within a group of colleagues, when even our position within an organisation, i.e. our job and financial security, when all these are at stake, and given the pressures we all experience in any circumstances to conform, is there not too great a conflict of interests for us to be an advocate for our patients? Surely there are so many situations where our patients' interests and our own diverge that we cannot, even in principle, be advocates?

Nolan (1993) characterises a view of nursing taken by some RMNs that 'It is nurses who are the patients' advocates and the . . . service they provide differentiates them from all other health care workers' (p.8). One may place this change in nurses' self-image in the context of several decades of change in society's view and treatment of mental illness. It may well be that in comparison solely with psychiatrists (and as often as not in opposition to them), nurses much more frequently take a position of speaking up on behalf of their patients and appear much better advocates. But at the same time, mental nursing is much more closely allied to psychiatry than other disciplines, and has less power to affect the course of treatment than many of them, *especially* psychiatry. As Nolan describes, psychiatry and psychiatric nursing have grown alongside each other and have a historical tie stretching back over more than a century. Although nurses' position as '24-hour-a-day' carers (Nolan, op. cit.; Strang, 1982) certainly gives them a potentially more intimate and therapeutic role, it does not mean they are divorced from the views and powerful influence of psychiatrists. Social workers, occupational therapists, psychologists and others may be in much more independent roles in this respect, and often much better able to identify and speak out about occasions where patients' rights and preferences are being over-ridden.

However, there may be a much greater obstacle in the way of practitioners from any of these disciplines being able genuinely to take the role of patient advocate. That obstacle relates to the political implications and ethics of working in the field of proffesionalised care itself. Bringing such ideas to a personal context, Sandra recalls:

> At first I wanted to go back to the ward . . . I'd have probably tried to lay the blame on [the tutor's] shoulders. But I was taken off the ward straight away. [My boyfriend] was friends with [people on] the ward. It was really difficult, him relaying messages between me and the ward manager. I was just so afraid of what might happen. I felt very intimidated by [the staff I'd been working with], that they might try and hurt me in some way.

In interview Sandra was explicit in describing her intuitive sense at the time of the incident in question that it would be this way if she complained formally, and her subsequent reluctance in blowing the whistle. She went on to identify a number of ways in which she had failed to advocate effectively on the patient's behalf as a result:

If I'd been acting as patient advocate I'd have made sure that man got disciplined. I would have written a more accurate statement. I wouldn't have been so afraid of what I was doing. As it was I just wrote the woolliest statement I could so that this man got off, because I was so afraid of him losing his job. In the disciplinary the statement was so woolly that they threw it out, not enough evidence. He stayed on in the job because I didn't want him going on the dole queue.

In addition, we may recall from Sandra's earlier comments that she wanted to belong to the group and didn't speak out in relation to various other incidents, or if she did, other staff members' ridiculing her soon stopped her doing so. Also, she avoided noticing other situations for a while afterwards as she had 'enough on [her] plate'.

I spent a couple of months in absolute fear. I felt abused. I can remember a couple of times being asked if I was depressed, people advising me that I should go and see my doctor, they thought I was depressed. It was incredibly lonely. I was just so afraid of what might happen. On the next ward where I worked only very few staff knew what had happened and only after I'd been there a while. I thought if they knew they'd be suspicious of me.

It is not by any means surprising that Sandra's ability to act as advocate was compromised in this way. As Sandra was only too aware, conflict of the sort she eventually found herself engaged in leads to stress and depression. With the best will in the world, knowing what the results of such conflict with the group will be like, it is difficult to act in a way one may know to be right.

It is clear that in any particular battle we enter into with colleagues or institutions on behalf of patients, it is likely to be painful to go out on a limb and there are powerful social and intrapsychic forces at work which keep us in line, no matter how dedicated we are to being advocates or to the cause at hand. With this in mind one wonders why anyone would want to put themselves through such trauma at all. What sort of impetus and strength of feeling is involved here?

A personal agenda

peering out . . . at a world of my own invention, I mouthed this word: schizo-phrenia. . . . I did not and do not know for certain that I have that disease. This much I knew and know: I was making myself hideously uncomfortable by not narrowing my attention to details of life which were immediately important, and by refusing to believe what my neighbours believed.

(Vonnegut, 1975, p. 180)

My own inclination has always been to see dissent as a spirited, righteous crusade, particularly in relation to psychiatry. I have always found appealing the sort of stance epitomised by Joseph Berke, for example, in Chapter 6, clearly able to have fun in circumstances that anyone would find challenging and stretching, but also taking away from the power of the establishment through his activity. For me, making someone else's experience that dissent is not a spirited, righteous crusade, the centre of a piece of writing, is curious and novel. Indeed, making myself explore the fact that sometimes and from certain perspectives conflict with the group is not a positive experience at all, but a trauma, has been quite a shocking experience. Not that it is new. A theme in *One Flew Over the Cuckoo's Nest* that strikes me afresh however many times I read the book is MacMurphy's growing sense of despair as he realises the immensity of the task he has taken on in fighting the system. But I am temperamentally much more inclined to denigrate any experience of difficulty in this area and act like the heroic role is the only option. So why have I courted the opposite experience here?

Perhaps my own experience of psychiatric nurse training has led me to this gestalt of perspective. I came into psychiatric nursing from a range of different pursuits and life experiences, in particular hot on the heels of a separation from my partner and child and a business failure. I decided to come back to some unfinished business.

On and off for some months at age 16, I had been psychotic. Sometimes during this period I would experience beatitude and love to a transporting degree, and felt in contact with God. Other times it seemed I was overwhelmed with the negative experience of threat from others who meant me harm. This ranged from a physical sensation of pain, resulting, as I experienced it, from voodoo practitioners trying to induce a heart attack, to an ongoing and terrifying experience that aliens in a space-ship were trying to track my thoughts and would be able to take over my mind if I did not manage to stop thinking about them. On my sixteenth birthday I awoke to the experience of walls and ceilings bowing and music from the radio visibly bouncing around the room. I have still not checked my suspicions out with my father, but I became convinced at the time that he had spiked the tea he had woken me up with with LSD as a birthday trick. Unlikely. Shortly after claiming I had to return to bed as I felt like I had the flu I ran out of the house, much to the puzzlement of my parents. I felt terrified and tempted to jump under a lorry.

My sister, 15 years older than me, babysat me while I was disturbed. She told me it was natural to be experiencing what I experienced, to see it if I could as a mystical state. Perhaps the odd things happening were paranormal phenomena where I was very sensitive to interpersonal vibes, sensitive maybe even to the extent of having experiences as described. And after all, there *is* always love around and there *is* always fear and threat around. Metaphorically my experience could be made to make sense.

Even though my sister had herself experienced emotional crisis at the age of 18 in a form that caused her to be sectioned for a while and force-medicated, she had managed to keep hold of her experience and maintain her own understanding of what was happening to her. Thus, thirteen years on she maintained the same fierce faith for me, that my experiences were real and intelligible, and she helped me through my psychosis unaided by medical intervention.

Around this time the seeds of my current project were planted, to take on psychiatry and show how its tendency to pathologise what might otherwise be constructed as meaningful experience is misguided and wrong.

A personal experience

The waitress brought me another drink. 'Can you see anything in the dark, with those sunglasses on?' she asked me.
'The big show is inside my head,' I said.

(Vonnegut, 1975, p. 187)

With this background and attitude, my training was, predictably, a struggle. Or rather it was a spirited crusade. I took patients' sides, believed what they said was valid and formed what seemed to me to be therapeutic relationships with even the most resistant and withdrawn. Wherever I went I argued for their right to have their experience taken seriously. On most of the placements out of the ten I did during my two and a half years training I made some innovative change and impressed, sometimes annoyed others with my dedication and work.

The story I tell myself now is how because of this I was a thorn in the flesh of the hospital, how I made too much noise, appeared 'agressively anti-authority' (Berke, 1994, personal communication). On reflection, the noise I made was rarely critical, it was mostly encouraging and energetic. But I had a lot to say. Sandra made much of my tendency to be long-winded in the group. Others probably found me similarly overgenerous with my opinions on my placements. People had a job to get on with, not endless time to listen to the pronouncements of a student. I can much more easily empathise with them now and see what I was probably like, from my current perspective of *ennui* with conflict. It seems though, associated with the role I took then, conflict was somehow often around. (I just opted not to see it that way at the time. It felt exciting.)

At the end of my training I was twice told that I would not qualify as a nurse until I had rewritten and represented my final dissertation. The others in the group read my dissertation and could not believe it had failed. The marking criteria we had been given was flagrantly disregarded by the hospital manager who marked my piece and subsequently refused to meet with me to discuss it. By way of explanation by her assistant marker, a junior tutor in the school of nursing, I was simply told, sorry, but we have added another marking criteria which supersedes all the rest, and that is 'professionalism'. I had fallen foul of this criteria particularly by attempting to convey a sense of the atmosphere of demoralisation at the day hospital where I was placed when I set up and ran the reminiscence therapy group that was the subject of the dissertation. To have passed comments of this kind apparently went against *professionalism*. The organisation's response was to withhold my qualification as a nurse.

In the end, after having to extend my period of training by three months to give me enough time to rewrite the dissertation, after having it turned down again, and then after writing another different dissertation, I qualified. I complained about the way I had been treated to the ENB who wrote and told me it was 'an internal matter between you and the school of nursing' (personal correspondence from ENB officer, 1993). It transpired that the dissertation was not a formal requirement for my being a nurse. I had already qualified as a nurse so far as the ENB were concerned, the moment I had worked the required number of clinical days, about three months earlier. The ENB did not appear to be worried that my school of nursing had misrepresented the facts to me, prejudicing my chances of employment.

The personal toll of this experience was greater than I realised at the time. Three years on, certainly I am still writing about psychiatry, but, then again, the conflict in which I am engaging with psychiatry in so doing is from a distance. I am not, at the time of writing, working *in* psychiatry. (I am in retrospect quite happy to have been turned down for six jobs at my training hospital and now to be employed by a Social Services department.) Writing something that goes against the grain of conventional belief is the sort of conflict where I can use my strength in thinking through things innovatively, creative reframing. I am not actually in personal conflict with my colleagues or employers, for example, in doing this. If anything, the opposite. Just as well; I am weary of personal conflict and feel like I would maybe now tend to avoid the stress of such a situation again, as Sandra has described.

In these circumstances it would be trite to prescribe that mental health workers should stand up for what is right, advocate and dissent, and it would be unrealistic to make such activity sound romantic and heroic without emphasising any of the problems involved. I did originally intend to construct this chapter around a single notion of heroism. In fact I was surprised when interviewing Sandra as I had remembered the incident she has described here in much more heroic terms, as though she had decided what was happening on the ward was wrong and straight away stood up against it, initiating the complaint and disciplinary procedure herself. Such a tale would have been much more in keeping with my initial plan for this chapter. But the above gestalt described in my own outlook and experience is why finally I have ended up with a much more cautious emphasis.

When I advocated furiously on behalf of patients during my training it was as a result of my own agenda. I was still acting out my desire to take on psychiatry, tell them they're wrong as a result of my sister's and my experience. Now that I feel a good part of that battle is over for me, I am less inclined to play that part. At the time, the quite large personal agenda that I was playing out appears generally to have been in harmony with the interests of the patients I was working with. I maintain though, that our interests are often not complementary, or even sympathetic, to our patients' interests, as exemplified by Sandra's story. In these circumstances any self-styling as patient advocate is far from honest.

Beyond advocacy

Whether self-importantly calling ourselves advocates or not, and whether or not we are compelled by our own agendas to act, if we are aware of professional malpractice or some other abuse or matter that we feel we should speak out on, even if we just feel that people's experience is not being taken seriously by other professionals we work with, then what, as psychiatric nurses or as mental health workers in other disciplines, can we do about it?

In their own small ways, all of the writers offering the case studies and experiences detailed in Part 2 will be giving responses to this question. Not, and I wish to emphasise this, that their stories represent pure advocacy or altruism. No doubt many have had their own agendas (see also Chapter 8) as I did in taking the stands and effecting the changes described. Many of our authors make this quite explicit. None the less, in many of the following chapters a clear account of the improvement of patient care comes through. All of the experiences and activities described probably speak both of altruism and personal gain, and there is no blame attached to that, so long as it is acknowledged.

I maintain then, that pure advocacy work is not possible working as an RMN. Nevertheless, it is possible to end on a positive note, because after all, Sandra in the above case study did blow the whistle; I have channelled my energies into putting together this text; and all of the other, ordinary practitioners contributing to Part 2 of the book have made a difference to their environment and their clients, as will be apparent. It is important not to underestimate the personal toll though. Joseph Berke has spoken publicly about suffering through a depression that lasted a number of years in the context of the battles he has had to fight, both within himself and in the outside world, while he worked to establish the Arbours. Sandra, myself and doubt-less many of the other writers collaborating in this text have experienced a personal drain and insecurity from the activities described, due to a great extent from our leaving

> the established culture of psychiatric nursing . . . [which] confers on [nurses] the security they need to work with the very sick . . . Theorists have failed to recognise how deeply embedded this tradition is and how valued by psychiatric nurses [who] gain their security from the *status quo* no matter how unsatisfactory.
>
> (Nolan, 1993 p. 159)

Nevertheless, while part of the culture of psychiatric nursing may be to gain security from the *status quo* in order to cope with the massive anxiety involved in working with people's turmoil and distress, another force at work is a more creative one, allowing, for example, a book such as this to be produced and the work described in it to take place.

> One . . . observe[s] the hair-trigger nervousness and violence with which people and societies react to threat, and the quite appalling terror and oppression which they will resort to in establishing and protecting their interests. But . . . the kinds of threat to which we respond so violently and brutally are built into our society more than into our selves . . . Given a safe enough environment . . . where [anxiety and] threat [from external sources] is absent or minimized (there can be very few of these – the nearest I can think of are some of the artificially constructed 'therapeutic communities' which were created in the sixties for the treatment of 'mental illness') or where people are united in opposition to a *common* threat (as in war) . . . most people are glad of an opportunity to love their fellows . . . . Though it is not a fashionable view, . . . I do have a sneaking feeling that, given half a chance, most people would . . . conduct themselves towards each other with concern, interest and affection.
>
> (Smail, 1987, pp. 100–2)

CONCLUSION

I suspect, like Smail, that people will always find it preferable to do something altruistic if a safe opportunity is there. What we can do will depend on three things: First, as stated above, on the strength and relevance of our own agenda; second, on the more 'personal' resources at our disposal as a result of our past and present experience of support and solidarity; and third, on the leverage we can exert in power hierarchies, e.g., through access to structures such as the media.

However, the opportunities afforded within hierarchies of power to speak out against prevailing ideology seem to have been reduced in recent years, as a result of developments in the political culture of our society. One area of unprecedented change during the Thatcher years was in the area of civil liberties, particularly free-dom of speech.

The British political system, despite its reputation abroad as the 'mother of all parliaments', has no bill of rights. Ewing and Gearty (1990) have showed how the traditions of trust in politicians and the judiciary have left us with a set of freedoms 'by default'. That is, whatever freedoms we have are not declared as our positive rights, but comprise the leftover, the residue, of activities not specifically legislated against. Thatcher legislated widely and with little heed to any need for consensus. In this she was supported by a judiciary no longer seeing itself as upholding the rights of the common man. The upshot was an ever decreasing ability to speak out freely and a number of cases where individuals in the civil service who felt unable to support what they perceived as wrongdoings, had to speak out clandestinely. To their detriment. They were pursued in a spirit of almost McCarthyite witch-hunting.

The trial of Clive Ponting, ending with his acquittal in February 1985 from charges brought under the Official Secrets Act, acquired major significance in this respect for both practical and constitutional reasons. Ponting had been an assistant secretary in the Ministry of Defence, and leaked some confidential documents proving that the Prime Minister, Margaret Thatcher, took her decision to sink the Argentinian vessel the *General Belgrano*, during the Falklands War, *while it was sailing away from* the Exclusion Zone. This was in contrast to her parliamentary claim that the ship had been on an attack course and was sunk in self-defence.

The prosecution argued that, under the Official Secrets Act, a civil servant who was privy to actions by his Minister had a duty to obey orders, even if his conscience told him that those orders were wrong, even if Parliament and the public were being deceived. However, as Tony Benn describes,

> Ponting made a spirited defence of his own position and was acquitted on the grounds that what he had done was in the public interest. This constituted a landmark in constitutional practice which led to changes in a Protection of Official Information Act, which marginally modified some of the absurdities the Official Secrets Act, without making any substantial change.
>
> (Benn, 1994, p. 401)

Some would argue that the case of Sarah Tisdall, a junior clerk in Michael Heseltine's Ministry of Defence (MoD), was dissimilar from Clive Ponting's in at least one important respect. Although she certainly took a principled stand when she leaked a copy of a confidential MoD paper to the *Guardian*, there had been no blatant attempt by Heseltine to mislead Parliament. Others would highlight the fact that while Parliament had not been *mis*informed, neither had they been informed, which was, morally, just as reprehensible. Tisdall blew the whistle in the early 1980s on the fact and the date that cruise missiles were arriving on British soil at the United States Air Force base at Greenham Common. Tisdall, a member of the Campaign for Nuclear Disarmament, felt that this represented a policy development about which the British public *should* have been informed, particularly as it put Britain at the front of any firing line should nuclear war break out. Although she had championed an important civil liberty (i.e. the right to information about major nuclear defence decisions), this was not seen as a principle of sufficient importance to override the state's right to secrecy and the duty of its public servants to preserve oficial secrets. Tisdall received a six-month jail sentence for having broken the oath she took under the Official Secrets Act, and became a *cause celèbre*, particularly for the Greenham Common protesters.

John Stalker's case was different again, in that he championed no particular cause; he simply insisted, to the embarrassment of the Powers above him, on doing his job as a policeman with great efficiency. Too great. He had been the deputy chief constable of Greater Manchester, assigned to head an official inquiry into allegations of a 'shoot to kill' policy being implemented by the Royal Ulster Constabulary (RUC) in relation to IRA suspects in Northern Ireland. He showed greater tenacity in carrying out this task than was required, and lodged a number of complaints against officers of the RUC for hampering his work by failing to make available to him information and files. More a professional insisting on doing his job properly than a 'whistleblower' in the sense that the word is normally used, he nevertheless ended up being made something of a *cause célèbre* by the media, and subsequently, after his resignation from the police, publishing an account of the way he had been treated. Of particular interest was the way in which great influence was exerted to have him drop some of the leads he had been pursuing, and how, when he refused to bow to pressure, Manchester's chief constable, James Anderton had had Stalker charged in relation to alleged association with a known criminal. Stalker was subsequently taken off the inquiry and suspended. After lengthy and unusually protracted police and court proceedings Stalker was acquitted. Meanwhile the inquiry he had headed gathered dust and was completed by another officer whose inclination was clearly not to lead the inquiry as Stalker had done. Although some of these events rebounded on Anderton, Stalker sacrificed his career for what he felt was an important principle, the truth.

A fourth case which springs to mind was that of Marietta Higgs, the doctor who diagnosed sexual abuse in a number of children in Cleveland by way of a controversial technique, claimed by some to result in physical trauma similar to that which it purported to detect. Higgs had not pioneered this technique, but took it upon herself to ensure it was implemented, and all suspected cases of child sexual abuse followed up thoroughly and fully. While the technique, involving the internal examination of children, may strike any ordinary person as unsavoury, and was implemented perhaps, as some claim, in an atmosphere of 'mass hysteria' among social workers and other staff convinced that 'Satanic Abuse' was all around them, it was nevertheless a principled and courageous stand that Higgs took. The sexual abuse of children has long been a subject of such taboo that it has appeared as though society would rather have the victims left damaged and unbelieved than seriously address the issue. As a result of Higgs's testimony, some fifteen children were taken to places of safety on the orders of Cleveland magistrates, and left there for nine months without contact with their families, before the family division of the High Court, in response to the parents' plea for judicial review or for the children to be made wards of court, overturned the orders, returning the children to the care of their parents. While Higgs appeared, and may indeed have been, unduly sure of her diagnoses, and although the media coverage of her case left an impression that she had been discredited, her career seems not to have suffered and evidently her stand has led to a far greater readiness on the part of professionals, the media and the public at large to accept that sexual abuse of children happens, and is a problem that needs addressing.

Lastly, it is worth mentioning the case of Duncan Campbell, the *New Statesman* jounalist, who wrote and produced a television documentary about the Zircon affair, focusing on the government's secret £500 million expenditure on a surveillance satellite, despite a firm undertaking that any such projects above £250 million would come before parliamentary scrutiny. The government went to extraordinary lengths to have the documentary banned and injunctions issued preventing publication in any form of the details of the case. Pressure was even put on the Speaker of the House of Commons (successfully) to prevent Campbell showing the documentary in a private screening to MPs, through which he sought to prove there was no Official Secrecy issue at stake. After the failure to serve an injunction on Campbell personally, the *New Statesman* was able to publish details of the case to the embarrassment of the government, and subsequently Campbell's home was raided by Special Branch Officers, using tactics reminiscent of Eastern European regimes, 'the knock on the door in the night,' as one MP described it (Ewing and Gearty, 1990, pp. 147–9).

All of these episodes of 'whistleblowing', and others, including the 'Spycatcher' affair, took place in the 1980s. They may have appeared at the time to demonstrate how Thatcher's political machine could not silence dissension or truth. With hindsight, though, one might be forgiven for suspecting, along with Benn, that they made small real difference and perhaps represented merely the death throws of a liberal political culture in which participatory democracy was something more than rhetoric. It might not come as a surprise that, a decade on, civil servants appear to be refraining from taking the sort of risks that Pontin, Tidsall, Stalker, Higgs and others took in going public and/or taking stands. It may be even less of a surprise if, as Hutton argues (1995), the several hundred topmost positions of bureaucratic and strategic power in the land are now occupied almost exclusively by government appointees, sympathetic to right-wing political philosophy. The climate now is one in which one covers one's own back first and foremost. It has reached a point where, more than ever before, the government is understood to influence even supposedly unbiased media reporting, for example leaning heavily on the BBC as to what documentaries to broadcast, despite the dire political implications. In one example, *Death on the Rock*, in which a *Panorama* team sought to show how the government had essentially arranged for and then tried to cover up the assasination of IRA suspects on Gibraltar, by its own secret security forces, the government attempted to have the programme banned with court injunctions dispensed by a willing judiciary, without any sense that such interference in free debate may be unjust.

The oxygen of such publicity is evidently not to be allowed to an organisation labelled terrorist. Such has been the argument rehearsed repeatedly by politicians on mainland Britain in recent years. Television and radio broadcasts concerning the IRA had, during the years 1989–94, under the provisions of the Anti-Terrorism Act, to disguise the voice of anyone suspected of membership of Sinn Fein, the political organisation representing IRA views, by replacing their voice with an actor's. The government has not wanted to be seen publically to be censoring views (despite preventing certain social statistics from Northern Ireland getting 'the oxygen of publicity' for years), but it achieved the next best thing, creating an impression that the public was being protected from a very serious poison in the form of Gerry Adams' or Martin McGuiness's voice.

Dictators have always kept a tight hold on the press and other communication media, to maintain a firm hold on dissent. In military coups throughout the world, we notice how early reports invariably describe soldiers taking control of the television and radio stations and the newspapers. We were familiar during the years of the USSR with the ominous description of the Moscow-based newspaper *Isvestia* as The State Press. And those who like to publish satirical or critical poetry, cartoons, songs, etc., have always incurred a particular wrath and vengeance at the hands of the regimes they disdain. Closer to home, gagging clauses in the employment contracts of NHS staff have in recent times made specific reference to the likely disciplinary outcome of disclosures to the media about the internal business of the organisation. And even in a London borough that has boasted the most socially aware and empowering mental health policies of any local authority in the land, the present author was recently threatened with the sack by his otherwise progressive manager if he went to the press with information about a prospective multi-million pound cutback in the Social Services budget and the likely implications of the resource reductions, proposed to comply with this new budget, for mental health provision in the locality.

The media is powerful and feared. As recently reported on television President Clinton believes that the Internet, the so-called 'Information Superhighway', is providing unprecedented opportunities for communication, dialogue and democracy. As such, it has to be seen as a potential threat to the powerful if its potential cannot be harnessed by them. Of course, this is merely a further development in a process that has been happening for decades, if not centuries. The revolution in media technology that embraced the world as a 'global village' was a revolution akin to the development of the printing press, about which there was apparently also a great deal of fear and controversy. It was considered by the worthy and powerful that by putting information and the means to disseminate unorthodox views into the hands of the untutored and unwashed, one was playing with dynamite. Any beliefs, however wild, unauthorised or dangerous, could be shared quickly and freely with large numbers of people. Lord, it was the sort of thing that could lead to revolution. But as with the printed word, and despite the rhetoric, the threat is easily harnessed by those with power. Power has a way of employing a variety of means. It transpires that

> Television is a much more powerful form of ensuring uniformity of belief than was the Inquisition. . . . it is still quite an eerie experience to walk round any residential suburb after dark and to note the extent to which people are imbibing exactly the same impressions and information from glowing screens.
>
> (Smail, 1987, p. 87)

At the time of the development of the printing press, at the start of the telecommunications era earlier this century and now with the communicative potential of the Information Highway, the conservative fear engendered by anticipation of change is often disproportional, and the worst nightmares of authoritarians and repressors have not been realised. Freedom of information, even when guaranteed by legislation and the enhanced communication potential of such developments, seems always to be more than matched by the potential for greater uniformity of belief, regimentation and social control afforded by technological breakthroughs. Perhaps no structure guarantees freedom of speech or access to ideas or information, and maybe equally the withdrawal or absence of structures cannot prevent such access.

In this context, one must look much more to culture than technology to ascertain whether structures are in place that support freedom of speech and dissent. And as argued above, culture has changed over the last decade dramatically in this respect. Our culture is one in which someone seeking to publicise iniquities they have experienced is more likely to have their motives challenged than their case taken up. One calls to mind the Soviet dissident, Shiranski, who dissented in the USSR very publicly in order to return to Israel, facing up to the full force of the state machinery of repression to keep him in line. His case was taken up on a world-wide basis and he was finally allowed to emigrate to Israel. Then he dissented there. Is there such a thing as compulsive dissenting? Dissenting personality disorder? The treatment meted out to Soviet dissidents at the hands of state psychiatrists, dramatically portrayed by Rubens (1985), would no doubt have used such a label. We may like to think of psychiatry in Western Europe and North America as more progressive and less 'state-sponsored' than that of the 'evil empire'. If arguments presented already in this text have not disabused the reader of such notions, it may be worth considering the definition of a form of psychiatric illness recognised by psychiatrists as a kind of 'litigious personality disorder'. In trying to trace this definition, an interesting passage came to hand in the pages of the newly released *Oxford Textbook of Psychiatry* (1996), showing clearly the potential for pathologising political dissent:

> *Querulant delusions* were the subject of a special study. . . . Patients with this kind of delusion indulge in a series of complaints and claims lodged against the authorities. Closely related to querulant patients are *paranoid litigants* who undertake a succession of lawsuits; they become involved in numerous court hearings, in which they may become passionately angry and make threats against the magistrates. . . . *'reformist delusions'* which are centred on religious, philosophical, or political themes. People with these delusions constantly criticize society and sometimes embark on elaborate courses of action. Their behaviour may be violent, particularly when the delusions are political

> (Gelder *et al.*, 1996)

This sort of label (paranoid/litigious personality disorder) came to mind on reflecting on the a well-known whistleblower who, it was hoped, might contribute a chapter similar to this, based on his own experience of blowing the whistle. The nurse in question had apparently lost not only his job as a result of going public on safety issues and appalling standards of care in the hospital where he looked after elderly patients, but also his ability to work in partnership. A potentially powerful chapter on the experience of blowing the whistle was finally withdrawn in somewhat acrimonious circumstances that left me with the impression of someone who had grave difficulties in developing collaborative relationships with colleagues, and was much more ready to escalate differences into some sort of terminal conflict.

But that is the point, isn't it? It is so much easier for all of us to look at the individual who wants to upset the apple cart as having the problem, rather than seeing the apple cart as a disaster that needs upsetting. And perhaps there is a lesson in this for future whistleblowers, that there is, as argued above, a personal toll to pay for going out on a limb, and it is important to be realistic about that before taking on the heroic, martyr's role. I have based the experiential part of my discussion mainly on the experience of another 'whistleblower', Sandra, who seems to have found it easier to own and integrate the personal impact of her experience, but none the less that impact was evidently no less powerful than my paranoid and litigious friend.

And it is with that less infamous whistleblower, Sandra, that I shall finish this chapter. I asked her what final comment or advice she would like to see in a chapter such as I was writing, and she returned to a subject that has perhaps been the main theme of this piece: Support. Although the trade unions' role in society has lessened, they are as important a source of support, encouragement and backing in speaking out, as the more informal networks and the other power bases in which we live and work. It seems evident that at some level all of the contributors to Part 2 of this book will have established these sorts of formal backing (e.g., through trade unions), informal support (e.g., through friends) or structural influence (e.g., through their organisational power base), in developing the work and taking the inspiring stands they describe.

Sandra

I wouldn't want anyone to go through the same experience as me unprepared. I want to emphasise how difficult and scary it was. Words of advice? The union was incredibly important to me. That's a plug as I am now a union steward. And make sure you've got support, a good support network.

REFERENCES

Arendt, H. 1963: *Eichmann in Jerusalem: a report on the banality of evil*. New York: Viking Press.

Atkinson, R.L., Atkinson, R.C., and **Hilgard, E.R.,** 1983: *Introduction to psychology.* 8th edition, New York: Harcourt Brace Jovanovich.

Benn, A. 1994: *End of an era: Diaries 1980–1990*. London: Arrow.

Ewing, K.D. and **Gearty C.A.** 1990: *Freedom under Thatcher.* New York: Oxford University Press.

Gelder, M., Gath, D., Mayou, R. and **Cowen, P.** 1996: *Oxford textbook of psychiatry.* 3rd edition, Oxford: Oxford University Press.

Kesey, K. 1973: *One flew over the cuckoo's nest.* London: Picador.

Milgram, S. 1974: *Obedience to authority: an experimental view.* New York: Harper & Row.

Nolan, P. 1993: *A history of mental health nursing.* London: Chapman & Hall.

Rubens, B. 1985: *Brothers.* London: Abacus Books.

Smail, D. 1984: *Illusion and reality: the meaning of anxiety.* London: J.M. Dent.

Smail, D. 1987: *Taking care: an alternative to therapy.* London: J.M. Dent

Smail, D. 1993: *The origins of unhappiness.* London: HarperCollins.

Strang, J. 1982: Psychotherapy by nurses: some special characteristics. *Journal of Advanced Nursing.* 7, 167–71.

Thoreau, H.D. 1984: *On the duty of civil disobedience.* Harmondsworth: Penguin.

Vonnegut, K. 1975: *Breakfast of champions.* St Albans: Panther Books Ltd.

Wittgenstein, L. 1958: *The blue and brown books.* Oxford: Basil Blackwell.

Part 2

Individual Struggles

Much of what goes on between nurses and their patients may involve no more than the exchange of words. Depending on the phrasing, however, such words may fulfil healing or damning functions. To the extent that we try obstinately to remain alive to such nuances, we can actively cease to do evil, strive to do good and purify the heart, all of which is, it has to be said, a struggle. The struggle to live a 'good' life and to do what is 'right' is essentially a struggle with oneself to develop integrity: living wholeheartedly the kind of life we think we should for the reasons we think are important. Of course, most of us know that it is easier to lecture on integrity than to practise it. Too often the 'ethical life' amounts to no more than a largely transparent injunction 'Don't do as I do – do as I say!'.

Integrity, however, seems to be important at some kind of fundamental level. Something at a deep level of intuitive understanding tells us that we *should* return a lost wallet – it could be *our* wallet; we *should* support people down on their luck – it could be *us*; we *should* leave our patients after an interaction feeling somehow better off as a result of having been with us – they are likely already to have suffered enough damage (and of course it *is* what we are being paid for); and it is especially 'good' when people are nice to you for no obvious reason. If such examples ring any bells for the reader, they probably also suggest the everyday status of ethics – as distinct from the dusty subject filed under 'philosophy'. Any such resonance suggests, moreover, that it is impossible to separate the professional role from the person occupying it. It is not possible for us 'as nurses' either to tuck our ethics away in some metaphorical drawer, or to draw them out on an 'as required' basis. *You* – the person – keep getting in the way with your intuition that you should be doing something more holistic. *You* – the person, keep stamping all over the rules and regulations, ignoring the codes and *pro forma*, exercising subtle revenge on patients for the bad mood life has left you with today. Ethics is a live issue and people *live* their ethics.

Every day, we live on the brink of our own personal freedom to conduct ourselves in any which way we choose. In any choice we make, although this fact may be too frightening to countenance, we are obliged to confront the risks of the unknown – it is impossible to *know* if one is doing the *right* thing, or what the consequences and karma will be, even when the morality we espouse and follow appears, by virtue of the fact that it is socially sanctioned, to yield security. Virtually everything we do is, in some way, dependent on ethical decision-making, with uncertain outcome. If the truth be known, decisions are rarely easy. Moral dilemmas, problems, challenges require us to decide between *this* and *that* action. With time for reflection we wonder 'why did I do *this* rather than *that*'. The ethical life path is rarely smooth; rather, it is bumpy with doubts and rutted with guilt.

These everyday ethical dilemmas – with their acutely personal dimension – are part and parcel of the working context of psychiatric nurses. The failure to reach agreement on what ought to be done; or the secreting of doubts or masking of guilt over what has been done, can pull a team, or a person apart. Rarely do we suspect that ethics lies at the root of such strife, that it is our unwholesome conduct that occasions such interpersonal or psychic *dis*integration. So, naturally, we rarely ever get around to discussing what is really the problem. The health care system often reinforces this. Health care is rarely a human place. It is riddled with numbers, forms, red tape, rules, targets, costings, unanswered questions and often ridiculous ambitions.

None the less, the practitioner in the ordinary, workaday world of psychiatric nursing may wish to cultivate whatever humanity there is in their work setting and relationships. We assume, by virtue of the fact they are reading this text, that the reader will count themselves among such ethically-minded practitioners. And we hope as editors that the following accounts of how some practitioners have tried to cultivate the humanity of their work and of the context in which it takes place, will encourage, guide and inspire the reader in this respect.

Part 2 focuses on individuals' experience of quite immediate ethical dilemmas arising as part of everyday working experience. We have sought, as editors, first, to allow our contributors in this section to role-model how the exploration of such dilemmas is an important social practice. We have ensured, second, that consideration is given by these authors to the means by which, as individual practitioners or teams, they construe and resolve such dilemmas. Although the two main themes explored in Part I are often evident, the current section emphasises the direct experience of confusion and uncertainty about conduct in particular situations.

From a potentially limitless variety of client groups, of types of mental health problem, of approaches to treatment and of clinical settings, we have had to select a limited number to present as typical contexts in which are found the sort of ethical issues faced generally and constantly by practitioners. Inevitably, the results of our selection may appear piecemeal. However, we hope that the following accounts, taken together, may offer a useful sketch of the way in which the editors' two main threads of ethical critique manifest in any situation. At the risk of repetition, these threads comprise, first, ethical problems concerning the immoral abuse of power in the psychiatric treatment we dispense; and, second, ethical possibilities concerning our obligation to heal by offering to share with clients their pilgrimage on a quest of personal (re)discovery and growth.

While our selection of subjects for this Part may appear *ad hoc*, we are aware of a certain organic quality manifest through the original selection of issues to be included, in the development of the chapters (the format has undergone many revisions as the project has progressed) and in our final choice of author and topic. In struggling to elicit the circumstances and refine an explanation for our selecting *this* and not *that* client group (or type of illness), or *that* and not *this* approach to care (or clinical setting), perhaps we miss the point somewhat. Our final selection is as much about the issues that impinge *on us*, that have made an impact on *our* work, that have never been adequately resolved in *our* own understanding, as about anything else. We should perhaps make no apology for this, as this text is much more the product of the editors' quest for ethical growth and the preparedness of potential contributors to join in with that quest, than it is an attempt to offer a definitive guide to ethical issues in mental health work. In which case, let it stand, as an incomplete choice, but one informed by experience of our own and our colleagues' and friends' work, as well as being influenced by our own and our colleagues' and friends' idiosyncratic but hopefully representative preoccupations in establishing an ethical practice.

Specifically, though, the thread develops as follows. Chapters 10, 11 and 12 highlight the tension between two approaches. One approach seeks to impose upon patients an alternative, more orthodox and more socially sanctioned 'reality' than the one they currently experience; the other approach validates and seeks to help articulate the other's 'reality' for what it is, however hard it is to do so. The client groups in question may be taken to represent particularly disadvantaged groups in general (although of course, all those suffering 'mental illness' are in a considerably stigmatised and disadvantaged group in their own right). The three groups comprise the elderly in Chapter 10, minority racial or ethnic sub-groups in Chapter 11 and women in Chapter 12. The thrust of the work and argument presented in each case is that there are great difficulties, and also ethical advantages in an approach which helps individuals and groups to elicit and assert their own reality. Not least of these advantages is the enhancement of one's own growth and authentic sense of self as a worker in this situation. In each of these three chapters the author describes an innovation they have made in working with (or training others to work with) the group in question, based on their own reflection, study, and individual struggle in-conscience with the issues at stake. In the case of Chapter 10, a reminiscence therapy group initiated by a nursing auxiliary is described, touching on issues of loss, mortality, trauma, organic illness, therapeutic touch, the mutuality of the therapeutic process, aggression and violence and the importance of helping people tell their stories. In Chapter 11, the experience of being racially different is elaborated, together with an account of how its impact for service users and providers in the experience of the author, a newly qualified psychiatric nurse, gave rise to a successful training initiative. In Chapter 12, a women's group initiated by the author, a social services day care worker, in response to deficiencies in service provision at the inner-city day centre where she worked, is described. Issues of disempowerment, being needs-led and tackling the interpersonal and political power issues with colleagues and the larger institution in which the work takes place are explored.

In Chapters 13, 14 and 15, more detailed attention is given to a variety of means by which one may scrutinise one's practice and the practice of one's colleagues, namely, writing, reflection and supervision. In Chapter 13, the usefulness of writing as a tool of reflective practice is elaborated, in relation to understanding complex group dynamics and developing a useful role working on an in-patient unit. The particular client group in question suffer eating disorders. The perspective is that of a student nurse attempting to make sense of an overwhelming experience. In Chapter 14 the merits of a Buddhist reflective approach to craving are enumerated, in relation both to patients' and to clinicians' desire for gratification and aversion to suffering. The particular groups in question are drug addicts (and others attempting to condemn unpleasant experience to oblivion) and mental health clinicians in out-patient, casualty and acute setings, each in their respective ways dependent on things being a certain way. The perspective is that of a psychiatrist using meditation skills to catch himself out in the game of trying to control the world around him, rather than appreciating and helping it to be. In Chapter 15, the advantage of intensive supervision (and the concommitant need for attention to staff dynamics) is emphasised, in relation to ensuring that one's practice remains respectful and collaborative. The work described takes place at a day centre and concerns an array of issues including institutionalisation, dysfunctional relation-ship, transexuality, chronic dependence, violence and long-term neuroleptic use. The per-spective is that of a psychiatric nurse in a day centre, using 'live' supervision to maintain and offer a point of grounding and balance, so as to restore equilibrium to a couple in crisis.

Part 2 concludes with Chapter 16, an account which focuses both on a particular area of psychiatric nursing practice, family work, and also on the means by which ethical practice may be enhanced, through structures that allow the whole team to reflect together on what may be occurring in the interaction between nurse and patient. The central issue addressed is that of informed consent to treatment, using the example of a collaborative style of family work to make the general point that negotiation, rather than domination, should be the touchstone of our relationships with clients.

It is said that life is the shortest distance between two points — life and death. What, exactly, are we doing most of the time, as we journey from one point to another? Searching for 'quality time'? Trying to separate the dross of existence from the 'jewels of satisfaction'? We know that, by and large, people do find these jewels — meanings, and bits of quality time — for human life goes on. We continue to struggle, and most of us find the struggle for meaning, satisfaction and wholeheartedness, overall, a worthwhile pursuit.

We, as editors, wish to underline the importance of allowing space for people (both clients and clinicians) to experience their feelings of turmoil in relation to ethical issues. With such 'space' we are able to make some headway in sifting the dross from the jewellery in our conduct and our experience. We hope that we have been effective in constructing such a space for (and with) the contributors to this section of the text, also in highlighting the link between such an experience of moral doubt and growth. If we were to specify one theme emerging from the following accounts to be seen as crucial, it would be the importance of encouragement and facilitation to enable people (both clinicians and clients) to *tell their stories*.

10

WHOSE REALITY IS IT ANYWAY?

Sally Cameron

It is exceptionally hard to negotiate with clients a view of their problems, equally hard to agree a treatment plan, without some degree of coercion by the clinician towards a particular outcome. The clinician has authority and will use it. Clearly, however, the practice of explicitly defining others' reality can be a recipe for much more overt abuse. A wide range of radical therapeutic approaches where 'reality' can be manipulated present ethical dilemmas. Here Sally Cameron describes her developing sense of abusing others by denying their reality in her work with the elderly. She writes about her experience of increasing alienation from reality orientation work. Sally describes how she managed to open a forum in which patients could talk about their lives and tell their stories, as well as detailing the interpersonal battles she had to face to do so. She underlines how unsettling it was for her to face her own fear of mortality and her inability to talk honestly about death. Finally, Sally emphasises the mutuality of the therapeutic process. She relates the struggle she underwent in allowing patients to share their life experience with her own growth, and the development of her subsequent work as a writer.

This chapter is based on my experiences working as a nurse in a new mental health unit in London from 1984–87. I had recently left university with a degree in psychology and no particular career plan, and the job seemed like a good start to something, of what I was unsure. While I had dismissed most of my degree course with the utmost contempt, I had always been somewhat drawn to the area of mental illness. I was 22 years old and had, as yet, made no connection between my attraction to madness and my own internal confusions.

I arrived at the hospital with a lot of enthusiasm and a head full of academic theory, excited by the prospect of my first encounter with real-life insanity. So I was rather disappointed to find not a single sign of madness in the huge, sparkling new building with its spotless expanses of beige carpet and pristine furniture. But there were plenty of professionals there with a lot to say about what was going to be our radical new approach to mental health, and we spent quite a few weeks discussing key issues and getting used to working as a multi-disciplinary team.

WHERE ARE ALL THE OLD PEOPLE?

The unit was divided into two sections called 'acute' and 'elderly', situated on opposite sides of the building. The two sides were like parallel worlds. On the ground floor the elderly day hospital was sited below two elderly wards and, on the other side, the acute day hospital was sited beneath two acute wards. The two halves of the unit had separate facilities and different staff, so there were in fact to be two multi-disciplinary teams working with two sets of patients who would have no contact with each other. At the time I never thought to question this separation which now seems to me so pertinent to the ethical dilemmas I later encountered. It is interesting that the sole criteria for placing patients was age and, with hindsight I would suggest that this separation served to reflect and reinforce the alienation of old people in our society. Another interesting point is that the younger section was named 'acute'. The definition of 'acute' is critical, serious, coming to a crisis, thereby implying that the 'elderly' patients were somehow not so serious, nor experiencing crises. Moreover, because the opposite meaning of the word 'acute' is 'chronic', the implication was that the elderly were somehow not going to change, were not able to be helped, were indeed 'no-hopers'. So both the physical separation and the linguistic definitions provided a good basis for the negative attitudes which were apparent from the start.

Such negative attitudes fed my own reluctance. When the Senior Nurse allocated me a position in the elderly day hospital my heart sank. I had bad memories of living with my grandfather's progressive senility and besides, how was I going to practise my newly-learned Rogerian client-centred therapy with some old fossil who thought that World War 1 had just started? My unspoken disappointment was in no way dissipated by the other nurses who joined me in the elderly day hospital. Interestingly enough most of them were black. They quickly explained to me that the rule in psychiatry was that white nurses did the glamorous jobs, the therapeutic chatting with the nice young neurotics, while the blacks cleared up the excrement. The memories of my grandfather's incontinence grew suddenly more vivid.

However, there were a few of my new colleagues who were obviously pleased with their new placements. Some told me clearly that they could not face the distressing confusions of the young, but were perfectly happy with the simple physical needs of the elderly mentally infirm. I liked listening to the stories that the other nurses told me. Before the unit officially opened we had plenty of time to sit around discussing our previous experiences and, because mine was entirely limited to the printed page, I was fascinated to hear experienced nurses talking about their work with real people, and over the first few weeks I learned a lot about what to expect. The two major themes which emerged were *chaos* and *control*. So I was prepared, so I thought, for the arrival of the patients.

THE CHAOS OF OLD AGE

Three months on. Let me give you a typical scene from the brand new up-and-running elderly day hospital. As you open the swing doors of the main entrance the first thing that hits you is the smell of disinfectant battling with the pervasive undertones of urine and faeces. The recently immaculate beige carpet is now badly stained and as you approach the large day room you can hear shouts, crying, and a low mumble of confusion. No one appears to notice your entrance. Several old people sit silently in wheelchairs, some distance from each other. One man crouches in a corner, wringing his hands and muttering to himself; another holds a radio to his ear, listening intently to the crackle between stations. An old lady with apricot hair methodically paces a circle around the television, barefoot and carrying a pair of pink, plastic sandals. From the bathroom you can hear the sound of intermittent screams. Shouts fly from the kitchen, and from the art room a high-pitched sobbing reaches a crescendo, just as a flustered nurse emerges from the bathroom wearing rubber gloves and a plastic apron covered in talcum powder. She has a deep scratch on her cheek which is dripping blood. Her first words to you are: 'Jimmy's just eaten the goldfish!'

I think that one of the major practical problems in the caring professions is that there are never enough carers. Even before you start analysing the quality of care there is always the issue of quantity. I found myself busier than I had ever been in my life. In just a few weeks my working day had transformed from a series of cosy coffee-orientated planning meetings to a constant routine of cleaning, tidying, washing, toileting, feeding and medicating. Sitting down for a chat with someone was a luxury, it was usually interrupted, and there was little time to think about what was said. And perhaps a part of me was relieved, in the beginning, not to have to listen to what I was being told. Because what I was being told was just too painful. It is pretty distressing to see a chaotic group of chronic no-hopers, but what is even more distressing is to realise that these people are actually a chaotic group of frightened individuals who are trying to deal with the major crises of old age.

It is not so hard to see why the emphasis was on keeping their bums clean. An enormous amount of time and energy went into cleaning up excreta, leading people to the toilet and changing endless wet and soiled clothes. There was a 'no nappies' policy, implemented supposedly to preserve the dignity of our patients, but serving only to make everyone obsessed by what was coming out of our patients' bottoms. We could deal with that end of things. Somehow, ironically, it was the other end that was more unpalatable. What came out of their mouths, and I'm not taking about the vomit, dribbling and ill-fitting dentures – we could deal with that too. It seemed to be the words that everyone was avoiding – the emotions.

GETTING INVOLVED

I was told right from the start that I should not get too involved. Another thing I was warned about was to avoid encouraging morbid thoughts. One-to-one work was rare, except in the area of personal care, and I had an instinctive feeling that it wasn't right to discuss emotions with someone when they had their knickers round their ankles. The emphasis of activity in the day hospital was on group work – cooking groups, art groups, craft groups and reality orientation. But the work I enjoyed most was listening to individual patients telling me about their lives. I can safely say that I got too involved. I spent a lot of time worrying about patients. I thought about patients long after I had finished work. I even dreamt about patients. It was the individual stories which made up the sum of my experience: each and every one seemed to throw a different perspective on my work but, limited by space, I shall focus on just three patients whom I believe are a good representation of the vast diversity I encountered.

Jimmy – dementia

Jimmy was a 72-year-old Irish man, tall and muscular with a grim expression. Looking at pictures of his brain scan the consultant psychiatrist marvelled at how Jimmy even managed to remain alive, let alone function as he did. The way Jimmy functioned was to pace very rapidly around the building all day long, thumping anyone who came near him and shouting, 'Fuck off, you fucker!' He was a patient on one of the elderly wards. Some of the patients on the wards were considered able enough to attend day hospital activities with the elderly patients from the local community. Jimmy was not considered appropriate for the day hospital, but he came anyway. Nobody really knew how to stop him, strait-jackets being out of fashion. I was scared stiff of him.

Elisabeth – definitely not dementia

Elisabeth was a 78-year-old woman from the East End of London. She dressed immaculately in bright sequined clothes and wore a lot of gold jewellery. Polio in childhood had left her with a withered leg and she had always worn a caliper, but a recent stroke had confined her to a wheelchair. She had been referred to the day hospital following an overdose of sleeping pills. Elisabeth said very little during her first visits to the day hospital. She sat silently tense in her wheelchair, refusing to join groups and chain-smoking Benson and Hedges. She regarded the other patients with an expression of horror and disbelief. Very occasionally she would beckon me with a jerk of the head and whisper in my ear, 'For God's sake get me out of this place!'

Millicent – is it dementia or isn't it?

Millicent was an 84-year-old descendant of the aristocracy. She was a tiny, frail woman with fine dark curls framing her enormous blue eyes. She looked as though she might have been a heroine in the old silent films. Millicent was brought to the day hospital each day by her elder sister, Henrietta, and there was usually a tearful parting lasting up to an hour. From then on, and for the rest of the day, Millicent would sit curled into an armchair, watching the door for Henrietta's return. Whenever I approached her she would clasp my hand, gaze into my eyes and say the words that she repeated constantly, the words that had become a familiar background murmur in the day hospital, and the words that had been driving her sister to distraction for the past year:

'I don't know what to do and I don't know what to say and I don't know where to go.

'How do I stop this? I didn't want this to happen. I never thought this would happen. You must understand that I *don't know what to do or what to say*.'

From the start I identified completely with Millicent. I didn't have a clue what to do or what to say either.

REALITY ORIENTATION

On one wall of the day room was a large white board on which information was written each day. For example:

TODAY IS MONDAY
IT IS 31st OCTOBER
THE YEAR IS 1986
THE WEATHER IS WET AND COLD
THE NEXT MEAL IS LUNCH

I had always had a problem remembering the date, so this was a godsend when it came to writing reports.

First thing in the morning the patients were sat around in a circle for a reality orientation group. Led by an occupational therapist they were given certain information and encouraged to participate in simple discussion. It went something like this:

O.T.:	'Good morning, everyone!'
	(a few mumbled hellos)
O.T.:	'Isn't it an awful day? Look outside' (points to the window and rubs her hands together) 'Brrr it's cold isn't it?'
Millicent:	'How can I stop this? I didn't want this to happen.'
O.T.:	(Ignores her) 'Who can tell me what day it is today?'
Millicent:	'I don't know what to say.'
O.T.:	'Look at the board, Millicent, and then you'll be able to tell us what day it is.'
	(Millicent stares at the O.T.)
Millicent:	'You don't understand. Please understand *that I don't know what to say.*'
O.T.:	(sighs) 'Elisabeth – can *you* tell us what day it is today?'
	(Elisabeth ignores her and stares out of the window. At this point Jimmy comes running in wearing only his pyjama jacket. He stares around the group.)
O.T.:	'Good morning, Jimmy. I was just asking everyone what day it is today – can you tell us?'
Jimmy:	'Fuck off, you fucker!' (runs out)
O.T.:	(brightly) 'As I was saying – Elisabeth!'
	(Elisabeth sighs and looks at her.)
Elisabeth:	'What?'
O.T.:	'I'd like you to tell us what day it is.'
	(Elisabeth raises her eyes to the ceiling.)
Elisabeth:	'Oh for God's sake, it's Monday the 31st of October.'
O.T.:	'Well done, Elisabeth! Now, can anyone tell me what's special about today?'
	(Silence)
O.T.:	'Elisabeth – I'm sure *you* can tell us.'
Elisabeth:	(staring at her with disdain and speaking very slowly and precisely) ' It's Halloween – and if you try to get me making pumpkin lanterns I'll stick one up your bloody arse.'

I was frequently required to join in with these reality orientation groups, mainly to encourage participation and to stop people wandering off, and from the start I felt uncomfortable with the situation. The patients reacted to the reality orientation groups in a variety of different ways. Elisabeth was clearly insulted by being asked to state the obvious. Jimmy was obviously not interested in the information and not at all happy with the method of communication. Millicent wanted to talk about something else. What was clear was that for all of them, the information being discussed was irrelevant. It was true that most of them did not know what day it was, but what was more important was the fact that each and every one of them *did not care what day it was*.

This is not to say that reality orientation does not have a place in the nursing of the elderly. But as Morton and Bleathman (1988) have pointed out, a blanket application of reality orientation is not only futile but can be damaging. I witnessed many times these groups develop into grotesque power games where patients were constantly reminded of their inadequacies by focusing on their inability to remember, followed by coercion into repeating facts and figures which bore no relevance to their present predicament. Also I was uneasy with the staff's apparent satisfaction at the end of a 'good group', where the patients had successfully repeated the information like parrots. Everyone now knows it's Monday. So what?

From the start this approach disempowers the patient by setting the agenda of *what is important*. It is the staff who choose what to talk about, not the patients. I believe that reality orientation has become popular mainly because it gives the staff a sense of effective working when confronted with the frustrating intellectual deterioration of the elderly. It is a good way of imposing structure on chaos. It makes *us* feel better. But where reality orientation becomes abusive is when it *negates* what the patient is actually telling us. There is an assumption that the confused elderly talk 'rubbish' and therefore they should be helped to talk 'sensibly'. I would argue, however, that there is always an underlying meaning in the nonsense of old age. This is hardly a new idea. Shakespeare's *King Lear* (1987) is a fine example of the breakdown of reason in old age, whereby a foolish king gains insight and moral redemption only by going mad. Anyone working with the confused elderly must have witnessed the patterns of Lear's own insanity – the incoherent chatter, the domination of a fixed idea, the strange attire, and the regression to a child-like state. But in Lear's nonsensical rantings are the seeds of truth and perception, and if we study the words of our patients as closely as the scholars study Shakespeare, we may find the beginnings to start making sense.

MAKING SENSE

In America Naomi Feil (1982), disillusioned with reality orientation, developed an alternative therapy for the disorientated called 'validation therapy' which focuses on the underlying meaning of speech and behaviour. So, instead of dismissing the nonsense we *listen* to the nonsense and try, together with the patient, to make sense of it. For example,

Millicent: 'I don't know what to say or where to go or what to do.'
Nurse: 'You look very worried.'

Millicent: 'Yes, yes, I am worried – because I don't know what to do.'
Nurse: 'What to do about what?'
Millicent: 'Everything! I don't know what to do about anything. I'm completely lost.'
Nurse: 'That sounds very frightening.'
Millicent: (clutches Nurse's hand) 'Oh it is! Yes, I'm terrified.'

Working with Millicent was not easy. She irritated everyone with her constant repetitions and refusal to take part in any activities. The other nurses dismissed my attempts to talk to her as a time-wasting exercise ('Off to do a bit of psychology on Millicent – ha, ha') but I tried to spend just ten minutes on my own with her each day, listening to what she was saying and trying to help her make sense of the intolerable reality she had found herself in. These sessions were for a long time almost identical and I found myself becoming increasingly exasperated by this woman's ability to say the same sentence fifty times in one conversation. Nothing seemed to change except that the other nurses stopped laughing at me and became quite angry that I wasn't pulling my weight. I was very aware that I was in danger of becoming one of those 'lazy nurses who sit around chatting'. The occupational therapists felt that my time with Millicent should be spent on task-orientated activities, developing cooking skills, etc. and participating in groups. And the clinical psychologist, while encouraging one to one sessions, advised me to take a more behavioural approach.

I did have doubts about what I was doing but something kept me at it. I found myself repeating Millicent's words to myself, like a mantra, until they became meaningful to me, and I began to realise that the fears she expressed, of being lost and confused and unsure, were feelings that all of us must have at one time experienced, feelings that are often hidden after childhood and which none of us like to confront.

Millicent: 'I don't know what to do.'
Sally: 'Sometimes I don't know what to do either.'
Millicent: 'Don't you? Don't you know what to do?'
Sally: 'No, I'm feeling a bit helpless. I want to help you but I don't know quite what to do.'
Millicent: 'I don't know what to say. Do you know what to say?'
Sally: 'Not always.'
Millicent: 'Isn't it awful? It's so frightening when you don't know what to say.'
Sally: 'Shall we try and find out what to say?'
Millicent: 'Can we find out? I don't know. I don't know what to say. How do we find out?'
Sally: 'We can try. We can help each other.'
Millicent: 'I'm scared.'
Sally: 'What's scary?'
Millicent: 'I'm scared I'll say the wrong thing.'
Sally: 'What would happen if you said the wrong thing?'
Millicent: 'You might go away.'

The staff were not impressed by Millicent's progress. She still spent her entire time in the day hospital waiting for her sister to return, and saying the same things over and over again. But no one noticed that what she was saying was completely different. Now, what Millicent said was:

'If we just keep trying. If we just pull together. If we keep on trying we'll pull through. If we just keep holding on we'll pull through.'

I saw this as a very positive step and I was pleased with myself, but at the case review it was unanimously decided that there had been no change in Millicent's condition. She still wasn't eating, she still refused to join in activities, and she still didn't know what day it was. The next step was ECT.

'So much for your *psychotherapy*,' sneered a staff nurse.

I was firmly put in my place.

NO PSYCHOTHERAPY FOR THE ELDERLY

Although a small number of people have acknowledged the benefits of psychotherapy, for example Hanna Segal (1980) it is widely believed to be of little significance for EMI work. Freud believed that people over 50 did not possess the elasticity of mental processes to cope with treatment, and certainly this view is reflected in the allocation of the limited psychotherapy services to the elderly in the National Health Service. The word psychotherapy possesses a mystique which has limited it to a narrow field: for many it still conjures up an image of a patient lying on a couch under the eye of a bearded man with a Viennese accent, and the nearest many mental health professionals have come to experiencing psychotherapy is watching a Woody Allen film.

During my period in the mental health unit, prompted by the dictum, 'Physician heal thyself', I began to see a psychotherapist, and this proved to be invaluable in my work. I firmly believe that anyone working in this field should have the opportunity to experience being a 'patient' themselves. I found my own therapy essential in understanding the power relations between the 'helper' and the 'helped', and in recognising transference and the importance of the relationship itself in the therapeutic process. I became increasingly interested in the importance of the past, an issue which was most relevant for many of the elderly patients I encountered who would talk of nothing else; and the increasing awareness of my own unconscious processes helped me to be aware of some of the unconscious processes underlying the behaviour and speech of my patients. I would also suggest that being the patient of a skilled therapist is the best way to learn effective communication, for me better than any counselling course, in-service training, supervision or textbook.

Psychotherapy is viewed by many as a 'special treatment' whereby the therapist *does* something *to* the patient. I think it is important to explode this myth so that all nurses and carers can practise psychotherapeutic intervention. A psychotherapist acts not so much as a skilled mechanic working on a machine, but as a caring and skilled gardener offering a nourishing environment in which living things are helped to do their own growing. A therapist therefore acts not as *controller* but as *facilitator*, and this involves having the courage to take the lead from the patient, no matter how chaotic and seemingly senseless that may be.

After another three months Millicent began to approach me for our sessions, rather than the other way around, which I felt strengthened my lonely assertions about therapeutic intervention. I was told, however, that all I was doing was creating a dependence which would lead to further problems when I left the job. I insisted that Millicent would be leaving the day hospital before I did, but even to my own ears I sounded arrogant and unconvincing. Millicent was expressing the same doubts herself:

Millicent: 'If we just hold on. If we just pull together we'll be alright.'
Sally: 'What else do you think we have to do?'
Millicent: 'We have to hold on together.'
Sally: 'What are we holding on to?'
Millicent: (looks worried) 'Are you going to go away? Are you going to stop holding on?'
Sally: 'No, I'm not, but what would happen if I did?'
Millicent: 'It would be so much worse.'
Sally: 'What's the worst it could be?'
Millicent: 'I'd be lost.'
Sally: 'What does it mean to be lost?'
Millicent: 'I'd be alone.'

It took me an inexcusably long time to make the connections between Millicent's fear of losing me and her obvious distress each morning when she was left by her sister. With a bit of persuasion I obtained permission to meet with Millicent and Henrietta together, and then things began to fall into place. It emerged that Henrietta, who was nearly 90 and had always taken care of her younger sister, had been having increasingly severe angina attacks, a fact which she had concealed from the staff at the day hospital, from her own GP and, so she thought, from Millicent. But over the past year Millicent had sensed that something was very wrong and had become paralysed by the fear that Henrietta was going to die. Henrietta had suffered alone, not wishing to burden anyone and wanting only to protect her little sister, while Millicent, unsure of what was happening and unable to verbalise her fears had gradually regressed to an all-consuming state of repetitive, obsessional worry – a state not dissimilar to many manifestations of dementia.

Through talking to the sisters together Millicent's abstract ramblings began to make perfect sense, and eventually she was able to verbalise her fears that Henrietta would die and leave her to cope alone for the first time in 84 years, a prospect which she found terrifying. The three of us began to meet regularly, a situation where I often felt quite out of my depth, but always with a sense of the great privilege it was to be witnessing these two extraordinary old ladies sharing their fears for the first time, remembering incidents from long ago which they had never discussed, and affirming their great love for each other. All this made me very aware of my own feelings of impotence, and my denial of what was so very obvious. Even with the new tablets prescribed for Henrietta's heart she was still 90 years old and that was well above the average life-span. Millicent herself was a very old lady. Increasingly I became aware that either of them could drop dead at any moment.

THE BIG D-WORD

It is interesting that in my long induction period to working with the elderly, during all the planning meetings, training sessions and informal chats, there was one word that was never mentioned. Death. Yet it would seem logical to suppose that in old age, when considering the future, *death* would certainly be on the agenda. The subject was frequently mentioned in the day hospital by patients and always avoided by the staff. For example,

Patient: 'I feel so ill. Am I going to die, doctor?'
Doctor: 'No, no, plenty of life in the old dog yet!'

Patient: 'It won't be long before I'm six foot under.'
Nurse: 'Now don't be so morbid – come and have some lunch or you'll starve to death!'

It was common practice to joke away any mention of dying, to 'boost morale' by positive thinking and to discourage 'morbid thoughts', but I felt dissatisfied with the avoidance of what was so obviously a vital issue. I also felt totally uncomfortable talking about the D-word myself, and it was through examining my own reluctance that I became aware of the enormity of the task. For it was not only the accepting the proximity of death to the patients whom I liked so much that was difficult. It was also accepting my own mortality, something that at the age of 24 I just did not want to consider.

One incident springs to mind particularly. A young doctor and a staff nurse were examining an old lady who was dying of cancer and had developed a urinary tract infection. After the examination I found them in the office, the doctor white-faced and drawing heavily on a cigarette while the nurse flirtatiously teased him about his 'new girlfriend'. When I asked what was wrong he laughed and told me,

'Sorry I'm just recovering from a nasty encounter with Rose's fanny. You should have seen the state of it!'

The nurse giggled and I was struck not so much by the callousness of their response, but by the obvious anxiety which 'Rose's fanny' had provoked. What was the nature of this anxiety? To my mind there was something very symbolic about the ancient, dying, reproductive organs of an old woman which triggered deep unconscious feelings in both doctor and nurse, and it was these intolerable feelings which were displaced into repulsion and humour. Nurse and doctor had thus bonded in a defensive alliance, asserting their youthful sexuality while detaching themselves totally from the patient as a person.

Isobel Menzies Lyth (1988) wrote an excellent paper on the primitive and intense anxieties aroused by nursing, and the defences used to contain this anxiety. As other contributors to the text have acknowledged, these defences all represent ways of creating distance between us and the person who evokes this anxiety. Throughout my time in the elderly day hospital I was constantly aware of the evasion of feelings and the general reluctance to confront the issues which seemed most pertinent to working with patients in the last stages of life. The emotions produced in this situation are wide and varied, but I would suggest that a major factor in our detachment from the elderly is an unwillingness to accept these people as like ourselves or, more importantly, like our future. For, after all, we will all one day die, and most of us will experience some degeneration of old age. On an unconscious level, then, working with the elderly cannot but trigger our deepest, most primitive fear, the fear of annihilation.

DON'T DWELL ON THE PAST

After death, the second big taboo was history. The basis of reality orientation lies firmly in the present, yet I began to notice that the patients were at their most interested and animated when telling me about the past. The memories, naturally, were often distressing – the deaths of loved ones and other traumatic events figured strongly in conversation, and I was very aware of the constant urges of the staff to 'forget'.

'Come on now, cheer up, you can't live in the past', was a frequent response to a patient's tearful reminiscence. There was a general feeling that to think about past pain was not only futile but could make the patients even worse, and I was frequently told that opening up old wounds was a very dangerous business.

Six months on Elisabeth was still attending the day hospital and still refusing to do anything but chain-smoke and touch up her scarlet fingernails. From our brief conversations I felt that Elisabeth had a lot to say and I got the impression that she just needed the right environment. I was convinced that the right environment was in the reminiscence group which I was running with an occupational therapist, a new group which I was very excited about. I felt that I had found a kindred soul in Jenny, the occupational therapist, and for the first time since starting the job a year before I felt confident that I was doing something worthwhile – enabling people not only to tell their stories but, as Gerald Egan (1990) advocates, helping people to *understand*, *accept* and *share* their stories. The group had been going a month and was held once a week on a Wednesday, a closed group for eight patients whom Jenny and I had thought might benefit, one of whom was Elisabeth. So far Elisabeth had adamantly refused to attend.

One Wednesday I was trying, as usual, to encourage Elisabeth to join us. She had run out of cigarettes and was extremely angry that the staff had refused to go to the shops for her to buy some more.

Elisabeth: 'I'm not going to your group – you can't make me.'

Sally: 'I'm not trying to *make* you do anything – you can choose what you do here, but I'm just telling you about the choices.'

Elisabeth: 'Okay – you've told me. I'm not going.'

Sally: 'Why not just give it a try? You can always leave if you don't like it.'

Elisabeth: 'Look I don't want to come to the bloody group – I just want a fag. Will you get me some?'

Sally: 'I'm sorry I can't do that.'

Elisabeth: 'Why not?'

Sally: 'I'm not allowed to.'

Elisabeth: 'Why not?'

Sally: 'Because this is a hospital and it's considered unethical for staff to buy cigarettes for patients.'

Elisabeth: 'You agree with that do you? You smoke yourself, you bloody hypocrite.'

Sally: 'Well – I –'

Elisabeth: 'Look what I'm saying to you is if you want to help me go and get me some fags. You know I'm stuck in this bloody wheelchair and I can't get to the shops. You're the one who's always talking about choice – well,

I'm choosing to smoke, and if you don't get me my fags then you're denying me the choice of how to live my life.'

It was a truly ethical dilemma. I thought about it. Elisabeth winked at me.

'If you get me my fags I'll come to your stupid group,' she said.

The dilemma was solved, and I ran off to the shops.

Later, when I was being disciplined, the Charge Nurse reminded me of one of our foremost rules – never use bribes as a means of getting a patient to do something. He did not seem to understand that it was I who had been bribed.

Elisabeth came to the group, sat rigidly silent throughout, and pretended not to be looking at the old photographs we were passing around. The group was run by letting the patients take the lead. We provided stimuli, in the form of old objects and photos, and then followed whatever conversations emerged. One of the patients, Eva, who had been diagnosed as having Alzheimer's, was vividly remembering the war, describing how she had sat in an air raid shelter, listening to the bombs fall and holding hands with her brothers and sisters in the candlelight.

'It was awful,' she was saying. 'Ooh, it was terrible, but when we all held hands I felt alright – I wasn't scared then.'

'Yes,' agreed Millicent. 'If we just hold on we'll be alright.'

'Shall we do that now?' suggested Jenny. 'Come on, let's hold hands.'

Everyone tentatively reached out, except Elisabeth.

'What are you then?' she asked Jenny. 'Some kind of lesbian or what?'

'Oh that's it,' said Eva 'Don't we look funny – but it's ever so nice.'

Everyone agreed.

With a look of disgust and a sigh of resignation Elisabeth slipped her hand into mine and stared intently out of the window. I was surprised at how much her hand was shaking. Everyone else carried on talking about the war, and the circle of hands remained intact until the end of the group.

The following week Elisabeth came to the group again and once again kept silent for the most part, except for occasionally correcting people on the dates of certain notable events. Towards the end of the group, however, she began to fidget, and I could tell she wanted to say something. The other patients were animatedly discussing ration books and Jenny asked Elisabeth what she remembered missing during the war.

'Are we going to hold hands again?' asked Elisabeth.

BEYOND WORDS

The importance of touch cannot be underestimated, particularly for the elderly who have perhaps lost intimate relationships, and who are often acutely aware of the degeneration of their bodies. It is sad that in our culture old age is so often equated with ugliness, and the simple joys of stroking and caressing are often not on offer to the elderly. Much has been made of the benefits of animals for old people and a local resident in the community frequently brought her pet labrador into the day hospital for the patients to pat. But I think this can only be a substitute for the human physical contact which is missing in so many elderly people's lives.

Jenny, the occupational therapist, developed a very successful 'hand massage' session as part of a gentle exercise group, basically just stroking and rubbing the fingers, hands and wrists, an activity organised in pairs which was so popular that it frequently became a part of the 'talking groups' too, at the request of the patients. Obviously touch is very emotive and can produce both pleasant and unpleasant feelings, so one must always be cautious in instigating physical contact, but I found Jenny's hand massage work to be extremely effective and acceptable in an unthreatening way to most people across different cultures. As a two-way exercise it gives the patient not only the pleasure of receiving, but also of giving, and, for ourselves, there's a lot to be said for the experience of really *seeing* and *feeling* a hand that has worked through a lifetime.

Elisabeth became our top hand masseur and progressed quickly to necks and shoulders. She still said very little, except when she needed cigarettes, or to put one of us in our place with her caustic wit, but she consistently attended the reminiscence group, which Jenny had eclectically re-named 'talking and touch'.

It was a long time before Elisabeth told her story. There is an uncomfortable feeling about silence, but for Elisabeth, and for many of the patients I worked with, silence can be a powerful form of communication. I was a little nervous of Elisabeth: she had a sharp tongue and a knack of homing into people's weaknesses, but I began to make time to sit with her for short periods. I always asked her permission and she always gave it, with important reservations.

Sally: 'Can I sit with you for a while?'
Elisabeth: 'If you must.'
Sally: 'Does that mean you'd rather I didn't?'
Elisabeth: 'You can sit next to me but don't start asking me any of your stupid questions.'

So Elisabeth and I spent many times together sitting in silence. The odd thing was that Elisabeth did not show the least anxiety about this. Often when I went into work she would nod at me and then at the empty chair next to her, but when I went to join her she would not say a word. The anxiety was all mine. I was confused about my role but I felt somehow that what was happening was important. Here was a woman who was in such great pain that she had tried to take her own life. I concentrated on my own feelings, what was making *me* uncomfortable in the silence, and gradually I was able to relax with Elisabeth. I need not, however, go into the immense derision I received for going to work, sitting on my arse and saying nothing. It was many years later that a supervisor in the social services pointed out to me that this was probably my greatest skill, and he wasn't being sarcastic. I think what many professionals find difficult is simply to *be with people,* and to allow them to be as they are. When confronted with extreme emotional distress I think there is a natural urge to *do* something, to *say* something, to *change* something, and we can so easily forget that the first step is to hold what is there.

For Elisabeth I think both silence and touch were important factors in allowing her to feel safe enough to tell her story, which eventually she did. And I cannot begin to do justice to that story, which was the stuff of great novels, and yet which was sitting there before me, very much in reality. Gradually over the first six months of the reminiscence group Elisabeth began to talk about her life, not just to me but with other staff and patients in the reminiscence group. She was an incredibly bright woman with a great deal of insight, and her observations ceased to be vindictive and began to be useful to herself, to other patients, and to me.

Something that had always interested me was how the reminiscence group always ended up talking about the war. It had always seemed to me that the war was remembered for being a happy time when people bonded together with united purpose and great camaraderie, but Elisabeth shed more light on this. We were passing around an old ration book.

Eva:	'Ooh, yes, I remember that – look, two ounces of butter – you had to spread it on thin, but it tasted like heaven. I used to cycle 15 miles up to the farm for a single egg.'
Elisabeth:	'You really appreciated it, didn't you? Not having so much.'
Eva:	'Oh yes. But you always wanted more!'
Elisabeth:	'Well, we're on short rations now, aren't we, love?'
Eva:	'Rations?'
Elisabeth:	'Well, life's rationed isn't it – and we've nearly used up all our tokens.' (Everyone nods.)
Elisabeth:	'I mean, it's a bit like the war now, isn't it? That's what it was like. Never knowing if you'd be blown up, or if you'd see your brother again. I feel like that now – I could go any minute.'

So it was that Elisabeth began to make connections between the stroke she had recently suffered and her subsequent suicide attempt. Although she had never talked about the stroke, and brushed it off to her friends and family, the threat of illness and death had been terrifying for Elisabeth, and had thrust her into a deep depression. Noel Hess (1987) has written about this fundamental anxiety of old age: the dread of being abandoned to a state of utter helplessness which can easily be triggered by the catastrophes of old age, such as stroke and dementia. Again I feel that Elisabeth would have benefited enormously from talking to a trained psychotherapist, but what struck me most was that, given time and the space to interact *as she chose*, she naturally progressed to identifying her internal turmoil and resolving her conflicts. For Elisabeth, as for everyone I worked with, the past was essential in understanding the present.

EVERYONE HAS A PAST – EVEN JIMMY

The reminiscence group was eventually grudgingly accepted by the staff as being beneficial but only, it was stressed, for those patients who were 'intelligent and articulate', i.e. those not suffering from dementia. Jimmy, meanwhile, continued to rampage around the hospital, despite his ever-increasing dose of tranquillisers.

One day, as we sat looking at some favourite photos of the war Jimmy stormed into the reminiscence group, kicked a chair across the room and told us all to fuck off and fuck ourselves. Never one to miss an opportunity Jenny silently showed him a photo of Hitler. Jimmy stared hard at the photo and then snatched it from Jenny's hand.

'Fucker!' he shouted at Hitler.

Jenny handed him another photo, this time of a group of British soldiers in uniform. Jimmy took the photo and looked at it intently. Then he looked up at the group. We waited. Jimmy looked back at the photo and then turned to us – and saluted. It was the first time I had ever seen him smile. Suddenly everyone was saluting and Elisabeth started singing 'Pack up your troubles in your old kit bag and smile, smile, smile.' Jimmy was laughing a deep throaty chuckle and saluting us all and there was such a commotion that the Charge Nurse came in to see what all the noise was about. Jimmy saluted the Charge Nurse, and the Charge Nurse saluted Jimmy, and from that moment on everyone always addressed Jimmy as 'Sir!'

The change was both immediate and extraordinary. From a situation where it had taken two large male nurses an hour to get Jimmy dressed in the morning we found that now a single small member of staff could greet Jimmy with a salute, hand him the appropriate clothes and leave him to it. Of course sometimes he got it wrong. Jimmy still appeared for lunch with his jumper inside out or his shoes on the wrong feet, but given a salute and a prompt he would laughingly rectify the situation. The quality of Jimmy's life could not but improve. No longer afraid that he would smack a passer-by in the mouth, we were able to go out for walks with Jimmy, to the park and to shops. Jimmy had somehow found his passport to the outside world. He didn't talk but everywhere we went he made friends. It's amazing how many complete strangers will salute you in the street, given half a chance.

I had always been told that it was important never to collude with patients in their delusions, so our new way of working with Jimmy certainly posed some ethical dilemmas. Suddenly all the staff were behaving in an ostensibly bizarre manner, reinforcing some distant memory of another time and place. But the change in Jimmy seemed to justify it all, for not only was his care now easier to manage, but also for the first time in his hospitalisation he appeared to be happy.

No one will ever know what was going on in Jimmy's head, but by a stroke of luck and coincidence, something had triggered a resolution within him. A salute – that small gesture of respect – seemed to symbolise an entire agenda of interaction and communication which for Jimmy had been almost lost. Was our new mode of interaction patronising, infantilising and dishonest? I think rather that Jimmy had found a tolerable reality of his own, and that it was our duty to accept that reality as a peaceful end to his journey.

CONCLUSION

Everyone has a story. The way people tell their stories is infinitely varied and often the means of communication is very different to our own. I hope to have shown that certain ways of working with the elderly may actually deny patients their own reality and thus hinder what Elisabeth Kubler Ross (1969) sees as a natural resolution of conflict before death. I would suggest that the role of the nurse, therefore, should be as facilitator, enabling patients to define their own reality, to tell their own stories, to make sense of their own unique experiences, and to find peace at the end of their lives.

I found that working with the elderly was a two-way therapeutic process whereby I learned to value the wealth of the near-complete life cycle, and so gained insights into my own life. I no longer work in mental health, but this experience informed and enriched my current work as a writer, for I was given the gift of more stories than one could write in a lifetime. There are stories everywhere, all around us, better stories than any Hollywood movie or soap opera. All we have to do is stop and listen.

REFERENCES

Egan, G. 1990 *The skilled helper: a systematic approach to effective helping.* 4th edn, California: Brooks Cole Publishing.

Feil, N. 1982 *Validation – the Feil method.* Cleveland, Edward Feil Productions.

Hess, N. 1987 King Lear and some anxieties of old age. *British Journal of Medical Psychology* **60**, 209–15.

Kubler Ross, E. 1969 *On death and dying.* London: Routledge.

Menzies Lyth, I. 1988 The function of social systems as a defence against anxiety. In *Containing anxieties in institutions; selected essays.* London: Free Association Books, 43–85.

Morton, I. and **Bleathman, C.** 1988 Does it matter whether it's Tuesday or Friday? *Nursing Times* **84**(6), 22–7.

Segal, H. 1980 Fear of death: notes on the analysis of an old man. In *The work of Hanna Segal: delusion and artistic creativity and other psychoanalytical essays.* London: Free Association Books, 173–82.

Shakespeare, W. 1987 *King Lear.* Harmondworth: Penguin.

11

ASSERTING DIFFERENCE: PSYCHIATRIC CARE IN BLACK AND WHITE

Karla Boyce

As argued in the previous chapters, the negotiation of personal reality is a vital part of the therapeutic process. Our culture and our race are critical components of the 'reality' we experience. The positive acceptance and exploration of difference in race and culture between clinician and client are thus vital. Equally, attention to these issues in other areas of their experience is crucial. Clearly, any sense that particular cultures are 'alien' thus has enormous implications for the clinical work. Similarly, the sense that all cultures are the same will adversely affect the work. Here Karla Boyce reflects on her experience as a black student nurse and as a newly qualified black clinician in London. She describes the alienating effect of a system that expects assimilation without acknowledging difference. Developing a case study in which she was involved with the restraint and seclusion of a black woman, Karla explores the implications of this experience of alienation both for clients and clinicians. She discloses her own response to working in such an environment. Karla describes her attempt to change things locally, including involvement with a black women's staff group, a challenge to the procedures in the institution where she worked and the introduction of a course she devised on race, ethnicity and mental health.

When Ben Davidson trained with Karla as a mental health nurse they shared a trip to Friern Barnet hospital in North London, where the process of deinstitutionalisation was progressing apace. Nearly all of the patients, many of whom were lifelong residents of the institution, had been decanted into the community. Two striking pieces of history emerged from the visit. One was that the hospital boasted the longest corridor in Europe (substantially more than a mile in length), to which all the wards were connected. The experience of walking down that echoing, ghost-ridden tunnel from nowhere to nowhere else is unforgettable, and must be an endlessly recurring image in the mind of any former patient. But also of note was the institution's history, particularly to Ben Davidson as the grandson of East European Jewish immigrants who had come to England in fear of their lives around the turn of the century, escaping from pogroms in Russia and Poland. It appeared that the vast majority of the madfolk catered for by the institution in its early decades were Jewish émigrés, diagnosed mad but presumably responding to the impact of their oppression, dispossession, cultural and geographical dislocation and an experience of savage anti-Semitism in their new 'home' country. Presumably their presence was the reason the asylum had been located in this area.

Here the experience of racial discrimination and the impact of stereotyping on mental health and mental health care is discussed only in relation to black people. It may be objected that this is an omission, as the experience of racial and cultural prejudice, discrimination and disadvantage is far more universal. Which is true; of course the issues addressed apply to other groups, and are of universal importance. But the point which this chapter emphasises is how we may, individually or in groups, try to remain true to our experience and work with it to make a difference. Karla speaks from experience and if her experience conveys something of a practitioner at the start of a career, taking the greatest interest in issues that affect her personally, or if the reader is left feeling as though an oppressed minority may not be allowed much space for concern about other oppressed minorities, so be it. What it is hoped the chapter will also display is the possibility that one may use one's experience to make a positive difference, by asserting that *this is* the reality one is experiencing, in black and white terms or otherwise.

I am a black woman and a psychiatric nurse. This chapter is the product of reflection and study arising from my sense of being in a system that expects me to assimilate and accept it, but does not easily accept or acknowledge me for who I am. The ethical dilemma addressed throughout will be as follows: How differently should black people be treated in the psychiatric system and by psychiatric nurses?

In the first part, I shall reflect on my experience as a black psychiatric nurse, emphasising my training, but also as a newly qualified practitioner. Second, I shall explore the implications this has for a system that provides a service to black users. Third, I shall explore the dilemmas I face, describing how I try to use my experience to make a difference.

I shall conclude by emphasising the continuous nature of ethical strife, elaborating the problems in effecting change both practically in one's practice environment, and also within one's own experience and prejudice. I shall propose that a black person within a fundamentally white system can, nevertheless, assert one's difference to challenge assumptions and develop a more balanced interaction of cultures.

For my purposes here, I wish to use the following definitions of the terms used in the text:

BLACK PERSON	any person whose skin colour renders them liable to racism.
WHITE PERSON	any person whose skin colour does not render them liable to racism.
CULTURE	those ways of life including religion and spiritual practices, values, art, food, play, customs, which are shared with others of one's own race or ethnic group.
ETHNIC/ETHNICITY	an individual's identification with a group sharing some or all of the following – nationality, history, geographical origins, culture (including religion), skin colour, language.

(London Borough of Lambeth, 1992)

BLACK IN A WHITE SYSTEM

Black visibility: 'Do I belong here?'

As a black person in a mainly white society, I am acutely aware of my difference, and regularly question whether I belong here. It is important for me to find other black persons with whom I can identify and relate, who share and empathise with my experiences and with whom I can discuss common issues and obtain support and advice. As Fannon noted:

> To many colored intellectuals European culture has a quality of exteriority . . . the negro may feel himself a stranger to the western world. Not wanting to live the part of the poor relative . . . adopted son . . . bastard child . . . he feverishly [seeks] to discover negro civilization.
>
> (Fannon 1993 p. 203)

The experience of living in this society provides a constant reminder that I am part of a minority. When I was an undergraduate student, I was one of three black people in a group of more than 80. When I undertook nurse training, the picture was similar, where I was one of two black people in a group of ten. In my training hospital black nurses were 'thin on the ground', of the three wards where I was placed during training, only one had one black Registered Mental Nurse. One ward employed a black enrolled nurse on night duty and two black nursing assistants on days. The third had only one black nursing assistant. There was only one black nursing manager and one black ward manager in the whole hospital. There were, however, three black tutors and many black cleaning and catering staff. During two weeks of working night shifts, I noticed that there was a 'black network' on night duty. I did not reflect on this situation consciously at the start of my training. Indeed, I felt privileged that I had been let in to an exclusive club. Later, I reflected on the health and transport industries' recruitment drives in the West Indies in the 1950s. I wondered if that was still the lot that black people inherited in the Health Service: to do the jobs that others shunned – the 'nigger work'. I felt that black staff at my training institution were greatly undervalued. I could not understand why the organisation accepted a situation of apparent separation of staff by race, or why black people themselves accepted it. They were either token 'senior workers', or were located in less attractive positions. In this respect I was particularly struck by the numbers of black workers – more than half of them women – on permanent night duty. Here, there was no supervision, little or no opportunity for training, even less opportunity to develop clinical skills, and a metaphorical space where, significantly, black workers could be invisible.

Those black nurses on permanent night duty seemed to be alienated and excluded from the daily routine; powerless, in the sense that they did not have the opportunity to participate in decision-making, for example, in ward rounds during the day. In general, they had less opportunity to develop professionally and move up the career ladder.

Those other few black people in positions of power appeared to have been elevated as 'tokens', they were in a minority and isolated from their ethnic groups, and they thus ran the risk of being used as scapegoats in times of difficulty. Somewhat demoralised, I left the prestigious training institution where I had first become a nurse to seek employment elsewhere.

Needs: 'I am not the same!'

He who is reluctant to recognise me opposes me

(Fannon, 1993, p. 218)

In my training, neither race and cultural awareness, nor transcultural psychiatry were addressed. It was apparent that working with black people with mental health difficulties was a topic which warranted a place on the teaching agenda, given the significant presence of black people in the patient population. I and my other black colleague took it upon ourselves to use (some would say hijack) some of the peer group teaching sessions, which students took turns in leading, to fill the gap.

Our tutors coached us extensively before we embarked on the project. They prepared us for the possibility that we might be activating 'white liberal guilt', anger and resentment. We were left with a sense that the event had to be handled with the utmost delicacy. All this fuss made me angry. I was angry that I had to be gentle with a culture that has been oppressing and dominating black people for years. It felt as if I was being forced to say 'Excuse me, I'm terribly sorry but you've just slapped me in the face'.

> What then did you expect when you unbound the gag that had muted those black mouths? That they would chant your praises ? Did you think that when those heads that our forefathers had forcibly bowed down to the ground were raised again, you would find adoration in their eyes?

(Sartre, cited in Fannon 1993).

In attempting to address race and culture, I and my fellow student focused on the West Indian culture that we knew. Since it is based on my experience, this chapter, similarly, is biased towards exploring the dynamics of race as they affect Afro-Caribbeans. However, there are many cultures and disadvantaged groups that come into contact with the mental health service, for example those from the Asian sub-continent, Arab-speaking countries and, much closer to home, the Irish community. All these peoples experience similar issues of oppression, alienation and exclusion. I trust that while my account will be based on my own experience, the universal themes relating to race and oppression will become evident.

What I had hoped to get from my tutors was positive support, nurturing and a sense of their own enthusiasm. I was frustrated because, instead, I sensed their fear and apprehension about what might be brought up by addressing these issues. They may have felt they were supporting us (the black minority), even protecting us from an unexpected angry reaction from the group. It seemed, however, as if the (white) group were offered support (through us) in dealing with their (potential) anger, rather than us being offered support with our feelings.

From tutors – both black and white – there was no real commitment to exploring and providing for the very different needs of black student nurses, nor to exploring and providing for the needs of the black users we served. Supervision by black tutors, and environments where we could talk openly and honestly about our experiences with other black students and professionals, were rare. I struggled to find a space where we could explore what we had to offer the organisation as black people.

As we were trying to arrange our placements I was informed of some mental health projects specifically requesting black students. I was not quite sure what was the agenda. Did the organisation have something specifically to offer black students, or did they wish merely to use us to give the appearance of a multi-cultural team, thus tokenising and exploiting us? It was unclear whose needs were being met. Our curiosity got the better of us, though, and my black colleague and I accepted one such placement. Our fears were not realised. Instead we found a supportive and racially aware staff team, who accepted us as black people and encouraged us to assert our difference. The team were also sensitive to our special needs and keen to learn from us as we were to learn from them. This experience, however, was the exception. More commonly during our training, as I have described above, I felt that the emphasis was on assimilation into the institution, without much exploration of the tension between the psychiatric system and those people from different cultures whom it purported to look after.

High expectations

One hundred years ago, some black people were slaves, and there were commonly held assumptions that their intelligence was inferior to that of white people. This has left a legacy, the echoes of which I believe live on in the psyche of all black people. There is a common assumption made by black people that they have to be one hundred times better than a white person to make progress in 'their' world.

> There is a fact: White men consider themselves superior to black men.
>
> There is another fact: Black men want to prove to white men, at all costs, the richness of their thought, the equal value of their intellect.
>
> (Fannon, 1993 p. 12)

I sometimes feel ashamed to say 'I don't know' or 'I don't understand', for fear that my ignorance may be interpreted as stupidity. Asking for help or making a mistake are dilemmas, because I am validating commonly held stereotypes of the stupidity of black people. I feel reluctant to show any sign of weakness sometimes, because it makes me vulnerable and inferior and I am anxious to prove otherwise.

After completing my training I needed to get a work permit. The criteria stated at the time that, as a citizen of Trinidad and Tobago, to be given a job in the United Kingdom, my employers had to go to elaborate lengths to prove they could not find a British person or someone within the EEC to do the job. I was warned that when applying for jobs, some employers would not even consider my application because of this inconvenience, and, indeed, I had many rejections. My present employers waited three months for me to start work as the permit application was processed. I felt very grateful to them and was keen to show my gratitude by giving 101 per cent to my job. I felt that this was also necessary to ensure that my employers felt I was worth the trouble when the work permit needed renewal. The notion of having constantly to prove myself better than white peers is not simply my black fantasy. Government legislation dictates that if I am to continue to get employment in this country, I have to prove that I am better than professionals in Britain and Europe.

Cultural bilingualism: 'leading a double life'

Cultural bilingualism refers to the balancing act of living in two cultures. For many black workers in the NHS this means maintaining a balance between participation in the dominant, white culture at work and the minority culture which is the individual's own. Making the shift to a new culture involves fine tuning one's psychic antennae to the norms and aspirations, and sometimes the language and dress of the other culture, to show one is willing to fit in and establish oneself as able to do the work. It also involves making similar adjustments in attuning to clients' needs in a service that provides care mainly for white Europeans. Adopting the values of another culture can cause conflict within the individual, as they begin to lose sight of who they are and where they come from. One has to attempt to maintain a complicated balance of attempting to belong, yet asserting one's difference.

From a black perspective, evidence of this double existence is sometimes very visible, tangible and obvious. We may wear different clothes or speak a different language or with a different accent at work. I heard recently from a white Welsh colleague, whose manager had instructed her to get rid of her Welsh accent, when presenting material at conferences for the institution. Evidence of this double existence is often less visible, tangible or obvious. But the difficult balancing act of cultural bilingualism is always there for a black worker in a white institution, and real conflicts arise for black professionals working with both black and white service users, and also other black, as well as white staff, as they attempt to represent a white European service. Black workers may be viewed with suspicion and ambivalence by both staff and clients, both black and white. On the other hand, black service users may have increased expectations from a black worker.

IMPLICATIONS FOR SERVICE USERS

Psychiatry, power, control and oppression

Psychiatry is rooted in European culture. Its methods may not be universal to all the world's peoples. We must remain aware of culturally different idioms of distress, and the implications they pose for psychiatric diagnosis. Culture influences the way in which distress is conceptualised, communicated and resolved with others. Being encouraged, or even coerced into forgetting your own culturally-derived methods of coping is a facet of psychiatric treatment for black people. People who find themselves distressed in an alien culture are unlikely to find it easy using the symbols of the dominant culture to articulate their distress and obtain help. At such times it is particularly hard to express oneself in another tongue. Under stress, we all resort to patterns of communication that are most natural to us.

The cross-cultural variability in diagnostic patterns, and the political and racist implications of this variability also need to be highlighted. Littlewood and Lipsedge (1989) suggest that the frequent diagnosis of black people with schizophrenia, and the infrequent diagnosis of depression, validates cultural stereotypes. The images associated with schizophrenia suggest the bizarre, the irrational, what is outside and scary. Some 20–30 per cent of black patients are in hospital involuntarily compared to 8 per cent of white in-patients (ibid). This phenomena, some argue, is because blacks are regarded as more anti-social and dangerous, and the police are more likely to be involved in their admission. I have also known psychiatrists to teach that illness in blacks is organic and therefore the symptoms are more toxic and less responsive to social context. The perceived uncooperative nature of blacks may determine their transfer to secure units, a phenomena which does not necessarily reflect that they are more violent than whites. What is taken to be confirmation of irrationality and lack of insight may be no more than refusal of unfair treatment and physical resistance to a situation of unequal power.

Historically, psychiatry has been used to justify atrocities. It was suggested that it was acceptable to enslave black people as it suited their natures, they were happy in that state. 'Drapetomania' was an illness afflicting black slaves, the 'morbid desire to run away from the slave colonies'. In the absence of evidence of criminal activity, police may even today use sections of the Mental Health Act as a means of arresting someone for being racially or culturally different, expecting psychiatric endorsement for this practice.

Away from psychiatry *per se*, black people are less likely to be referred for psy- chotherapy through stereotypical perceptions of them as non-compliant, irrational, aggressive, emotional and non-verbal. Also, psychotherpay is a 'talking cure', and people who speak with a different accent may be thought to have a poor command of English. And again, as Kareem and Littlewood (1992) suggest, the power relationship that exists in therapy may be unacceptable to blacks, who are naturally already sensitive to such power imbalances.

Psychotherapists work with the patient's inner world, while psychiatrists work with his body and behaviour, both typically reluctant to address outer realities. In each case, by not acknowledging a person's race, culture, gender and social circum- stances, they effectively fragment the person. The general assumption is that overall responsibility for distress lies with the patient. In reality, there are socio-political and economic factors over which the individual has little control, affecting their inner world, for example prejudice, poverty, racism, sexism and social disadvantage. Not taking these into account denies a fundamental characteristic of the person and a crucial aspect of his problems.

Case study

I met Beatrice when working in an inner London acute admissions unit. Beatrice was a 55-year-old black Afro-Caribbean woman with a long history of mental illness, and had often been a patient on the ward. On this occasion, she was admitted informally, because her family were having difficulties coping with her at home. Six days after her admission, Beatrice assaulted two members of staff. She had run out of money to buy cigarettes, and she felt that the staff were withholding her money. She was put into seclusion for eight and a half hours. I met her when I agreed to do an overtime shift as a bank nurse. My task was to stand outside the seclusion room. Under no circum- stances was I to enter the seclusion room alone or open the door (although I was given the key). I could, however, communicate with Beatrice via an intercom and we could both see each other through a window in the door.

When I first saw Beatrice in the seclusion room, she was walking around, dancing and singing loudly, banging on the door, demanding to be let out and to speak to her doctor. She was ripping paper off the walls, attempting to break the mirror and smash the windows. She responded to no attempts at verbal engagement by me, except for shouting at me to 'open this door!'. One of my first thoughts was that this woman could be my mother. I also realised that, apart from Beatrice, I was the only black person around (a black male agency nursing assistant appeared later on). I empathised with some of the powerlessness and helplessness that she must have felt. As I was a bank nurse I was principally an extra pair of hands. I was not involved in the decision-making processes, and I had to be fairly tactful. I remember asking the ward staff a lot of questions about Beatrice and why the situation had arisen. It became important to me to make some sense of this situation. The more I questioned, the more irritated the staff seemed to become. There was a sense of frustration and a feeling that Beatrice had got what she deserved. It had become increasingly difficult and eventually impossible to manage Beatrice's behaviour on the ward. But what was glaringly obvious was that there was a complete breakdown in communication between Beatrice and the staff. One of the nurses commented after an interaction with Beatrice through the intercom: 'I've lost any rapport I had with her.'

There was also fear. There were several people milling around outside the seclusion room door discussing the case, and occasionally observing the 'mad black woman', as they appeared to view her. Beatrice was really putting on a show. She seemed to be expressing her distaste at being confined in seclusion. On three occasions during my shift, the room was entered by staff. Once, for an independent psychiatrist assessment for possible detention under a section of the Mental Health Act; second, for a social work assessment as part of the same process; and third, to offer some food and medication. Beatrice was co-operative. She was told to sit on the floor as four nurses and the independent doctor entered the room, while other onlookers stood at the doorway. Everyone stood while interviewing Beatrice. Beatrice was co-operative in answering questions. Although she began to get quite angry towards the end, she did not once rise from the floor. I could feel the nurses' anxiety as they shuffled to get out of the room, pushing people in front and complaining that the black male agency nurse had stayed in the room too long. I began to wonder how much of a chance this woman had been given to express what was going on for her before she was secluded. I wondered whether it was a case of assuming that black meant violent!

Beatrice continued to demand to be let out. She continued to damage the fabric of the room and urinate and defecate on the floor. The registrar on the ward commented on her 'mad behaviour' in a jovial way. I felt very irritated with him and made a sarcastic remark about his ability to comprehend madness as opposed to an expression of frustration – he ignored me. Her periods of pacing and shouting were interspersed with periods where she sat on the floor. At one point later on in the evening, Beatrice was sitting crying. I struggled to establish, in my own mind, the therapeutic benefit of this intervention. As far as I could conclude there was none. It was clearly a punitive measure designed to frustrate, humiliate and intimidate. I felt angry and ashamed to be taking part in such a practice. Later in the evening, Beatrice's son arrived. The nurses spoke of trying to 'bring him round to our way of thinking'. This spoke volumes. Clearly, they felt their way of proceeding was best and had little respect for what he might have to say. The family had opposed the use of the Mental Health Act in the past, and were unhappy also about Beatrice's being medicated. Previously, she had experienced adverse reactions to psychotropic medication. On one occasion she had been unable to walk. Beatrice's son was briefed on the situation and allowed to visit her in seclusion with one nurse. Beatrice's son found his mother reasonable after his visit and asked for her to be removed from the room. The staff cited her dancing and singing and damaging the seclusion room as evidence of her mad behaviour, to which the son replied: 'She's frustrated.' This discussion escalated into a stand-up argument between one of the nurses and the son, in full view of the other patients, with little regard for confidentiality. Soon the hospital security guards appeared on the ward, followed by the police! Beatrice's son finally asked if he could take his mother home, because he felt that the seclusion experience was unacceptable and was in no way therapeutic. The nurse in charge said that, if the consultant agreed, she would allow it.

When my shift ended the police were trying to convince Beatrice's son of the need for psychiatric care, as the nurses had washed their hands of the situation. They were no more prepared to hear his point of view than the nursing staff. Instead, he was obliged to accept theirs. I phoned the ward the following day to find out the outcome. I was told that Beatrice was detained under a Section of the Mental Health Act at ten past midnight. She had been in seclusion since midday. Later on her relatives had allegedly 'assaulted staff and busted Beatrice out of hospital'. I felt rather amused and delighted by the family's intervention.

Lessons to be learned

When black people come into contact with the psychiatric services, the relationship which develops may replicate the power dynamics of racist oppression. On a very basic level this occurred in the above scenario, in relation to Beatrice and interactions with her family. The development of a collaborative relationship is crucial to psychiatric nursing and, of course, relationships are based on communication. This case study shows the poor quality of the staff's relationship with a client who, supposedly, was well known to the service. An assumption is commonly made that black people are non-verbal, dangerous, violent and uncooperative. Beatrice appeared to be viewed this way. However, defiance, or other related defences, are predictable responses from people who expect to be abused or neglected, whatever their background. I had asked the staff whether anyone had explained to Beatrice that her money had run out, only to be told that she was too 'mad' to engage in such an exercise. However, the Beatrice I saw interviewed by the independent psychiatrist was able to account for what she had done with her money, to the last pound. What seemed to be occurring was some form of misunderstanding about extra money, which Beatrice thought the staff were withholding, which they had not bothered to explore with her.

Communication with Beatrice's son was equally appalling. Before he arrived, there was talk of 'bringing him round to our way of thinking'. It was obvious from the start that his views were not going to be held in much esteem. The racist fears and assumptions of the team were apparent by the call for the hospital security and the police. The failure, or reluctance, to establish any kind of productive rapport was demonstrated by handing over to the police the task of convincing Beatrice's son of his mother's need for hospital treatment. The staff's efforts to 'shout down' the son, resulted in an all too public breach of confidentiality, which served only to ridicule Beatrice's son in front of the whole ward. His powerlessness was reinforced when faced with two agents of social control, the hospital and the police. His concern for his mother, who in his culture was someone to be respected and valued, was ignored. Instead, he was faced with a situation where his mother was being humiliated, frustrated, punished, neglected and misinterpreted. Instead of an exploration of these issues, he was encouraged to accept passively the team's perspective, that his mother was 'difficult to manage on the open ward'. This situation illustrated clearly white workers' fears and expectations of a black client (and her family). It also shows how their subsequent conduct, based on these fears and resulting from their inability to deal with the difficulties of the situation, reinforced oppression due to their poor communication. Their response to the situation from the outset appeared to involve no more than the exercise of power to deal with a client whom they found difficult, for their own reasons.

Young Afro-Caribbean males are more likely to be diagnosed as schizophrenic than the indigenous population (Cochrane, 1977). Black patients are more likely to be perceived as aggressive, irrational and violent, therefore needing to be controlled and kept passive, as they may be dangerous or unsafe. Racist mental health practice reinforces stereotypes of difficult, unmotivated, non-verbal, dangerous black clients. These stereotypes often avert appropriate responses. One thing that was clear from the above scenario was that seclusion was not the best response to the situation. Apart from its punitive value, seclusion served only to frustrate and anger Beatrice further. It destroyed any working relationship between staff and client, however tenuous. It served to reinforce in Beatrice's son's mind any suspicions he had about the service's inability to care for his mother. No attempt was made to address issues of racism.

The reaction to the fantasy of black violence was shocking, as it manifested both in the seclusion and in relation to Beatrice's son, when the staff felt it necessary to call security, then the police, when he began to argue his mother's case. No attempt was made to give myself or the other black agency nursing assistant an opportunity to advocate. In that sense, our specialist status as black people was devalued. We might have been used to communicate with Beatrice's son. Instead, the black agency nursing assistant was criticised for his attempts to get involved and establish rapport with Beatrice. I was given the job of gaoler, and was excluded from any of the decision-making processes. My skills as a health care professional were ignored. Although I was part of the racist organisation, I myself felt trapped, excluded and alone. I struggled to find a useful role for myself. I wanted to empower Beatrice's son in his struggle against the organisation. I wanted to be involved in working towards a productive solution to Beatrice's predicament, rather than a punitive, oppressive and anti-therapeutic one, which was operating. Yet, as a representative of the organisation, I had a responsibility to carry out the decisions made. Additionally, because of my status as a bank nurse, I had to accept exclusion from the decision-making process. I felt as if I had sold out on my race, and I was angry with the organisation for putting me in such a position.

THE WAY FORWARD

There are complicated dynamics in operation when a dominant cultural system works with peoples from other races or cultural backgrounds. When dealing with something we are not familiar with or do not understand, we all rely on our own assumptions. Today, many of those assumptions are influenced by the media. Difference sometimes makes people afraid and anxious. For 'the Other' in the dominant society, blending in and invisibility may seem to be the easiest option. Could this be a reason for the unfortunate scenario discussed above?

Challenging prejudice requires energy and vigilance. Sometimes such a sense of shock is felt by a racial attack, that one is not always able to respond immediately. Also it may be easier to pretend that nothing really happened. On many occasions, I have had the 'you should have said something' battle with myself. But what does one say, and how does one say it? Do you express the unacceptability to you of the person's comments? Do you react angrily and abuse them as they have abused you? Is it always possible to overcome the hurt and anger and formulate a clear constructive response? Or does one need to learn to hold on to those unpleasant feelings? Sometimes a sense of confusion is the only outcome.

Experiences of racism are often obvious. But at other times, they may be very subtle, and the recipient may just feel a sense of injustice and shock, but is unsure or unable to pin it to one specific thing. Sometimes there is confusion about whether you are being oversensitive, or whether there is a real issue. To deal with these uncertainties, I felt that I needed to take action. This resulted in three main areas of change. First, learning to accept, hold on to and project my blackness. Second, joining a group of black women whose aim was to review the position of black women in the organisation; and finally, introducing training on race and ethnicity and mental health to my training institution.

Holding on to my black self

To survive in a system which has difficulty in integrating difference, I felt that I had to develop a strong sense of my different self. It involved constantly fighting a desire to conform, giving myself permission to be different, accepting and being comfortable with my difference and projecting it as positive and acceptable. Part of this struggle was reflected in my hair, which I had straightened and worn in a European style for years. In the past few years, I have made a conscious decision to wear it in a natural style. I have made a conscious decision to hold on to my Trinidadian accent, which is unique to me and the culture I come from. Sometimes people may not take time to tune in and understand different regional or foreign accents. Indeed, some people may devalue what is said, because it is presented in a different accent.

It is important for me to continue developing an awareness of cultural differences and making them known to white colleagues, so they too may understand. I work hard at examining what it means to be black and work towards developing self-love and self-awareness. Mixing with other black professionals and reading literature by black authors is also important. Reminding myself of the things we have in common as black people and giving myself a sense of identity and belonging are crucial. It is easy to become fragmented and out of touch with one's cultural group. Or to feel one's experiences of racism are isolated, or the result of some form of 'paranoia'. In response to experiences of racist stereotyping and discrimination it is important to make a statement to the person about how the experience of racism or discrimination makes one feel, thus facilitating a discussion on reasons, motivations and different ways of proceeding.

Black people have come to internalise and expect discrimination, and in some cases may accept it passively because they feel they have no choice. It is important to demand respect and the right to be heard. Crucially, one has to constantly make an attempt to speak up for ones-self and one's needs, and empower black clients to do the same. It is important to recognise discrimination and challenge it assertively and constructively. Sometimes it may feel awkward and uncomfortable to be different and the need to blend in may be far greater than one's ability to focus on the value diversity can bring to an organisation.

Joining a group of black women

At the group of hospitals where I was employed I became involved with NHS FEW (New Horizons for Ethnic Women), which comprised over 100 women from the service. One outcome from this involvement was the identification, and presentation to management, of what we had to offer the trust specifically as black women. I got involved in FEW after it was well underway. However, I was able to gain much from the experience. One of my first impressions was the sense of ease and comfort I felt in being around other black women. There was a feeling of support, common ground, shared purpose and belonging. People spoke freely and comfortably and I became aware of an unconscious process that goes on when I am in meetings with my white colleagues. I never say spontaneously what I am thinking, but I go over things in my head several times for appropriateness and accuracy, selecting only those which my colleagues might understand.

FEW also provided training for its members and we generated clear recommendations to the Hospital Trust about what we saw as priority developments. Among the recommendations which emphasised the special needs of black staff and patients were:

- Training in the management of diversity for the trust's managers.
- Training that specifically targets black and ethnic minority women.
- Managers working towards harnessing the benefits that cultural diversity could provide and rewarding it financially.
- Using black staff in the planning and provision of services for black people and rewarding this financially.
- Attempting to reflect the multi-cultural composition of its workforce and customers.

Given that 25 per cent of the Hospital Trust's clientele were black, it was evident that the Trust needed to listen to the voices of its 18 per cent black staff. This might make all the difference between customer satisfaction and dissatisfaction. NHS FEW showed that that black women had, and could use, a voice. One year after its inception, NHS FEW opened its doors to black men in the Trust.

Introducing training on race, ethnicity and mental health

Following my involvement in the construction of a course dealing with the planning of psychiatric care for women, it became clear that there also was a need for a programme which dealt with racial issues in care planning. The group leader felt that, as a white woman, she was unable to write a course on race, and invited me to develop a module on 'Race Ethnicity and Mental Health'. The programme aims were:

1. To enable practitioners to consider cultural differences and their impact on interactions when working with clients from culturally different backgrounds; and
2. To facilitate practitioners, both black and white, to become aware of their own cultural biases and assumptions and how these may influence their interactions.

The programme began with an examination of the history of black cultures and their encounter with European cultures. Issues like slavery in the West Indies, colonialism, immigration and the 'Othello experience' – being black in a predominantly white culture – were also addressed. Growing up in the West Indies, I studied West Indian history and have a reasonably firm grasp of such topics. It is surprising how many people in this culture, both black and white, have little or no knowledge about these topics. These issues have been forgotten, perhaps because of feelings of embarrassment and shame about the atrocities inflicted on the New World by the more 'civilised' peoples of the Old World.

The programme also looked specifically at racism, exploring definitions and people's experiences and feelings, especially in relation to stereotypes, such as the 'Big Black Man'. It is assumed that black men are large, strong and violent. This assumption may result in black men being sedated almost as soon as they enter the psychiatric setting. This stereotype was implicated in the case of Chistopher Clunis, where professional fears of holding such views appeared to lead to an abdication of responsibility for his care.

Psychiatry sometimes appears to work against the interests of people in general, dealing largely with concepts of normal and abnormal behaviour. Black people are often described in terms which emphasise their 'otherness' or alien status. Alternatively, European culture and Europeans are often depicted as 'normal'. Often this leads to black people – by their very blackness – being subjected to pathologisation. The programme emphasised examination of the power relationship that exists between patient and practitioner. Exploration of the potential this experience had for ressembling an experience of racism and oppression common to all black people was therefore addressed.

The programme suggested the importance of exploring misinterpretation. Mental health services are not set up to cater for black users. Rather, they have come to meet the services. This has the potential for despair being misinterpreted. The course also looked at the importance to black people of coping and 'keeping it in the family'. Finally, I hoped the course would allow students to explore some culturally specific ways of dealing with madness, with practitioners becoming aware of their own values, beliefs and assumptions, when working with users from culturally different backgrounds. Value judgements do not only take place in workers, both black and white, but in the user of the service also. There is a need, therefore, to look at the dynamics of black workers and black service users and white workers and black service users.

The module is growing in popularity and is constantly subject to revision. The students so far are mainly, although not predominantly, black. Some white people take the view that: 'I don't need to attend, I'm not a racist'. There is often a feeling that we may be 'preaching to the converted' or avoiding the more explosive issues. However, students do come with many fears and expectations about undertaking this sensitive, emotional work. Some have gone on to set up black groups in their clinical areas, and to share teaching with their peers on certain aspects of the course that may have been particularly important to them.

CONCLUSION

The struggle towards ethical conduct in the area of multi-racial work is complex, dynamic and constant. It is full of dilemmas for professionals, both black and white. For the black professional, they must decide when, if ever, to confront or challenge racism and discrimination. If they decide to do so, they run the risk of being seen as militant or aggressive. This response is likely to have the effect of devaluing their experience and making them anxious or reluctant to ever articulate their feelings again. They must bear the pain of living in a culture that has little respect for difference.

Black staff must be constantly fighting a battle inwardly and outwardly to determine their real value. They must fight to prevent 'cultural dissolution', and defend themselves against the pain of devaluation. This struggle can be difficult and frustrating, and some black people find it easier to 'turn a blind eye', perhaps being aware of what is going on and doing nothing, or perhaps even altogether denying the existence of any problem. When I first came to school in this country, I remember going home and being asked about racism in England. I remember replying that there was no racism in England and in fact I had never experienced any.

For some white professionals, there is a tendency to deny that racism or oppression occurs. They may refuse to recognise it, or make light of it, or become defensive. That is their defence. They may be afraid to acknowledge their fear of the Other, and react to this by trying to conceptualise difference in terms that are familiar. Thus they will make an opening for misinterpretation, frustration and sometimes a complete breakdown of communication. For those who are aware on some level, there is the shame and embarrassment which must be endured and the dilemma of deciding whether or not to take responsibility for the actions of their ancestors or forefathers.

Different cultures can live and work together in harmony, learning and growing with each other. In Trinidad and Tobago, Negroes, Indians, Chinese, Whites and mixtures of these races live together in harmony. This is not to say there is no racism or discrimination. But, on the whole, harmony is achieved. Different cultural celebrations are respected and recognised and on the whole, in the words of the Trinadadian anthem it is a place where 'every creed and race find an equal place'. With hard work and self-awareness, a more balanced interaction of cultures may be achieved and this might have important consequences for the relationship between differing cultures on different sides of the fence within mental health.

REFERENCES

Boyce, K. and **Preddie, S.** 1992: Nurse training. *The Bethlem and Maudsley Gazette: a cultural Issue* **39**(3). Winter, 23–4.

Fannon, F. 1993: *Black skin, white masks.* London: Pluto Classic.

Kareem, J. and **Littlewood, R.** (eds) 1992: *Intercultural therapy.* Oxford: Blackwell.

Kiev, A. 1964: *Magic, faith and healing.* New York: Free Press.

Littlewood, R. and **Lipsedge, M.** 1989: *Aliens and alienists.* London: Unwin Hyman.

London Borough of Lambeth Social Services 1992: *Good practice guide: working with black people with mental health difficulties.* London: London Borough of Lambeth.

12

WORKING WITH WOMEN

Dawn Thibert

Here Dawn Thibert looks at ethical dimensions of mental health ideology and care in relation to gender. She relates her discussion to clinical and personal experience. As with age, culture and race, so with gender and sexuality. Our experience of personal reality is inextricably bound up with our experience as men, as women, as gay, as lesbian, as heterosexual. Feminist critiques of psychiatry pay particular attention to such issues. They stress the effects of gender stereotyping in our reaction to bad experience e.g. men tending towards aggression and the penal system, women tending towards anxiety, depression and the psychiatric system. Having discussed these ideas, Dawn describes her experience of conducting a project to identify women's mental health needs in an inner city, community day centre. She looks at the impact of a women's project on the client group as a whole. Dawn conveys a sense of her own parallel struggle to find a space in the centre, both within the staff team and within the client group, as a lesbian woman. Dawn explores the difficulties in some aspects of this work, for example identifying needs, establishing realistic expectations and validating the right to be oneself. She then recounts the development of the project into an ongoing woman's group and concludes by discussing empowerment and the practical difficulties in encouraging women, herself included, to assert themselves.

To give the chapter some historical context Ben Davidson tried to find a passage which had struck him some years earlier in connection with psychiatry, gender and power. The reference was to the historical treatment of women in psychiatry. He asked the 250 members of an international psychiatric nursing list on the Internet for help. Did anyone 'recall reading a passage which describes a form of treatment being researched at an asylum in Britain, possibly last century, in which varying amounts of water were poured from different heights (I think through grills on successively high floors in what may have been a tailor-made tower) to establish the *therapeutic quantity* of water to be used and *correct force* to be applied, as well as the *optimum frequency* of treatment? I think the case in question was one where the patient, a woman, was sexually unresponsive, or possibly had unacceptable ideas of developing interests other than her husband, and the success of the treatment, her return to sanity, was evaluated in relation to the woman's readiness to resume her marital role.'[1]

---

[1] Two references came back:
Sklar, K. All hail to pure cold water! In Leavitt, J. (ed) 1984: *Women and Health in America*. Wisconsin: University of Wisconsin Press, 246–54 (thanks to Leana Uys, South Africa); and Hunter, R. and MacAlpine, I. 1970: *Three hundred years of psychiatry*. Oxford: Oxford University Press (thanks to Joseph Berke, London).

A number of interesting comments came back, three of which are reprinted below. First, two from a contributor in the US:

'BEN . . . While it can hardly be [disputed] that any system that has the power to define mental health can misused as a form of social control I HOPE you are not going to make the case that women are the gender most affected . . .

'In response to your earlier post asking why I cared if you were making the case for women being the most oppressed by psychotherapy . . . I was reacting simply to the whole notion of women being oppressed in the western world (probably the biggest myth EVER perpetrated in civilized society). Right now the whole psychotherapy field is rapidly becoming feminised . . . either by women themselves . . . or the "sensitive" guys who, raised in the 1950s and 1960s, saw their fathers disrespect their mothers and thought this to be oppression. Hell, I was one of them. I believed that since women defined their status as oppressed it must be so. HA!!! I'd give my eye teeth to have the range of choices western women have. IMO [in my opinion – ed.] it is MEN who are oppressed but taught to suffer in silence – the idiots don't have a clue. Sometimes it is possible to be so open-minded that your brains fall out'
    And then, a contributor from New Zealand offered the following:
'Ben, don't have a reference to help, just to say that even in today's world women still get cold water poured on their hopes and dreams. Good luck, Brenda.'

In this chapter I will focus on my experience of conducting a project to identify women's needs, and subsequently running a women's group at a Community Mental Health Day Centre where I worked for nearly six years. Prior to these initiatives I had been involved in several attempts to improve the service to women, as well as making a continual effort to welcome women individually, as women as a group were under-represented in their use of the service. The project, out of which the women's group arose, was a concentrated effort to get to grips with how we could better meet women's needs and improve the service offered to them.

    A number of ethical issues emerged in the course of this work. As my literature review will show, even just being a woman may be seen as problematic and unhealthy. I challenge these underlying perspectives in mental health service provision. As I shall describe, increasing 'women's space' disrupted the status quo at the centre, prompting a backlash from men opposing the women's group, which in turn contributed to the difficulty women found in accepting and using the physical space they were given. Ethical dilemmas thus arose: what is the best way to balance service provision for women and the client group as a whole? Should we collude with the oppression of women by allowing their needs to be put lower on the agenda; or risk disaffecting some men by insisting that women's issues are addressed? And, finally, from a therapeutic perspective, how should women be helped to explore their experience and be further empowered to make their own choices?

    I shall introduce the subject with a case history that describes the experience of many female clients I have worked with. Following this, I shall review some of the literature about women and mental health, relating some of the issues covered to the experience of the client introduced in the case study. I shall then describe the Day

Centre and women's use of it, and also the project I set up to identify women's needs and the women's group that grew out of this project. I shall then highlight some of the gender issues at play. Finally, I shall reflect on my experience of working with women, further elaborating some of the gender issues and dilemmas, and identifying key lessons learned.

Eva

Eva is a 60-year-old Afro-Caribbean woman. She came to live in England in her twenties. For most of her childhood she had been considered a troublemaker and hard to discipline. She had no friends and became quite isolated. From around nine years of age Eva was sexually abused by a pastor who had used his position to gain Eva and her family's trust. The attentions he forced on the child included sexual acts that Eva still finds too hard to describe. She experienced dread at the prospect of telling anyone what had happened. This resulted both from her family's reaction when she attempted to tell them what was happening and from the power of the pastor himself. He told her she must keep it a secret, that nobody would believe her anyway. Eva was afraid of him and had not made further attempts to tell anyone what was happening. The abuse continued to take place regularly over several years.

In the early 1960s, aged 24, Eva emigrated. She came to England alone, aiming to find work. Once in England, Eva trained as a dancer and travelled around Europe, especially Germany, with a dance company. She was raped twice during this time. She came back to England and had three children, not keeping contact with any of the fathers. Shortly after the birth of her first child, the pastor turned up on her doorstep unexpectedly. Feeling protective of her newborn baby, she found the strength to tell him to go away, but he continued to live in England. The compounded misery, abuse and turmoil of her life led to a series of breakdowns, episodes where she felt that she could no longer cope. As a single parent she had no alternative but to place her children in care each time she became 'unwell'.

Eva subsequently spent nearly forty years being treated by doctors and psychiatrists for depression. This was a major experience of her life. She was given medication and had many psychiatric hospital admissions. She tried to tell hospital staff during one such admission, possibly obliquely and no doubt hesitant about naming the experience, that she had been raped as a child. She did not feel believed. So, like the people caring for her, she once again forgot this experience.

When at the beginning of the 1990s she came to our Day Centre, Eva felt that staff *believed* her. The novelty of this experience for her was such that she expressed her gratitude openly. Over a period of some six weeks we met her regularly for hour-long sessions in which she told us some of her story. During these sessions Eva started to recover memories of her childhood sexual abuse, although she could not be sure it was not her fantasy. Staff suggested that the events plaguing what she called her imagination may actually have happened, and that it may help her to investigate this further. Accordingly, she began to see a specialist counsellor and we supported her in this.

Subsequently, we offered Eva a place twice a week in our drop-ins to make friends and be heard when she was angry, and we sometimes visited her at home if she was too depressed to make it out. She was angry frequently and in relation to all manner of conflicts she seemed to be involved in. For example, at one point she was in battle with the local authority over housing to which they said she was not entitled (she was squatting), with an airline over lost baggage they implied had not been lost or had not existed, with a shop over goods which they would not accept were faulty, with a removal firm over disputed damage to her furniture, with an insurance company over a refused claim. We were overwhelmed by the number and relentlessness of her battles, to the extent that a lot of her stories of day-to-day events took on an unbelievable character. An insensitive interpretation was once made, after she came in ranting about the latest event in one such dispute, to the effect that she might be bringing such battles on herself by taking the fighting stance she apparently always adopted. This prompted a dramatic reaction from Eva, including a relapse into depression. Like so many others, we had ended up symbolically replicating and reinforcing the disbelief she received on first trying to tell others what was happening to her as a child.

Eva has spent most of her life thinking that the abuse did not happen and she made it up. She feels she is bad. She is depressed. Through being diagnosed as mentally ill by the psychiatric system she has come to consider herself mad and her experience invalid.

When Eva recently found the strength to confront her abuser, an experience that made her feel thoroughly sick, he did not deny what had happened. Eva is at times angry both about the abuse and also about the treatment she received from the psychiatric system, where she sometimes feels her struggle to be believed and understood has been hindered far more than it was supported. At such times as these, when she has more faith in herself, she is relieved at the thought that she is reacting naturally to her childhood sexual abuse and other facets of a harrowing life story. However, Eva still finds it hard to trust her own memories.

GENDER ISSUES AND MENTAL HEALTH

I shall introduce the discussion by sketching some general themes that emerge from the current literature on gender and mental health. Following this, I shall represent in summary form some of the main areas, as I see them, where ethical strife is at the heart of our clinical practice.

It is well documented by many (Cooperstock, 1981, pp. 131, 137, 141) that women are more likely than men to use mental health services, be diagnosed mentally ill, be prescribed psychotropic drugs, and given electroconvusive therapy. Women receive the least serious and most poorly defined diagnoses, e.g., neurosis, psychosomatic illness, hysteria and depression, and they are more likely to attempt suicide. A lot of the literature concentrates on the dubiousness of these diagnoses, but recognises that women do tend to respond to disappointment or loss with depression rather than aggression. This could be a factor influencing women's higher use of mental health services, whereas men are more likely to be sent to prison for being aggressive and anti-social (Burns, 1992, p. 111; Weissman and Klerman, 1981, pp. 170, 174).

Explanations for this situation are scant, as hardly any psychological theories consider the issue of gender. Ussher (1991, pp. 116, 122), notes that psychoanalytic theory does consider gender, but reduces women to envious and inferior neurotics. Freud believed that women are biologically disadvantaged due to the lack of a penis, and have a difficult development through penis envy. Many female writers in psycho-analysis offer a different perspective. Indeed, Karen Horney, one of Freud's pupils, wrote about the implications of men envying breasts and the capacity for motherhood (Howell, 1981a, p. 4). The antipsychiatry movement, exemplified by Laing, was more notable for its concern about women, but had no coherent analysis to offer.

Bayes (1981, p. 83) describes how gender bias underlies theories and practice in the mental health field. And, as Howell (1981b, pp. 309–10) explains, treatment without regard to gender may not address women's particular issues, for example menstrua-tion, pregnancy, mothering role and mid-life transition. While women's reproductive processes from menstruation through to menopause have become the province of medicine, women are seen merely as at the mercy of their 'raging hormones' (Ussher, 1991 p. 249). Where mental health care is on offer, a knowledge of women's specific experiences and of how crises may be related to such issues is clearly needed to work competently and compassionately with their needs.

The defininition and treatment of women's distress: the feminine double bind

Inequality exists between men and women, where, on the whole, women are treated as a subordinate group and have lower access to power. Men as the dominant group have largely defined femininity and dictated its associated roles for women. Such stereotypes permeate structures in society (Howell, 1981a, pp. 2–26; Miles, 1988, p. 112). Having thus defined the traditional women's role, the dominant group have then devalued it: Women are looked down on as dependent on men and submissive. Subordinated groups such as women internalise the values of dominant social groups, and come to believe they are inferior and inadequate, developing low self-esteem. In addition, although prospects for women have greatly changed, accumulated changes in social organisation are now new sources of personal stress, as in the case of a woman managing a career, family and home commitments.

Replicating this general view of women as inferior, there are varying definitions of mental health between women and men. Broverman *et al*, (1981, p. 94) found that male and female clinicians applied an agreed general standard of health for adults only to men, and perceived healthy women as significantly less healthy.

Miles (1988, p. 11) notes that the aim of treatment can be to return women to their traditional role, which is often domestic, or to make 'bad' women 'good'. Women are seen as 'bad' in this respect when they deviate from their traditional, submissive role, e.g., when they are aggressive or violent, regardless of the circumstances occasioning such behaviour. Conversely, they are seen as 'good' if they adhere to such a role, even if this is a disempowered and therefore unhealthy position. Showalter (1986, pp. 120,145) found that women rebelling against their sex roles were in the past labelled with nervous disorder and hysteria.

While femininity itself is seen as inferior, women rejecting the devalued female role (and also women assuming this role *too much*) can be labelled psychiatrically ill (Chesler, 1982 p. 56), especially where behaviour is deemed mad because it breaks social rules. Thus, the medical and psychiatric understanding, diagnosis and treat-ment of women are all pervaded by the generally held stereotypes of what it is to be feminine; in turn, experts in mental health constantly reinforce such stereotypes

(Stephenson and Walker, 1981, p. 118). It seems that women are caught in a double bind, where both adopting and rejecting the feminine role are seen as pathological.

Medical versus social agendas

Ussher (1992, pp. 52, 56–7) notes that science in clinical psychology has developed as a masculine enterprise, top grades being dominated by men. Miles (1988, p. 131) and Ussher (1991, p.68) criticise the psychiatric model for treating women whose problems stem from social inequalities. Social, economic and legal problems, for example, can be defined as intrapsychic and misdiagnosed as psychiatric disturbances. Women's oppression can thus be defined as personal, ignoring sexism and disempowerment as factors in their distress, and avoiding any analysis of the social and political causes of women's distress. In Miles' (1988) study where women and men were interviewed about their psychiatric referral, more women than men felt their formulation of what was wrong was discounted and not believed, like Eva. More women than men felt their doctors minimised their complaints, lacked sympathy and were not taking them seriously, particularly when depression and neurotic problems were related to their reproductive processes (Miles, 1988, pp. 119–20, 126). Little wonder that many, including Showalter (1986, p. 125), consider the feminist therapy movement the best hope to meet women's needs. This movement has been instrumental, for example, in the creation of rape crisis centres and women's refuges.

As happened with Eva, treatment often does not begin to identify or tackle causes of unhappiness, merely medicating women in distress. After forty years of being treated in the psychiatric system, Eva thought that all of her problems were due to a medical complaint, 'depression' and downplayed the sexual abuse she had experienced as a child. As incest is rarely the problem women initially reveal, psychiatrists often miss this crucial factor, even though sexual abuse of girls and women is endemic in our society (Walker, 1992, p. 177; Ussher, 1991, p. 265). Indeed, until recently many psychiatrists felt that rape did not even create psychiatric issues. Although the negative effects of sexual abuse may not be obvious until a 'developmental trigger' occurs, these effects have been recognised to include personality and identity problems, difficulty with relationships, fear of attack from men, which can lead to agoraphobia.

Eva is constantly fearful of men, including male staff. When Eva first saw a black male student placed with us she saw the face of her abuser, she felt fearful and she shouted at him. She constantly fears men in the street and is ready to defend herself if she is approached. Recently she told us she had threatened someone who she believed was following her, with her walking stick. Such incidents raise so many feelings that she often feels depressed afterwards, possibly reflecting the helplessness, aloneness, confusion and powerlessness she felt at being sexually abused as a child. Linking her current feelings to her past experiences has helped her understand them better. It is not difficult to see how the effects of sexual abuse often get defined as 'mental illness'. Women may generally have learnt to express their distress in terms of symptoms of their 'illness', if this is the only way to feel heard.

Women as carers

Eva, like many women, struggled with family life unsupported. Motherhood is a difficult enough time, but psychiatric theory and practice blame mothers for their children's problems (Chesler, 1982, p. 74; Laing, 1967, p. 113). To exacerbate this, women frequently do not believe they have the right to put their needs on a par with those of their family (Brodsky, 1981, p. 615). It is not surprising that a poverty of supportive relationships is linked to depression in women.

The burden of care in the family, and also 'community' care, falls most often on women. As 80 per cent of carers are women, closing institutions without alternatives often throws patients onto unemployed female relatives. Carers are recognised as having needs in the 1990 NHS and Community Care Act, but it remains to be seen how well they will be met. The new Carer's Act 1995 gives carers the right to an assessment, but extra money is not being allocated to Social Services Departments to meet the needs identified.

Conclusion

The context of women's lives including sexism and racism needs to be taken into account, according to Westwood et al. (1989, p. 64), when trying to make sense of individual experiences and identify needs. However, much of the literature reviewed shows how the perception of women's needs and the way they are treated are distorted in mental health by an underlying sexist bias that devalues and pathologises women, whatever the social circumstances and whatever they do. Couple this with the fact that women generally do not expect their real needs to be met, and it is clear that it can be no easy task to identify or respond to what women need and want.

WOMEN AND THE DAY CENTRE

The Community Mental Health Day Centre is situated in one of the most densely populated areas of Europe and, according to Jarman (1983), the borough experiences almost the highest levels of urban social deprivation in Britain. The Centre has been open for over eighteen years, is run by a local authority Social Services Department, and has two sister Centres. At the time all three Day Centres were attracting predominately white, male clients, far exceeding the proportion of men or white people in the local and psychiatric hospital populations.

It was exciting to work in a non-problem-centred, health-orientated way, where strengths were emphasised and healthy aspects of a person encouraged to grow. A therapeutic service was provided where attention to and exploration of relationships were prioritised. The main features of the service were, an 'open door drop-in' (an open-access, informal, social environment used regularly by up to 40 clients with a range of psychiatric histories and mental health needs), and sessional work (i.e. focused psychotherapy) with individuals, couples and families. Women tended to use sessional work more often than men, but the drop-in was used predominantly by men. Their attitude to women was mostly to see them as a potential sexual partner. This made it an intimidating space for women. For example, on showing a young woman around the drop-in, she was welcomed by being asked to sit on a man's lap. I challenged the comment and tried to put her at ease saying that she did not need to expect such behaviour. She replied in a depressed way, 'It is the same in hospital'. She did not return.

This kind of welcome was also extended to new female staff. I often found myself feeling angry and protective of both female clients and staff being introduced to the drop-in. I had to control my anger at being referred to or treated as a sexual object. I faced the dilemma of whether to suppress my natural, angry reactions in an effort to engage with the men, many of whom did not seem to know any other ways to address women, or whether, more genuinely, to show how their conduct made me feel.

Even though the staff group gave a high priority to the exploration of gender issues and held anti-sexist values, men always held management positions and women made up the bulk of lower grade workers, reinforcing a sexist structure in the team. Female staff formed a subgroup to develop services to women, and immediately faced the question of how well this could be supervised and managed by men. This was not resolved, as when conflicts arose between female staff in the subgroup, our managers saw the need to take control. Nevertheless since November 1988, four initiatives for meeting women's needs were attempted, but attendance was poor and none of the projects continued to their end. The staff were left thinking that it would be difficult to get anything off the ground for women at the Centre.

When I looked at the Centre's current attendance statistics in April 1993, I was astounded to find that only 8 per cent more men than women had been assessed for the service in the previous four and a half years, but that at the time 43 per cent more men were using the Centre. Women were dropping out of the service at an alarming rate, clearly indicating that their needs were not being met.

THE PROJECT

Thus, when I had the opportunity to carry out a project in my workplace as part of an academic course entitled 'Innovations in Mental Health Work', I was keen to focus on women. My first task was to capture the imagination of the staff team and get them all involved. Fortunately this was not difficult and their enthusiasm helped to expand my initial aims, which had been to identify issues that were of particular concern to women and ascertain how they are regarded and dealt with in mental health care. I decided to involve male staff in the planning and organisation of the project, thinking that it would be more likely to succeed if we had their support. The final objectives were as follows:

1 To see what differences there were between the medical model and the model used at the Day Centre as a response to women's needs.
2 To see if in clients' experience any of these needs were addressed in the mental health care they received.
3 To consider whether the 1990 NHS and Community Care Act would address women's needs.
4 To raise the consciousness of women involved in the project about sexism and its effects, and empower both female clients and staff.
5 To identify areas of growth in service provision at the Day Centre to meet the needs of women.
6 To develop a women-orientated space at the Day Centre.

They sounded impressive in discussion and on paper, but in reality I felt daunted by the objectives, thinking it would be challenging enough to just run a women's group and motivate the participants to complete a questionnaire I had devised concerning their needs and whether these were met. A female colleague agreed to help me lead the women's group, which would meet fortnightly. We wanted to bring women using the Centre together, so that they could get to know each other. We were hoping to identify issues common to women and value their contributions, thus increasing their confidence and empowering them. We would demonstrate our appreciation for their participation in the project with 'treats' at group meetings and a free outing to the theatre, which would be a piece of groupwork in itself. We would encourage women to say what they wanted from the Day Centre in order to help improve the service offered to them. We hoped that awareness of women's issues would be raised as the women shared their experiences. Each group meeting would have the same structure, to provide continuity and boundaries. The main exercise or agenda for the next meeting would be planned by the staff in between each group, in a supervision meeting, responding to issues that had emerged. Informal time for the women to be together without staff was built in immediately before and after each group meeting.

The next task was to get women to come to the group! I quickly learned to adjust my language and the concepts I used. When I first talked about the 'project', women looked at me blankly, presumably because even with my explanations it just did not make sense to them. I then emphasised that the women's group would be fun, and 21 women showed interest! I kept them informed of our plans by letter, which turned out to be greatly appreciated. Subsequently letters were sent every fortnight in between the groups, describing how the previous group had gone and setting out what was planned for the next one.

The group, which met nine times for the project, attracted 16 different women (six black and ten white), over half of whom were older than 50 and most of whom had long psychiatric histories. In the first two meetings we identified issues and needs to be included as items on the questionnaire. In the next 'house meeting' (a meeting in the Centre involving all clients and staff, held monthly) I talked about the project. Some men reacted very negatively, opposing the women's group. They asked for a men's group. This had happened before when a women's group was announced, but nobody attended the men's group set up at their request.

The next women's group meeting (attended by 12 women) was spent discussing how women had felt in this house meeting and how they wanted to respond to what was said. After a very lively discussion, some women were left feeling uncomfortable and uneasy at spending their women's group talking about men. In the fourth meeting we tried to address left-over feelings from the last group, acknowledging differences between us. We then talked about what we might want a women's group for. After this group we had an outing as a treat and a thank you for participating in the project, after which I sent out the questionnaire. In the fifth group we asked why women came to the Day Centre and what they would do if they did not come. As many women were asking for help to complete the questionnaire, we then looked at methods for gaining information, and found that an interview was preferred. We started to look at how we could make the extension, a relatively new part of the building in which the group was held, more inviting to women. This part of the building was subsequently designated as women-friendly space and the women's group continued to be held there. In the seventh group we focused on fun, playing a game of quoits (throwing loops on a pole for points). This was very successful, provoking a lot of laughter, and provided an outlet for competition between women. In the following group we agreed that the group should continue, as after the initial nine sessions, 'the project', was over. The last group was spent giving each other feedback. I was touched by how much love and appreciation was expressed.

By the last meeting, staffing at the Centre had decreased leaving just me and a relatively new deputy manager. I was left struggling with a massive agenda devised by a full staff team, which felt overwhelming at times. My involvement was important as a focal point for the project, which I had to balance with the huge amount of other work. I was aware of how important my attitude was in encouraging enthusiasm, and a lot of commitment was shown to me by the women who attended the group.

I had been nervous about running the first session, feeling very daunted by the prospect. Gradually though, I came to feel more comfortable, relaxed and better able to work with the group. I learned to take more leadership and responsibility and took time over issues of trust and safety. I found it both useful and difficult to be open and willing to discuss the issues raised. I tried to facilitate in such a way as to ensure that all the women might contribute and sum up points made. At the same time I tried to hold back and allow the group to have a life of its own when lively discussions took place. I encouraged fun.

It seemed important to the women that conflict would be managed and reassuring that staff were in control. None the less, some women did not return after being in conflict with each other or with us, or if they felt uncomfortable with what was being said, to the concern of those remaining. Clearly we made the group safe enough to continue, but not for all women to continue attending.

Women found it difficult sometimes to attend the group for other reasons, some requesting transport. As the literature shows, women often shoulder the burden to care for others, and they will thus be excluded without creche or respite provisions. When planning a women's group practical issues as transport, carer support and contact in the home, need to be addressed, to enable women to attend.

GENDER ISSUES HIGHLIGHTED BY THE PROJECT

The wide gap in expectations

The aims and objectives devised at the beginning of the project were way beyond what was possible to achieve. Client-identified issues such as coping with stress, safety on the street, and women being more likely to stay at home than go out, were identified on the questionnaire as more relevant and were more readily discussed than those issues identified by staff, highlighting a gap between staff and client expectations. Although the results of the questionnaire showed that the Day Centre is addressing a wider range of issues for women in our sample than was addressed within the psychiatric care they received, we found that we had to adjust our expectations. We may have been expecting that women would have very complex needs due to the effects of sexism, and then not heard basic needs being expressed, for example to feel safe on the street and to enjoy themselves. Women generally had very low expectations, possibly due to internalised sexism, resulting in the general presumption that they should be satisfied with their lot.

The difficulty in identifying women's needs

The issues identified by the literature review and by the women themselves were difficult to translate into needs, especially as most women said that their needs were being addressed well by mental health services. The literature shows how women's mental health needs are often redefined, simply not heard or disbelieved. I noticed a tendency of my own to reinterpret what women were saying, and had to make an effort to side step my preconceptions of what women might need. Women may be so used to having their needs reinterpreted that they may have learned over time not to express them directly at all. I certainly noticed a reluctance and hesitancy for women to say what they wanted in the project. It seemed hard for them to accept that their needs would be considered, perhaps because the expectation that they should put others first, e.g., husband and children, is so ingrained.

There are certain hidden issues which the medical model does not address, e.g., sexual abuse, alcoholism and violence. Women did not want to talk about these, possibly because they were too painful. It could equally be that they have learned to hide these issues, especially if they had not been taken seriously on past disclosure. Also, they may have completely blocked off these experiences, to the extent of not realising they had suffered such abuse. Sexual abuse has until recently been a taboo subject in society, which is reflected in the psychiatric system's reluctance to deal with it. The project revealed that over half of the women would feel unable to talk about sexual abuse with their GP or psychiatrist. Some ten out of the 16 women attending the group had made hints or disclosures of childhood sexual abuse.

The difficulty we had in discerning women's needs and understanding them in their own terms has implications for how well assessment under the 1990 NHS Community Care Act will do in this respect. Local Authorities have produced plans for implementing Community Care. However, gender issues have not necessarily been prioritised. For example, the Borough where I work initially highlighted race issues, while failing to mention gender issues in mental health. If gender issues are not highlighted, it seems doubtful that the full extent of women's needs will be addressed.

Women being seen as a problem

Much of the literature concentrates on what are seen as problematic aspects of womanhood, but the project showed that women wanted to talk more about how to cope, than focus on their problems. Women in the group talked about their experiences of being in other women's groups, where they had felt pressure to talk about problems, and how uncomfortable that had made them feel. I believe one reason for the women's group's success was that the participants felt better at the end of the session than when they arrived. They wanted encouragement, and were attracted by the thought of having fun. Jane summed this up, in her reply to my asking what she wanted from the group: 'I enjoy coming and I'd like to share confidences and support each other to help build my self-esteem and confidence and trust with the whole group'. 'Socialising', 'enjoyment', 'getting out and about' and 'sharing experiences' were requested far more than any discussion of problems. Could it be that women are fed up of concentrating on, and being seen in terms of problems?

Women working with difference in a group

Unstructured discussions were lively but often dominated by a few vocal women, leaving others uncomfortable. While discussing the men's reaction to the women's project in the third group meeting, attitudes to men were expressed ranging from hating to defending them. There was no possibility of a consensus of view, and in the heated debate, a woman reminded the group that I am a lesbian and so, she thought, I would not know about men. I wonder if they were trying to make sense of their differences by locating them between the group and me, at the same time looking to me to help resolve them. I became very aware of how much power I held in the group as a leader, and whilst it was tempting to join the debate, I facilitated as evenly as possible. I felt cautious and worried about influencing the group, trying to remain neutral. This was the only time that my sexual orientation came up in the group, but most of the women knew that I am a lesbian. Women may have felt more comfortable criticising men in the belief that as a lesbian they would not be risking my disapproval. My presence as a lesbian was balanced by my heterosexual co-leader who was married and pregnant.

Many of the women were angry at men they had been involved with and were assertive in expressing their views. However, some women, especially those with men in their lives, felt uncomfortable after this debate and did not return to the group. One woman thought that the group was 'anti-men', seemingly afraid of herself being labelled anti-men and/or a lesbian if she criticised men. Such labels can be used as a means of attacking women not deemed submissive to men or feminine enough. Jane told us that her husband and sons had been deriding her attendance at the group, claiming that 'they must all be lesbians'. This implies that no 'normal' woman would want to be in a group without men. It also reflects how lesbianism is often regarded as unacceptable by patriarchal society (Ussher, 1991, p. 84). It seems the fundamental definition of woman is in her relation to 'man'. She is not allowed to exist in her own right without men. Both women's groups and lesbians are, by this definition, not quite 'women', and challenge patriarchy.

As half the group were black, race was another visible difference. There were enough black women to gain support from each other, and it was important for us as leaders to acknowledge and value their experience, especially as we were both white. I was worried that any underlying racist assumptions in the group would discourage black women from attending. A difficult moment arose when a white woman claimed that she had been victimised by black people. I was tempted to respond and defend black people's experience, but feared this may have undermined the black women present. Instead, I encouraged black women to respond, and one woman talked of some of the racial abuse she has suffered. It seemed hard for the white woman to hear this, but at least a countering black perspective was able to be expressed. Since the end of the project, the group has had black female staff leading and black women continue to make up half of the membership.

We made an effort to acknowledge and value difference, but conflict remained an uncomfortable issue. We found women in the group sometimes competitive and unkind to each other. Brodsky (1981, p. 575) found women in consciousness-raising groups do not react in traditional female interaction patterns, but were often 'catty, aggressive and competitive'. The literature shows how women are expected to be submissive, unassertive, caring and thinking of others first. If we are surprised when women are unkind to each other, perhaps we too are buying into the stereotype of femininity. Perhaps, on the other hand, women grouped together might expect and need to emphasise their common identity and may fear that this is in jeopardy when differences become too divisive.

Conflict was also expressed between women with similar experiences. They may have recognised more clearly the effects of their own experiences of oppression or abuse in other women, finding this uncomfortable. Perhaps these women verbally attacked others who they actually wanted to be closer to. Because the experience of women is rarely recognised, potential acknowledgement from each other may have evoked difficult feelings such as hurt or anger at previous lack of recognition, which needed to be defended against. The view women are encouraged to accept, that their problems are due to their individual pathology, may have been challenged if they had realised they were not alone in the experiences they had suffered.

I wonder too if women are not used to being in conflict. In the past, traditional expectations of women were to support men's views rather than express their own. Women must be affected by this legacy and it is uncomfortable to change against such strong internal and external expectations. Most of the women were in their fifties, and would have been under greater pressure to fulfil a traditional female role, having grown up before recent changes to women's equality. This role had added implications for group members as black and white working-class women, where they may be expected to be strong and work hard, but denied power.

REFLECTIONS

The empowering aspects of the project

It seems to me that the psychological impact of creating women's space at the Centre led to a greater sense of achievement and power than any actual discussion of sexism itself. Establishing space provided recognition and gave a message that women had a place at the Centre and were welcome. We tried to empower the group further by offering some control in the way things were done, for example women were asked to state their needs, choose their treats and outing and say whether they were comfortable with my video taping sessions as had been planned. (No video taping was done as one group member was uncomfortable with this.)

The fact that the group was able to continue after touching on difficult issues, that some of the women were not daunted by many of the men's antagonistic attitude to the group and that women were requesting that they continue meeting, showed that they felt they had more power than previously. They were certainly more able by the end of the project to accept their need for separate space. I was surprised by the number of women attending group meetings for the first time, and how well they participated. Some, like Eva, could defend the women's group in the drop-in and other women too showed signs of being more assertive.

I believe that valuing women and their contributions was an empowering process in itself (see also Chesler, 1982, p. 123). Women's experiences and views are devalued in our society and femininity itself can be seen as unhealthy. Internalising these messages alone causes women to develop low self-esteem and a lack of confidence, without the additional disempowerment that comes with being a psychiatric patient.

Women liked being treated well by the staff and some said how valued and appreciated this made them feel. Perhaps feeling valued and cared for as a human being comes before any internal change, growth or healing is possible. We valued the women enough to ask them what they wanted out of the Centre, and whilst this seemed a difficult question to answer, they at least experienced being asked. The empowering quality of this experience is borne out in that by the end of the project they could make demands and decisions as described above.

It was important to respond to the needs being expressed in the language that the women used. For example, in asking what women wanted from the women's group and how to make a women-orientated space, crafts and sewing were requested. I thought that they had been unable to articulate their 'real' needs. In supervision I realised that they had responded in terms of their own experience of enjoying women's company around these activities, particularly appealing to women of that age group. It was disempowering if I could not hear the meaning they intended. Accordingly, I learned to change both my language and the way I listened. For example using the term 'women-friendly' space rather than '-orientated' made more sense to the women. Involving women in determining how the group would evolve was crucial to its success. They became allies and grew to accept that it was their group.

Staff empowerment

I became empowered through taking on responsibility for the group and project. It was a difficult and painful process finding myself managing a group of women after having myself always been managed by men. I struggled with taking responsibility, half not wanting to and still seeking guidance from my manager. I felt rejected and alone when he encouraged me to get on with it. I tried to distance myself by referring to 'the women', as if I were not involved. I feared success in case it raised my expectations. As I dared not expect too much it was harder for me to acknowledge or enjoy the strengths and successes of the group. I was used to carrying out others' instructions, usually a male manager's, and more comfortable assuming a disempowered position of feeling that I could not cope with the task.

Through my reading, I became more aware of how difficult it is for women to progress and be themselves. I found that I had internalised these messages in the same way as the women attending the group. In a fortnightly forum where staff discussed gender issues, we realised that women in the team generally did not have the same confidence in their work practice that was evident in men with less skills and experience. My female colleague and I began to acknowledge our own ability, never before having thought of applying for senior positions. We became empowered enough to gain management positions.

It seems that we had been following what Holland (1992, p. 75) describes as a reflexive model of practice, which assumes that what is so for the client is so for the practitioner and both are required to change. What I learnt about myself helped me perceive the struggles of female clients in a clearer way. Women working with women, don't just expect the clients to change; you will change too!

The impact of the women's group on the Centre

The main outcome of the project was to establish women's space at the Centre. The main room in the extension building is now a 'women-friendly space', with decoration and information about women's events displayed to reflect this. Women's meetings continue to be held there.

It has not been easy, however, for women to use the space created for them. This was highlighted by the outing organised for the group, where, although women seemed enthusiastic, five cancelled at the last minute. On the day of the outing, one asked where the men were, and another asked if male staff were going. This was the first women-only outing at the Day Centre and we were struck by how hard it was for women to accept a treat that the men were not getting. The literature shows how women are defined in relation to men, and how women do this to themselves too and have learnt not to expect or give to themselves. So a women-only outing threatened this learning. As women grew to accept their space, though, many felt that they could talk about things in the group that they would not be able to in front of men, for example how intimidated they felt by themselves in the drop-in. Jane commented that: 'It's a relief to come to a group with just women. I've been looking for one, and I don't feel threatened here. I feel quite happy saying what I said, I would not have had the courage in front of men.' Eva commented, 'How can you talk to a man about breasts, for example?' Generally, during the project we found women being more friendly and confident with each other in the drop-in. Women who had not attended much before started arriving at the drop-in and asking if other women were there, staying if there were and leaving if not. On occasions when a lot of women attended, we noticed the drop-in was calmer.

Creating women's space did not come without a struggle, an external as well as an internal one. When I first talked about the project in a house meeting, many men were antagonistic and derided the need for women to have separate space. Ussher (1991, p. 9), too, often found herself answering questions about men, when talking publicly about women's issues. She also noticed (ibid., p. 306) that women grouping together can help identify needs, but are reviled for doing so, because it is assumed they are excluding men. Previously, such reactions have meant the end for women's projects at the Centre. It was important for us to provide space in the following group for women to voice what they would have wanted to say in the house meeting. In a staff gender forum after this house meeting we noticed how female staff stayed silent in the discussion, mirroring what had happened in the client group. We then made sure that female staff took a more active part in debates on issues concerning women.

As the Centre was closed to new clients at the time of the project, it is impossible to tell if the project had an impact in attracting and holding more female clients. But the group is still going and on a recent outing, the first time the Centre held a day trip abroad, to France, only one man and seven women came. Day outings had in the past mainly attracted men. It was a first for the Centre to attract so many women to a day trip.

Reviewing the attendance figures for that period, it appears that a high white male attendance meant a drop in other groups and vice versa. This could indicate a struggle for space. We found men attempting to reclaim space created for women. I found a very sexist comic strip on the women's notice board, and although the extension had been open for some time during the drop-in, it only started to be used by men directly after the women's group meetings. One male client attempted to use his power on the client committee to turn the extension into a library. Some anti-women sentiments were aroused, for example a man stated loudly that he 'hates women', in front of women in the drop-in. These reactions suggest that the women's group was challenging, just by its existence, the dominance of men in the Centre (which replicated that in society and psychiatry). Some male clients were encouraging and we tried to increase this voice to counterbalance the anti-women sentiments being expressed. I decided to involve male staff in planning and supporting the project, providing a model that men can help promote women's issues.

CONCLUSION

My main recollection of the project is that empowering women enough to use a separate space, where they are valued and appreciated, proved to be a difficult process. It was important to try to work creatively with conflicts as they arose, and not to give up. Women in the group gained support and got to know each other better. It may have been inevitable that it took a long time for some women to be able to use the space, and to accept each other. But knowing that it existed had a psychological impact, and women at the Centre have steadily increased their presence and voice in all aspects of the service. As staffing shortages continued, women expressed concerns about the women's group and the Centre closing. They were not differentiating between the two, indicating that they now saw the women's space as an integral part of the service.

My commitment to anti-sexism should be obvious by now, and I was fortunate to work in a place where my views were welcome and the empowerment of women was desired. Even so, the project proved to be a difficult task. I imagine that it would be even more difficult in a place where the culture was not so favourable, for example where one had to face direct opposition and sabotage from colleagues. Apparently this can happen only too often to female staff attempting to put women's needs on the agenda.

On reflection I am struck by how much effort it took to put women's needs on the agenda and not to be put off by men's response, and the amount of support that I needed to maintain the group. I found that receiving support was not a straightforward process. Although I was offered much good quality support, in retrospect I found one or two aspects disempowering. Like the women in the group, I did not expect my needs to be taken seriously, which was reinforced whenever I felt that my fears were being dismissed. Even so this made me deal with my fears, worries and lack of confidence, like the clients did.

I did not realise at the outset how much I would personally be involved in the process of empowerment. This process has implications for all female staff, who of course belong to the same sexist society as their clients. Maybe change in clients would not take place if the staff involved in such projects were not also open to change. Internally I struggled against feeling that I was doing something subversive in changing the *status quo*. Like the women, I feared the male backlash. I was afraid of being accused of undermining my male manager, of favouring women and of neglecting men's needs. Fortunately I had a good enough relationship with many of the men using the Centre that they did not seem to feel neglected. But I was concerned about how the men would react. I did not want to disaffect and lose potential male allies, but neither did I want men's needs to take over the agenda, so colluding with the devaluation of women's needs. This was a struggle for me, even though I was really pleased to be concentrating on women. It was the same dilemma that women clients experienced, whether or not to feel alright about putting time and energy into women, and fearing the social code this breaks with men. I dealt with this dilemma by involving male staff in the project, to keep them as allies. But I was left struggling to incorporate the male agendas. It was a balancing act.

Women do need a separate space to work out issues for themselves, but it is a struggle to keep that space. I listened to the men's fears, but held firm about the women's space continuing. Sexist stereotyping also puts men into uncomfortable roles. It is unfortunate that, rather than seeing the benefits to them of challenges and changes in this area, they mostly react to their sense of losing space and power.

As I did not want to risk the disapproval of my male manager, (especially as we were proud of the anti-sexist values held in the team) I found it difficult to criticise him. I am still struggling with this issue, and have found myself appeasing male agendas again in writing about the project. I first wrote about the women's group as piece of academic research, adopting a writing style I did not feel comfortable with. I tried to make women's experience central, but felt constrained by needing to meet a 'male', academic agenda.

More recently I have worked with male editors in reworking the paper into this chapter. While the introduction of my own experience and focusing on women's experience in general have clearly been encouraged, I have, on occasion, none the less felt misunderstood by some of the editorial comments made. And, again, I have felt overly cautious about asserting my view. For example, the editors thought that 'giving the women treats and looking after them' made them sound like children. I had some particularly useful feedback on this from a feminist writer on social policy, who understood better what I was trying to say. She thought that looking after and treating, for a change, women who carry the burden for care was a really good point. She added, why shouldn't women whose lives are such a struggle, be treated, don't we all need it? Moreover, would the editors have challenged Joseph Berke in the same way when he advocates 'putting the "treat" back into "treatment"'? I would not have felt entitled to stick to my guns without this further encouragement. This highlights how difficult it is for women to free themselves of male constructs and do things in ways which feel best for them.

I am struck with how difficult it is for women to be themselves, be valued for it and to progress. It seems to me clearly wrong that simply being a woman is seen as problematic and unhealthy. In the mental health system, stereotypes interfere in the treatment of women, who have invariably been denied the opportunity of defining their own needs.

In the event, I found that initially women needed staff to lead, before they were sufficiently empowered by our validation and encouragement to take more control of their space. Women were too anxious at first to use the informal space we offered at all, without staff present. After about a year of having a staff-led and structured group, the group has become more informal as women are making links with each other and want to talk about things that concern them as they arise. Female staff are still available and help to organise enjoyable things like going to cafes and seeing films. More recently, female staff have co-ordinated an agenda set completely by the women themselves, and they have continued to concentrate on enjoyable activities.

There is a question being discussed at the Centre of whether the women's group should continue as it is now or whether the meetings should change to something more like a therapy group, where, for example, child sexual abuse disclosures could be made, as it is assumed that this might be 'better for them'. For my part, I do not see that having fun is incompatible with therapy. I wonder if what is being asked for in the name of therapy, is for women to get back to concentrating on their problems and for staff to hold more power and be more in control of the group. Having fun is an important part of the empowering process, which would in my view help to build up ego strength, making exploration and working through problems more possible. Some women may not want to expose their abuse, as such exploration can evoke painful feelings and a disruption in coping mechanisms such as denial. I think that space for focused groups and individual work should be available *in addition to* the existing women's meetings, as the need arises. It is a dilemma trying to decide the best way to 'help' women explore their experiences, but, as I have highlighted, women have rarely had the opportunity to define their own needs. Whilst women are struggling with conflicts in this area, it may be difficult for staff to just let the process develop in the way and at the pace women want, without interference, but it is important that they do so.

In attempting to identify women's needs, staff need to listen to (rather than define or redefine) women's agenda. The process of change might seem slow, but individually and collectively we make an impact, as evidenced by the project. Anyone finding it a struggle to address women's needs might feel like they are taking on the world, and in a sense they are.

REFERENCES

Bayes, M. 1981: The prevalence of gender-role bias in mental health services. In Howell, E. and Bayes, M. (eds) *Women and mental health*. New York: Basic Books. pp. 83–5.

Brodsky, A. 1981: A decade of feminist influence on psychotherapy. In Howell, E. and Bayes, M. (eds) *Women and mental health*. New York: Basic Books, pp. 607–19.

Broverman, I. *et al.* 1981: Sex-role stereotypes and clinical judgements of mental health. In Howell, E. and Bayes, M. (eds) *Women and mental health*. New York: Basic Books, pp. 86–97.

Burns, J. 1992: Mad or just plain bad? Gender and the work of forensic psychologists. In Ussher, J.M. and Nicolson, P. (eds) *Gender issues in clincal psychology*. London: Routledge, pp. 106–28.

Chesler, P. 1982: *Women and madness*. London: Harvest/HBJ.

Cooperstock, R. 1981: A review of women's psychotropic drug use. In Howell, E. and Bayes, M. (eds) *Women and mental health*. New York: Basic Books, pp. 131–40.

Holland, S. 1992: From social abuse to social action: a neighbourhood psychotherapy and social action project for women. In Ussher, J. and Nicolson, P. (eds) *Gender issues in clinical psychology*. London: Routledge, pp. 68–77.

Howell, E. 1981a: Women from Freud to the present. In Howell, E. and Bayes, M. (eds) *Women and mental health*. New York: Basic Books, pp. 3–25.

Howell, E. 1981b: Women's treatment needs. In Howell, E. and Bayes, M. (eds) *Women and mental health*. New York: Basic Books, pp. 309–10.

Jarman, B. 1983: Identification of underprivileged areas. *British Medical Journal* **286**, 1705–9.

Laing, R.D. 1967: *The politics of experience*: London: Ballantine.

Miles, A. 1988: *Women and mental illness*. Brighton: Wheatsheaf.

Showalter, E. 1986: *The female malady*. New York: Pantheon.

Stephenson, S. and **Walker, G.** 1981: The psychiatrist–woman–patient relationship. In Howell, E. and Bayes, M. (eds) *Women and mental health*. New York: Basic Books, pp. 113–30.

Ussher, J. 1991: *Women's madness: misogyny or mental illness?* London: Harvester Wheatsheaf.

Ussher, J. 1992: Science sexing psychology: positivistic science and gender bias in clinical psychology. In Ussher, J. and Nicolson, P. (eds) *Gender issues in clinical psychology*. London: Routledge, pp. 39–67.

Walker, M. 1992: *Surviving secrets*. Philadelphia: Open University Press.

Weissman, M. and **Klerman, G.** 1981: Sex differences and the epidemiology of depression. In Howell, E. and Bayes, M. (eds) *Women and mental health*. New York: Basic Books, pp. 160–95

Westwood, S. *et al.* 1989: *Sadness in my heart: racism and mental health*. Leicester Black Mental Health Group, University of Leicester.

13

WRITING AS A TOOL OF REFLECTIVE PRACTICE: SKETCHES AND REFLECTIONS FROM INSIDE THE SPLIT MILIEU OF AN EATING DISORDERS UNIT

Ben Davidson

Here Ben Davidson draws on experience as a student psychiatric nurse to sketch out some of the ethical dilemmas facing practitioners working within a culture that is split. The experience on which the chapter is based occurred on an in-patient eating disorder unit. The conflict between forms of physical treatment and psychological care is described as are a number of complicated dynamics within and between the staff and patient groups. Ben argues that by remaining alive to, and obstinately committed to communicating one's experience, by writing and other means, it is possible to find a role in such a situation.

The idea of the collaborative, healing relationship between nurse and patient is 'a cherished idea within psychiatric nursing' (see Chapter 8). Yet almost inevitably, it seems, patients act out, staff burn out and collaboration and empathy between them subtly drop out of the equation. What is left in these circumstances and how should we handle it?

During my RMN training, for the first six months, I was placed on an in-patient eating disorder unit, immersed in a milieu where I had to try to fathom just such a scenario. The ward was in many ways divided. On the third floor of a recently built 'L'-shaped block, there was an eating disorder side (ten patients) and on the other side another speciality service (about ten patients again), with a few general psychiatry beds on each wing, thrown in for good measure. A 60-year-old man occupying one of the latter beds suffered manic-depressive psychosis. At the time I worked with him he was destitute, following a huge spending binge in which he had blown his substantial life savings. He had clearly now swung to a depressive phase. Rather angrily, it always seemed to me, he would defecate where he sat, lay, or, on occasion, just where he stood, insisting he could not help it. He made the staff angry, in any event, whatever *his* motivations might have been. If it *was* 'overflow' from chronic constipation, as some argued, he certainly did not make the situation any easier by standing, for example, in the medication queue in his pyjamas and allowing diarrohea to spill down his leg onto the carpet, aware of the fact but disinterested. Yet I managed at times to find some relief in scraping him down and cleaning him off in the bath (he was too unmotivated and resistant to do it by himself), particularly after an hour-long session supervising the wrangling and antics of the anorexic patients at their meal table.

The ten of them would sit around the table comparing and disputing the size of their potatoes and the unfairness of their portions, distressed beyond measure at how much butter was spread on their toast, cutting peas into improbably small pieces before forcing themselves laboriously, torturously (and with considerable 'encouragement'), to swallow each bit. They would hide mashed potato in their trainers and knickers. After an hour's mind-warping effort to cope with this sort of experience, something as earthed as cleaning down Joe could indeed be a relief. It was an intense entry to psychiatric nursing. In at the deep end.

Although my main interest was in psycho-dynamic work I was struck by the importance of having a range of interventions to offer, particularly as many people we looked after were at a dangerously low weight and required quite focused 'behavioural' intervention in relation to their eating patterns. I participated in running the eating programme that formed an essential component of in-patient treatment, supervising meals daily and regularly eating at the table with patients. Twice I helped in 'force-feeding' a patient whose weight was at a dangerously low level. With the luxury of more time, once 'danger periods' were averted, and with help, I saw some patients change the patterns that comprised their 'illness', breaking through maladaptive habits into a greater understanding of their situation, into an experience of new feelings and into an ability to choose different ways of being.

A university lecturer in nursing lectured my set one day early on in our course about academic pathways and career development in nursing. The message she conveyed was that research is not distinct from what we do from second to second. It is merely a formalisation of the ordinary human process of activity and reflection. We had surely been thrown into momentous experiences wherever we had been placed, she told us, and should try to write about them. By writing we are reflecting. Regularly, daily, every evening after a shift if possible, reflect and write about what it had been like. Whether or not we felt interested in research, writing in this way could well keep us alive to the experiences we were involved in. All of us who were willing to write would be engaged in reflective practice. It was good advice.

This chapter is the product of some such writing. Both in terms of the ideas contained within it, and also in the fact of its existence, it is also one answer to the question posed above. In circumstances where patients act out, staff burn out and collaboration and empathy between them subtly drop out of the equation, what is left and how should we handle it?

Jeremy sits moaning and sighing, holding his head, complaining of a migraine as he stares at the mess on the table before him.

11.40 a.m. Evaluation time. The enrolled nurse, Ulrike, is coordinating. She hears a report that Jeremy has vomited again over the dining table and the other patients are complaining. Someone snorts contemptuously and there is laughter. It is agreed that if the vomit is still there after the meeting someone will offer him support in clearing it up. More contempt is allowed to haemorrhage into the air, for Jeremy, for the idea of giving him support, for the person who suggested it and for the system we all work in; this contempt is left to hang in the air as an animal noise while we leave the staffroom.

Two hours later, Liselle, a patient, interrupts the afternoon shift's planning time to report that Jeremy, still at the table, has again been sick. She is met with a courteous but abrupt response from a staff nurse, Jane, that we are aware of this, but busy at the moment. Liselle makes sure we know she feels something should be done. We let her know we have heard her. She leaves, exasperated, and the planning continues. The extent of our attempt to process Liselle's interruption is limited. It amounts to one of the nursing assistants, Daphne, wondering why Liselle 'don't go and sort something out, instead of bleating to us'.

More laughter.

Putting the most charitable gloss on these events, I privately observe that we probably do not get it across to Liselle that we want it to be an issue for the eating disorder patients to confront together with Jeremy, that they find his behaviour disgusting. But maybe there is no need to underline that; Liselle knows that it is ward policy for 'peer group pressure' to play an important part in treatment. I am a student nurse, anxious to understand before criticising, so I say nothing.

'Peer group pressure' seems to mean something like the process of Jeremy's peers making him feel bad for causing them distress by his vomiting. Accordingly, as Jeremy, like everyone else, needs to belong, to feel acceptance and approval, he will want to change his behaviour. Something as unsophisticated as this, however, seems unlikely to be effective with the in-patients here who are as low in weight as 4 stone and in some cases willing to starve themselves to death. The patients too seem unanimous in the view that for members of their group who do not want to eat, this sort of crude pressure is worthless. I want to find a meaning to 'group pressure' a little more convincing if I am to believe that this is the first and foremost treatment of choice. I think about the sort of understanding of group process I am familiar with from my recent background in group-analytic therapy.

From this viewpoint, eating disorders may acquire meaning seen against a background of complex intrapsychic, interpersonal and family dynamics (Lawrence, 1989; Crisp, 1980). For example there are five patients here in whom it has become clear there is a desire to punish, as well as anger towards one or both parents. Where there has been sexual abuse as a child, painful marital breakdown and recriminations, or persistent neglect by alcoholic parents, these feelings are understandable to say the least. There is, at the same time, however, such terror at losing control and expressing this wrath, such unwillingness to look at these feelings (which would after all involve some degree of re-experiencing the traumatic events associated with them) that this anger and desire to punish get expressed by way of a self-starvation programme.

The sense of control and self-determination afforded by adherence to such a starvation programme also figures in an understanding of eating disorders (Moorey, 1991). One young woman on the ward, Madeline, has stated this explicitly in describing how her parents and siblings attempt to control so much of her conduct and her mental world that the only area where she feels she can exercise any autonomy is in her eating.

In group-analytic terms, whatever the specific complexities of these family relationships, the patient's interpersonal patterns of communication, the style of relationships between her and the most significant other people in her life, will sooner or later become manifest in her conduct and in the relationships she forms with others on the ward. This process, with other patients and staff (or indeed with the eating-disorder group as a whole or with the entire ward) having foisted upon them a role or roles that the patient more or less unwittingly assigns in recreating her familiar relational world, is known as *transference* (Kreeger, 1987). From this viewpoint it is of the greatest importance to allow, or even better encourage relationships between patients to develop. And it is essential that difficult issues such as distaste with another patient's behaviour when he vomits over the dinner table, be aired and confronted. The hope is that this will contribute to the manifestation of transference, so that exploration and eventual resolution of the issues(s) underlying the eating disorder may take place in the context of the relationships on the ward.

This, then, I hope, is why Liselle is left, along with the other patients, to confront and deal with Jeremy's inability or unwillingness to keep his food down, even when he knows he will not be allowed to leave the table and must vomit there over his food while the other patients eat their meal and seethe, more or less silently, each in their own misery and isolation. They are developing relationships and allowing conflicts to arise which may eventually provide a basis for the understanding and resolution of whatever issues underlie the eating disorder.

I wonder whether Liselle understands all this. If she does she may just about be able to see Jeremy's being kept at the table to vomit as some sort of therapeutic agent – compelling her and the other patients to express their emotions and relate (as well as encouraging all of them to give whatever support or censure is necessary to help him stop, thus conditioning Jeremy not to want to vomit). Without such understanding, however, it is impossible to see the same episode as anything other than vindictiveness and insensitivity on the part of the staff. If Liselle and the other patients see it only in this way, presumably they will be less inclined generally to co-operate in their treatment, and less motivated in particular to engage in whatever therapy is available. One needs to feel safe before risking 'opening up' in a therapy situation, and a patient here is not likely to feel safe if she experiences the regime or staff as vindictive and hostile.

Here follows the sum total of formal explanation of the crucial 'relationship-forming' component of the theory behind our 'peer group pressure' approach, given to patients on admission in a general booklet explaining policy on the ward:

> If you should have difficulty in finishing your meals or in eating, we have devised a group therapy approach which relies heavily on peer support and peer pressure to assist you to overcome your problems in a supportive manner. The supervisor's role during mealtimes is to facilitate this process by calling on your fellow patients to support and assist you.

The idea of the staff's role as facilitative of 'fellow patients [mutual] . . . support and assist[ance]' is included, but, as can be seen, only in the context of mealtime protocol, and even then in such a muddy way as to leave the notion of patient interaction and trust and openness in the group as prerequisites for therapy, more or less obscure, so obscure in fact, that one may wonder if such issues are understood clearly by staff at all, let alone patients.

At the dinner table Ulrike is arguing again with Jeremy.

'So you're saying that because you've got a migraine you shouldn't have to eat, are you?'

'No, I'm not saying that.'

'And what about the last three days, then. I suppose that's your excuse for not eating then. If we listened to you, you'd never eat.'

'I'm not saying that, Ulrike. I know I have to eat. I'm just saying this migraine makes me feel even more sick. In fact I think its this food that brought the migraine on.'

'Jeremy, just get on with your food and stop arguing, or am I going to have to feed it to you myself?'

A staff nurse, Clive, is inducting a new student, Emma, onto the ward. This is her obligatory psychiatric placement within the training she is doing as a sick children's nurse. It is evening now, quiet, the bustle of ward rounds and meetings and appointments for patients and staff over for the day. The staff room is relaxed, and while I browse through some patients' files, Clive tries to reassure Emma, who is unsure of her role, scared of mental illness and extremely nervous about meeting any patients. His reassurance is addressed specifically at qualms that may well arise in response to the disturbing events likely to unfold at her first mealtime encounter here.

> They're a manipulative lot, these anorexics. Be careful about trusting your first impressions, you'll see what I mean when you've been here a while. They'll go on about how ill-treated they are, but take no notice. They're wrong. We don't care the way they'd like us to but we care enough to keep them from starving themselves to death, no matter how bloody difficult they are.

She has already been told by another student that 'They're very crafty; they'll take laxatives when you're not looking and make themselves vomit in the toilet, stuff like that. We have to inspect the contents of the bowl before they flush it away with some of them, and they have to ask us before they go to the toilet.'

Emma seems reassured. I too feel some reassurance but also a considerable degree of unease. I am invited, welcomed into an attitude that forms an important bond amongst members of staff; there is an impressive cohesiveness within the staff group, and amongst them in the staffroom I feel a great warmth and security. But this bond and warmth seem intricately linked to, perhaps even founded on, a kind of oppressive suspicion and antagonism towards the patients.

Neither the patients nor the staff, it strikes me, are initiated into the theory of the therapeutic milieu of the ward, and a picture emerges of conflict between the two groups, taking place in a void, in the context of which it seems unrealistic to expect the patients to feel safe enough to 'open up', or even comply.

I feel in an unreal space between two worlds, each one trying to shield itself from the insecurity caused by a hostile 'them' against 'us'. The patients are undoubtedly manipulative. Presumably, like most people, they try to get what they want through devious means, subtly controlling, manipulating others' responses rather than asking straightforwardly. No doubt people who starve themselves to get needs met could reasonably be said to be more manipulative than others, even if their conduct is 'the reasonable upshot of their life history' (Smail, 1987). But in *our* intense preoccupation with '*their* manipulativeness' I just wonder what else is going on. Why do nurses so want this aspect of patients' characters to be highlighted? Why does 'manipulativeness' need to be understood as a defining characteristic of anorexic psychopathology? And why does such an understanding form an intrinsic part of induction for new staff on the ward, to the extent even that an injunction is subtly made in the name of self-preservation to put aside all other perceptions? Why is there such neglect of the theory underlying this group psycho-dynamic approach, such lack of attention to the facilitation of patient-group cohesion, and such an obvious absence of a forum for the safe airing of feelings in staff brought up by the patients? The patients are sometimes and in some degree manipulative, no doubt, but equally, the staff are sometimes and in some degree angry and unsupportive to the people on the ward, particularly to those patients least in charge of their eating patterns and presenting the greatest management problems, as above. No one is perfect!

A short time on, after an evening meal, I help Jeremy clear the vomit from the table, restricting myself as much as possible to advice on strategic issues such as where the Dettol is kept, how to negotiate the doorway with a heavy bowl of water and when enough Dettol has been administered so that the table can be rinsed and dried. With such support, Jeremy manages to clear the mess without too much fuss and in reasonably good part. However, I am left somewhat jangled. Jeremy seemed in misery and I felt sorry for him. I was not very harsh with Jeremy, and even spoke to him in quite a kindly way. Have I thus exposed myself to staff and patients as too sympathetic and not sufficiently dispassionate to provide the firm boundaries necessary to become part of the team and to get these people better? Should I have shouted and bullied, just a little? Will I now be seen merely as a walkover and become a soft target for *manipulation*?

> Two months later, 1.15 p.m. an argument rages around the dinner table. This time, though, it is between me and the anorexic patients.
>
> 'Oh, c'mon, you two. Do stop playing with your food. What's the matter now?'
>
> The words are barked from the comfort of some newfound confidence after learning that I can manage a group situation without anarchy breaking out. I have run the psychodrama group on my own that morning never having done it before, standing in for the qualified nurse who is on leave, and I managed to get everyone participating in some trust-building exercises and role-plays learnt recently in school. It went well and I feel strong.
>
> 'Well, don't look so shocked. Tell me what's going on. What's the problem?' Irritation spills out. I do not want to be supervising the meal.
>
> The two girls who are making games, one of mashing up her sponge pudding with the custard and the other of chasing it around her plate, do not know quite how to react. The sad-looking girl, Sally, who has occasional moments of quite astonishing fury unleashes some of it in their defence:
>
> 'If you had to eat this mess like us you wouldn't be so bloody smug.'
>
> I am somewhat taken aback. I wonder whether she sported the same snarl just before she stabbed her mother with a pair of scissors. Normally such a forceful reaction would scare me, but, unusually, this time I do not much care. I have taken the plunge and may as well now start swimming.
>
> 'Oh do stop complaining and get on with it. Its not that bad,' I retort, unabashed.
>
> Liselle is as sharp as ever: 'I suppose you're going to say that because we are

anorexics our perceptions are distorted, are you, and really it's hot although we all think it's stone bloody cold.'

'I'm not going to say that, no . . . '

'Oh, yes, lovely this is,' says Sally. 'I suppose Amanda's is really appetising too.'

Everyone laughs and Amanda must feel the heat of it. She is faced with a plate of liquidised green mush, probably cold, and probably no easier for her to eat than the fish, potatoes and peas it used to be before someone got impatient with her complaints about being unable to swallow, and put it through the food blender. I feel a pang of protectiveness towards Amanda who is currently beyond anyone's help, psychotic perhaps, and does not need, I feel, to be caught in this crossfire. It becomes obvious it is more than crossfire though, when Nigel makes some reference to green cowpats, and the uproar continues. Very little guilt seems to be around, although Amanda's nose is really being rubbed in it; the patients are as angry with her as the staff, it seems, just as they used to be with Jeremy before his discharge. It is some time before the baying and cackling abate. I feel the hurt dam up inside Amanda and wonder that her frailty can withstand it.

'Harveys Bristol Cream,' she whimpers, unintelligibly, and I hear them laugh all the more. Take me on, you idiots, not Amanda, I want to tell them.

I become placatory. 'If you say its cold, you're probably right. I'm not going to argue.' Then, not wanting to seem too conciliatory, I quickly add 'So alright, its cold. So what?'

'Would you eat it?'

'I've just had some. It wasn't brilliant but it was edible.'

'I suppose our perceptions are distorted if . . . '

'Liselle, if you are going to say it's cold, no, I don't expect your perceptions are distorted. But if you say it's a cow pat then I think they are definitely distorted, deranged even. There's a difference between it not being very nice and it being inedible. Why don't you stop going on and eat the bloody stuff.'

Scott's plate is suddenly empty. He looks at me menacingly, defying me to challenge him, ready to protect Liselle's honour.

Two courses and a further ninety minutes on, Sally is still there, and wants blood: 'You've changed, just like the rest of them. You weren't like this when you started. Now you're bossing us around just like Malcolm and Sue. I think something must come over you, like you become power mad.'

Where can I go? Sally, the only reason I would be eating as much as you have to three times a day would be if I were anorexic, and if I was I don't know what I would feel. But I'm not. And unfortunately you are. But somehow I'm in it with you and someone is paying me a pittance to get you out of it and I am scared to see that I don't really know how to but I will try to love you and see it through together with you . . . I do not say this though. I've gone in far enough for now. I try to show I have had enough.

I shake my head as it rests in my hands, elbows on the table. I imagine how I look and recognise the posture Jeremy used to adopt. 'Do stop this. I've said I'm not questioning your perceptions. The food may not be particularly nice. But it is edible. Eat it.'

'OK, you've had one portion now, but if you had to eat it three times a day with snacks in between, you'd be complaining just as much as we do.'

Sally is a 19-year-old girl having a tantrum, her fury unleashed is precise and powerful and she rattles me. I retreat into a defensive retaliation, and putting on my pedantic tone, begin: 'Sally, does it occur to you . . . ' Then I decide to open the field again and go for safety with a brash attach on them all: 'Do any of you wonder whether it might not be you who have changed towards me?' After a moment's silence I soften my tone. 'Because it seems like this is the first time you've had a go at me personally for something to do with your food. The eating regime is obviously giving you a hard time, and these cock-ups the catering department keeps making must be infuriating. What was it the other day? Jacket potatoes with lentil filling and boiled potatoes to go with them? I'd be going mad. But today is the first time since I've been here that you have given *me* a lot of shit because of it, directed at me personally. I'm sorry if my attitude seems to have changed but I don't see why I should have to put up with a lot of shit when its not my fault.'

Which of course is partly not true, as it was me who drew the fire in the first place by being unusually brusque and petulant with Madeline and Jo who were playing with their food. This is not lost on Sally who no doubt senses some mendacity afoot, and directs a parting shot my way.

'Oh, let's just drop it, Ben, If I carry on you'd probably only go and tell Malcolm anyway, and then we'd all be in trouble. Just drop it.'

Not just caught in an unreal space between two worlds but wanting to be accepted and esteemed in both of these two camps engaged in the open hostilities described above, I am aware that I *have* changed. Two months back I would have held my counsel and bargained for everyone's approval, terrified of losing esteem or doing harm. Now I am willing to be drawn into these skirmishes and feel I have some grasp of what is happening. I try fumblingly to facilitate some willingness in the group to open up and talk, on this occasion, admittedly, more about food, but also about my relationship with the group. I am also drawing their anger and then showing I can withstand it. (If *I* cannot, then how can they be expected to trust in the safety of the group sufficiently to let out their feelings about each other?) I am modelling a willingness to engage in intense interactions in the group and survive. I am trying at some level to enhance group cohesiveness.

The theory goes like this: the more risk-taking is modelled and endorsed by the facilitator as a group norm, the more people engage in it in order to enhance their esteem and to belong. The more risks group members take in self-disclosure, the greater the esteem in which they are held. And the greater the ensuing mutual esteem in the group, the greater the cohesion. Yalom says that

> cohesiveness is a widely researched basic property in [successful] groups . . . In general there is agreement that . . . Group cohesiveness is not per se a therapeutic factor but is instead a necessary precondition for effective therapy, [and like] an ideal therapist-patient relationship [in individual therapy, it] creates conditions in which the necessary self-disclosure and intrapersonal and interpersonal exploration may unfold.
>
> (Yalom, 1985, pp. 49–50)

The cohesiveness which Yalom describes as a necessary precondition for effective therapy is in no small measure, within an in-patient group such as this, a function of the staff's willingness to disclose themselves and interact, as well as patients'. Indeed, perhaps the staff's input here is *more* important as their role is in large part that of role model; the limits they set for themselves are also the boundaries described for the patients in their eating and their interactions.

This highlights how nurses are in an odd no-man's land between patient and therapist. Although staff enforcing the rigid eating regime on the ward are caught up in the interpersonal dramas being reenacted and inevitably become participants to some extent, they clearly need to be some steps back from complete patient involvement in the group. And yet not quite so far back that they adopt the role of therapist. Maybe the ideal role nurses can adopt is that of 'facilitator of group cohesion' as a sort of preparatory step towards the work which a therapist might facilitate in more formal sessions. This work (at least to the extent that it takes place within the in-patient twice weekly group therapy sessions) is mentioned in the ward brochure:

> The group aims . . . to confront issues . . . which are contributing [to] and perpetuating your eating disorder in order that positive change may take place . . . The overall aim of the group is to provide a safe environment for you to explore . . . your behaviour in a way that meaning can emerge.

And of course 'a safe environment' in this context has to mean, if it is anything more than an empty cliché, an environment in which patients really do feel safe enough to disclose and explore their condition. Presumably an environment which patients experience as one where they are bullied by uncaring staff does not apply.

It should be emphasised that patients do not generally object to firm handling *per se*. Out of some six patients who I have heard complain at one time or another, all have confirmed that their treatment by the charge nurse Malcolm, whose reputation for noisy harangues is renowned, is not what they are referring to. All six have intimated this clearly, stating that his treatment of them is 'reassuring', 'it comes through that he cares', 'it doesn't feel like he's shouting for the sake of it', and, perhaps most significantly, 'its different with him because you feel he knows what he is doing'. Which apparently he does, being the only figure on the ward with experience of analytic psychotherapy and training. One is left with the suspicion that the patients' objection is to the sort of 'firm handling' characterised earlier in this chapter as being based on an antagonism towards them, which emerges as the only thing the staff group can use as a focus for their own need for group cohesion and support. And as suggested above, this may be in large measure a result of the absence of any proper dissemination of the ward philosophy from ward manager level, around which staff cohesion could more usefully develop, and the spelling out of such a philosophy in terms of specific roles and functions for nurses.

I realise how easy it is to be swamped and influenced by the culture of a place and by one's own inertia, resistance and bad faith, however much one would like it to be otherwise. My account above reflects some of my experiences and preoccupations over the six months in which I worked on the eating disorder unit, focusing mainly on group considerations, staff-patient dynamics and the procedures and structures of the ward. I have avoided in this account the worst excesses of pathologising patients with whom I worked, but I have nevertheless also avoided introducing any of them as people in the context of the distressing life stories they told. The final product centres, egoistically, on my recounting the story of my placement. As such, it is not just the culture of the ward or the permanent staff group that seems to have lost its empathic, collaborative heart, but myself too. I now wish to correct this imbalance.

While working on the in-patient unit I participated fortnightly in live, group supervision of a family therapist who would be seeing an eating disorder patient and their family for up to four sessions. Perhaps a good example of what is missing above is the material that came out of the family therapy sessions with patients, for example the sessions where the therapist saw Jeremy, his father and aunt.

Jeremy was 13, the youngest patient on the ward, transferred there after little improvement during his 3-month stay on a child and adolescent unit. His mother had recently died and his father was fast becoming an alchoholic. Prior to being admitted, Jeremy had had on occasion to look after his father, getting him to bed when he passed out from drinking too much. He had had to shop, prepare meals and the like. He did not want to go back to boarding school, where he was bullied, but, equally, the situation at home must have been intolerable.

None of this was discussed in the patient group, either during formal therapy sessions or elsewhere. His eating patterns were so extreme that it was hard to focus on anything but Jeremy and his weight and his food and his vomit. What emerged dramatically during family therapy was that Jeremy had not been able to grieve properly for his mother, partly due to family taboo and partly because his role had changed in relation to his father from child to parent, as a result of his father's incapacity through drink. When the supervision group got the therapist to pass over the family's preoccupation with Jeremy's eating and push against their resistance to discussing the loss of Jeremy's mother, a well of blocked emotion was thrown up, both by Jeremy and the others in the family group (considerable emotion was also expressed in the supervision group), and progress began to be made. Jeremy subsequently stopped being sick, gained weight and was discharged to his aunt's care, while his father accepted treatment for his alchohol dependency.

Madeline's family therapy sessions with her domineering brothers and father were also revealing. The supervision group had at one point to help the therapist withdraw from conflict with the men of the family, who were speaking for Madeline. The therapist himself, although endorsing ideas that we knew Madeline held, had been drawn into doing exactly what the other men were doing, speaking for her rather than allowing Madeline to speak for herself. In discussion between Madeline and her primary nurse after the session, it transpired that the men's dominance included unwanted sexual attentions. Madeline could not finally bring herself to tell the whole family that her brother had raped her. However, the fact that she had told *someone* and the threat she made subsequently to her brother that she *would* tell the whole family, including her father, if anything like it should ever happen again, seemed sufficient for her to gain the sense of control of her destiny that she had previously said was missing in her life except in relation to food. Our intuition that she would not relapse proved correct.

Scott's family dynamics, similarly, were revealing. The family meetings were attended by his mother, two aunts, sister and grandmother, all of whom, like many of us in the staff group, were influenced by this attractive 15-year-old boy's charm. The subject it seemed hard to discuss was his delinquency. Talk of his forthcoming court case on charges including aggravated burglary, talk also of its implications, was persistently pushed aside out of greater concern for his illness. The only contact from his absent father was when word reached him of an intervention from the nurse Clive. The father stormed onto the ward threatening physical violence if ever again anyone suggested that his boy needed parental disciplining. The picture we were given of family dynamics could not have been clearer. Discipline and control of Scott and criticism of the men of the family in general were taboo, while an idealising, doting love for him was powerfully endorsed. Attempting to restore some balance to this equation without jeopardising our relationship with him, we subsequently focused a lot in work with Scott on *the court's* likely use of its authority to 'discipline' him if he did not behave in a way that allowed us to report co-operation and progress, as we very much wanted to. We were surprised at how quickly Scott's eating disorder abated.

And what of the others? The 21-year old, Liselle's story remained unfathomed. Her parent's relationship never improved but her father's 'terminal' cancer went into remission. Liselle's forlorn devotion to him turned to anger when he announced that he was moving to the Far East with his new mistress. This turn of events, particularly Liselle's expression of hostility towards her father, seemed promising, but she had had numerous admissions before this one and it was felt, rightly, that there would be many more. Although many interesting facets of Liselle's relationships with significant others came to light, and possible links between these relationships and her eating disorder suggested themselves, we never quite found the key.

Sally went back to live with her mother in the Midlands. She had not gained much weight and, particularly as sexual abuse had been disclosed, it was felt that insufficient exploration or resolution of her distress had taken place. Somewhat to our surprise, none the less, we heard of no further eating problems. She even came to visit the ward with a present of chocolates, which she shared, when she attended a follow-up group.

Nigel never really gained weight sufficiently, but managed to convince everyone he would be alright out of hospital. Like Sally, he too had been a voluntary patient. The following year he relapsed to a dangerous degree, finally admitting when he reached 4½ stone that he was out of control. He asked for readmission. There were no beds. He died. As did the 32-year old patient I helped to force feed, who had, for some time in the months before admission, driven around the area in her car looking like a wraith and frightening passers-by who happened to look in the window.

I planned to 'restore balance' to this chapter by offering an empathic, collaborative account of patients' experience. However, in the last few paragraphs I have again told as much of the story of our work with patients as I have of their own stories. And in rereading my description of Angela as a wraith, frightening passers-by, I recall the same callous parody circulating the ward a while after I worked there. Yet she had died. Perhaps callousness is inevitable in response to such relentness misery and distress. It is painful to stay with the experience of pain, perhaps ultimately even more so when it is someone else's. I suppose this explains a range of phenomena. It explains staff's need to take a distant, hostile, 'us and them' stance *vis-à-vis* patients, such as in the situation described above. It explains the tendency to move away from the raw experience of a situation into abstractions regarding structure and philosophy, as to some extent in my writing. It is certainly a strange experience for me now, seven years on, to be recovering memories of my contact with such a disturbed group of people in such awful states of distress. And then I recall how my own eating, as well as drinking and sleeping patterns, went haywire during this placement.

The question with which I opened this account, and to which, in conclusion, I now return, concerns the sort of circumstances detailed above where patients act out, staff burn out and collaboration and empathy between them drop out of the equation. I asked what, in these circumstances, is left in the relationship and how should we handle the situation?

To summarise, it seems to me that through reflection and writing we can struggle to get a conceptual grip on the situation. With a leap of faith we can open ourselves to honestly experiencing what is going on in our relationships. Even if the resultant understanding and experience are partial, it should yield a point of leverage where something that we can *do* is revealed. And if what we do turns out not to have the desired result, then at least we have new information with which to enhance our experience and aid further reflection. In the above account a useful role to adopt suggested itself to me increasingly, the more I struggled to understand what was going wrong on the ward to cause the antagonism between staff and patients. As far as possible I tried to make a difference using this point of leverage, which was little more than the role psychiatric nurses should adopt anyway: helping people and groups to communicate their experience, in the context of an authentic, honest relationship.

When we find that in our own relationships with patients collaboration and empathy are largely absent, then I guess we can at least be honest about that. The influence one has on others is in any event marginal, and the only small corner of the universe over which one has control is one's own being. If, as I have tried to show, we can at least struggle to maintain an honest, authentic relationship with ourselves through reflection on and writing about our experience, then this in itself may make a positive difference to our approach and to the outcome of any intervention we make. We will have shown at least that we can communicate *our own experience*, and perhaps others will follow suit.

REFERENCES

Crisp, A.H. 1980: *Anorexia nervosa: let me be.* London: Academic Press.

Davidson, B. 1992: What can be the relevance of the psychiatric nurse to the life of a person who is mentally ill? *Journal of Clinical Nursing* 1(4), 199–205.

Kreeger, L. 1987: *Transference and countertransference in group psychotherapy.* Unpublished paper, available from the Institute of Group Analaysis, London.

Lawrence, M. 1989: *The anorexic experience.* London: The Women's Press.

Moorey, J. 1991 *Living with anorexia and bulimia.* Manchester: Manchester University Press.

Smail, D. 1987 *Taking care: an alternative to therapy.* London: J.M. Dent.

Yalom, I. 1985: *The theory and practice of group psychotherapy.* New York: Basic Books.

DOING AND BEING: A BUDDHIST PERSPECTIVE ON CRAVING AND ADDICTION

Paramabandhu Groves

Chapter 14 concerns addictions: clients' addiction to substances and other sources of security, as well as carers' need to intervene. It also concerns a set of means by which any of us may transcend such dependency and craving. Paramabandhu Groves relates these themes in his work to the Buddhist view of craving as a root of suffering, suggesting that as a result of the various forms of craving in which we all indulge, suffering arises. The Buddhist conceptualisation of ethics is introduced and Paramabandhu argues that through meditation techniques to enhance mindfulness and love, essentially through stillness and reflection, we may experience more fully what is going on in our own experience, allowing us in turn to respond more creatively to the difficult states our clients are in. In *being with* them rather than immediately trying to *do something* we can help them, also, to be with what is happening, rather than succumbing to craving for something else and aversion to what is there. This inaction, he argues, paradoxically, is the only way in which real change may evolve.

It may be of interest to consider the Buddhist view relating also to sanity and madness, in this regard. A pivotal stage on the Path for Buddhists is that of *Stream Entry*, where the degree of insight into reality (things as they really are) has reached a point where the disciple need make no further effort to progress, carried as s/he is inexorably towards the goal of Enlightenment by the sheer strength of the current. From this point onwards is said to be sanity, whereas up to such a point of insight is said to be one form or another of essentially *mad* experience. The fetters that one representation of the Path claims must be broken to achieve this state of Stream Entry, include *dependence* on a fixed view of oneself, that is as unchanging and static; and *dependence* on moral observances (and rituals) as ends in themselves, rather than as tools to be used to grow.

Working in the addictions, a not uncommon scenario goes as follows: I am counselling a woman who has been dependent on heroin and is receiving from me a prescription for methadone. She is trying to gradually reduce and ultimately stop taking the methadone to free herself from the grip of drug use. From time to time, perhaps feeling stressed or depressed or in the company of certain people, she buys extra methadone and starts using this on top of the prescribed methadone. This leads to a need to increase the prescribed methadone and so reverse the recent attempts to reduce the methadone. As part of the counselling we explore the reasons why she needs to buy extra methadone, what are the circumstances, what else she could have done and how it could be avoided in future. Despite exploring this together, it continues to happen. For a little while things are okay, we reduce the methadone and then she ends up buying extra methadone for very similar reasons to before – all the while insisting she does want to end her use of methadone and become drug-free. Eventually I notice myself becoming frustrated and irritated. Irritated that she will not make use of the work that we are doing together in the sessions. The irritation acts as a barrier between us. To the extent that I react to the situation with irritation, wanting her to behave a particular way, I am prevented from seeing what is really happening and responding creatively.

There are many ways in which our patients may not do what we want them to do. They don't turn up for appointments, they refuse to take the medication, they don't do their homework assignments or as in my example they don't make use of the work we have been doing together. The problem is not so much our preferences for our patients as the weight with which we want our preferences to be followed – which may be only revealed when someone doesn't do what we want them to do. Wanting someone to do a particular thing or be a particular way is part of a basic tendency which in Buddhism is called craving.

BUDDHISM

Buddhism originated with Siddhartha Gautama, a man who was born about 485 BCE (Before Common Era) into a wealthy family in an area which spans what is now the border between northern India and Nepal. As a young adult he became dissatisfied with his affluent lifestyle, seeing the inevitability of suffering (even despite his wealth). He left home and became a wanderer and after a few years through his own efforts reached 'Enlightenment', becoming a Buddha. 'Buddha' literally means 'one who is awake'. The Buddha had 'woken up' to the causes of human suffering and discovered means to transform himself, to completely free himself of suffering. This state of total transformation, characterised by profound wisdom, supreme compassion and boundless energy, is called Enlightenment. The Buddha spent the remaining 45 years of his life teaching others how they too could free themselves and gain Enlight-enment. He showed how we bring suffering upon ourselves through craving and he mapped out a path of spiritual development together with practices to traverse this path.

Thus Buddhism is essentially a path of personal evolution which transforms one's suffering and which is dedicated to the alleviation of the suffering of others. One becomes a Buddhist by committing oneself to the Three Jewels, which are the Buddha, the Dharma, and the Sangha. Committing oneself to the Buddha means taking the ideal of realising Enlightenment as the central goal of one's life. The Dharma refers to the teachings and practices whereby the goal may be realised. The Sangha includes all

those who are following the path and who provide essential support and encouragement. Committing oneself to the Sangha implies valuing this support and being
receptive to the influences especially of those more spiritually developed than oneself.

There are many formulations of the path. One of the most frequently cited is the
Threefold Way. This consists of ethics, meditation and wisdom. Each stage develops
out of the fullness of the previous one, although to some extent they may be practised
concurrently. Thus ethics forms the foundation for the successful practice of meditation. Meditation is a means of working directly on the mind with the mind in order to
transform it. From the depths of meditation arises the possibility of wisdom, which
when fully developed leads to Enlightenment. The rest of the chapter focuses on
Buddhist ethics and their relevance to working in psychiatry.

CRAVING

Craving is the urge or desire to obtain an experience other that the one we are
experiencing at present. This operates both in gross and in very subtle ways. Everyday
examples include the pursuit of pleasurable experiences such as good food and sex, or
the desire to have material objects such as a car, fine clothes, or the latest computer
model. It includes wanting to be in a different place or a different job or a different
relationship. The underlying assumption is that if only I had a new boyfriend/
girlfriend or when I get that promotion, then I will be happy. The values of our
society with its emphasis on hedonism and materialism back us up. Adverts promise
us that if we buy the latest product our happiness is assured. On a more subtle level,
craving is present influencing our behaviour much of the time. For example, if I enter a
room of people I don't know or a ward of patients I haven't met, in moments I will
have picked up impressions of the people and will tend to gravitate towards those I
like. Even if we try to be quiet for a few minutes, perhaps sitting with a cup of tea or
following our breath, our mind will be off, planning future pleasures or worrying
about how we can get what we want. It is very hard to stay simply with what is,
rather than being tugged off somewhere else, often into the future or the past.

There are a number of reasons why craving is unhelpful. First of all is the fact of
impermanence. Pleasure is fine as long as we don't expect it to last. We can eat our
food, savour it and enjoy it. But it is soon eaten, and if we are eating it primarily
because we are feeling a bit depressed, it won't work. The chocolate will give only
temporary relief, and if we keep eating we end up feeling sick. Or that experience of
thinking 'I'll just have a little bit more of that pudding because it was *so* delicious', and
afterwards, bloated, regretting it. If we try to get more out of our sense experience
than it can deliver to us, we suffer. Even with more lasting things – a television, car or
relationships – we cannot hold onto them forever. Sadly, sooner or later, we must let
go of them, or they will 'let go' of us by breaking down or leaving us.

Secondly, in order to keep the pleasure coming we have to keep on moving. It is like
skating fast enough over the ice so that you don't fall in. This works up to a point, but
it leads to restlessness as it is necessary to keep looking for new pleasurable experiences and to manoeuvre them our way. Not only does such a relentless struggle to
control our experience of the world, to obtain and hold onto what we want, at best
only partially succeed, it can also create a background anxiety. It may prevent us from

experiencing ourself fully, as instead we tend to superficiality. There may be attention to the process of obtaining pleasure, but an avoidance of experiencing either its inevitable loss or anything much else.

Thirdly, craving brings with it its flip side, aversion, which is not wanting to have an experience we are having. We push experience away from us, wanting to get rid of it. Aversion may also be thought of as frustrated craving. So when my client does not do what I want her to do, I become frustrated and irritated. In addition to the anger being unpleasant for my client if I let it out (or if it seeps out), it prevents me from thinking creatively about the situation. As well as pushing away our experience with anger or hatred we may try to get rid of it through distracting ourselves, for example with psychoactive substances, mindless television or busyness. Thus the 'difficult' patient on the ward may end up being unconsciously avoided or we end up being so busy seeing other patients that before we know it time has run out and we just don't have time to see that particular patient today. Apart from any actual damage these activities may cause directly, they prevent us from knowing who we really are and stop us from growing into what we could be.

Craving and aversion are doomed to failure because ultimately, as strategies for approaching the world, they don't completely work. Sometimes the objects of our desires may be within easy reach: we go to the fridge for the ice-cream, or a job just falls into our lap. However, we cannot completely control the world or other people in it. If we are attached to getting what we want we will suffer. Deriving pleasure from the objects of our craving is likened to honey on a razor's edge. It seems so alluring, but we don't see the razor. Just as the cocaine addict is impelled towards one more hit, despite its consequences, we too are attached to getting things to go our way and ignore or don't recognise the consequences of this attachment.

If our desires are frustrated, we may use various strategies to obtain what we want – through aggression, bullying or more subtle forms of manipulation. Sometimes it can be very hard to let go of what we want for our clients. For example, in recent years it has been increasingly difficult to find a bed for patients on a psychiatric ward. In particular I have noticed it is hard to admit a patient who might be given a diagnosis of personality disorder. Sometimes when working in general psychiatry I would see a patient in casualty about whom I was sufficiently concerned to want to bring them into hospital. I could easily find myself wanting to distort the truth slightly. As I discussed the patient over the telephone in order to arrange the admission, I could find myself dancing a wary path – the patient *was* suicidal (a good criterion for admission) but not *too much* so (which would mean the patient would need one-to-one specialling by a nurse, which might be difficult to arrange). I might play down any past history of violence (which would make difficulties for admission) and lean on anything suggestive of hallucinations or delusions (psychosis is always easier to admit). In this way I might get what I want – the patient admitted to hospital. But even apart from my own personal discomfort about not being entirely straight or stretching the facts of the case, it prevented me from passing on as clear a picture as I might otherwise have done and it glossed over the issue of the need for sometimes admitting someone with a personality disorder to hospital. A nurse might find herself facing the same dilemmas when wishing to transfer a patient onto another ward, e.g., to move a patient from a general ward to a psychiatric intensive care unit, or the reverse. Many pressures may influence the bending of the information apart from direct concerns for the patient's care, such as staff shortages, disturbance of other patients on the ward or simply the inconvenience of having the patient.

AN ETHICAL APPROACH

To the extent that what we do is motivated by craving and aversion, it will be confused and unhelpful. Confusion, also called spiritual ignorance, refers to an unwillingness to look clearly at our experience and what we are doing. It is like a veil, which we may not be especially aware of, that prevents us from seeing 'reality', how things actually are. We don't notice in our confusion that we are behaving as if something might last forever (through our craving, clinging on to it) or as if we might have complete control over the universe, thereby attempting to inhabit a bright world without any suffering (which aversion tries to push away). In a vicious circle, confusion is at once the cause of craving and aversion, and exacerbates them.

The unhelpful consequences of craving as detailed above include disappointment, anxiety, superficiality and hatefulness, as well as confusion; and these are just the effects on our own mental state. If we want to avoid these we can, according to Buddhist ethics, start by looking at our actions and in particular our intentions. For it is our intentions which will determine to a large extent the consequences. Our physical and verbal actions may be viewed as crystallisations of our mental volitions. We can attempt to adopt an alternative approach to one based on craving, aversion and confusion. If our actions are informed by contentment and letting go (as opposed to craving), by friendliness (rather than aversion), and clarity (instead of confusion), they are likely to have a beneficial effect.

Such a contrast between these sets of motivations (craving/aversion/confusion and letting go/friendliness/clarity) is not, in Buddhist ethics, a question of 'good' or 'bad' and all the judgements that these words imply. Instead an enquiry is encouraged into where on this continuum are our actions and how *skilful* are they. There is skill involved because it isn't always easy to know what is driving us to act and skill is required to be clear enough to see the likely consequences of our actions. It is not simply a matter of 'good intentions', since a skilful mental state is not just one characterised by apparent friendliness, but also includes clarity which enables us to see the likely effects of what we intend to do, or at least prevents us from ignoring otherwise obvious consequences. Thus there is a quality of wisdom – blind well-meaning activity is usually unskilful. If we want to be helpful, we need to bring full attention to what we are feeling and ask ourselves with great honesty what are our real reasons for acting (or not acting). For example, if we want to give more sedative medication to a psychotic patient, is this because we actually believe it would be helpful to alleviate the patient's distress, or is it to alleviate our distress or to make us feel safer or to punish the patient for 'bad' behaviour? Again, talking about patients at handover or discussing inter-staff difficulties – to what extent are we striving to be helpful and truthful or to what extent is resentment colouring our speech, or a desire to be accepted by our peers leading us to join in castigating the unpopular charge nurse or consultant? Our motives may well be mixed, but the more we can be aware of what mental states our decisions are coming from, the more we can strive to make helpful choices and act skilfully.

Seemingly compassionate activity may in fact be unskilful if we don't carefully discern the emotions we are experiencing. Particularly relevant to people in the caring professions are the two near enemies of compassion, which are sentimental pity and horrified anxiety. These may masquerade as compassion and are in danger of being confused with it. With pity we take a superior position that is condescending – 'oh poor you'. The essence of sentimental pity is that it appears to be feeling for and responding kindly to the person who is suffering, but in fact it is a way of distancing ourself from the other person's suffering. It may come from confusion in the face of pain or out of fear – fear of the pain itself or fear of what might be required to help the person if their suffering was truly acknowledged. Thus there is an element of hollowness about it, that the concern is not real. In a sense it does not take the suffering seriously, but trivialises it, partly by having a sentimental attitude towards it. With horrified anxiety, we are overwhelmed by the other person's suffering. We so completely identify with it that we are paralysed and are unable to act effectively to help the person. Compassion has its etymology in *com + pati* and literally means to feel with. However, with sentimental pity we do not really feel with the person's suffering, really touch into their difficulties; we do not get near enough to their suffering. With horrified anxiety we become too close and over-identify. Compassion treads a middle way in which we reach onto and stay with the edge of someone's suffering. Fine tuning our responses, we balance between cutting off from someone's pain, on the one hand, and, on the other, losing our sense of self in their pain – or, rather, the pain that is aroused in us but actually prevents us from truly seeing the other person.

THE DEVELOPMENT OF SKILFUL QUALITIES

I was called to see a man in casualty who had stabbed himself. The casualty officer told me he seemed rather cut off from his emotions. I went into the cubicle and began to ask him about what had happened. He started to relate how his girlfriend had left him and the grief he felt about that. Soon he became extremely distressed and tearful. He felt his life was not worth living and regretted he had not succeeded in killing himself. I felt uneasy about letting him go home – his wounds did not warrant admission to a medical ward – and broached the idea of him coming into a psychiatric hospital. He was clear he did not want to come into hospital. I felt at a loss as to what to do. But I just stayed there, with him, in his grief and anguish. I gave up trying to get him to do what I wanted and simply sat with him. After a time his acute distress had begun to subside and so I took my leave and told him I would come and see him again later after he had had his wounds stitched. When I returned a couple of hours later, I was surprised not so much by his decision now to come into hospital, but by him thanking me for helping him. At the time I felt I was doing nothing and of no help. However, in retrospect. I can see nothing was precisely what I needed to do.

When the casualty officer saw him I think he was probably still in shock and unable to connect with what he had done and why. How I think I helped him was to give him some space in which he could experience his feelings and anguish. Moreover, once I had stopped trying to make him do something – go into hospital to alleviate my unease – I was able simply just to be with him, neither being overwhelmed by his distress nor cutting off from it. In this space, which is friendly without any demands to be a particular way, things can be simply as they are. However, they are impermanent. Everything is in a state of flux. Giving someone this space with kindness can allow things to run their course, to complete. Thus the man could experience what was happening to him, without having to do anything with it and so the emotional current could run its course and settle, at least for a time.

I think as mental health workers it is very easy for us to want to *do* something. And of course it is natural and appropriate that we want to help to alleviate another's suffering. However, our wanting to help someone can be a form of craving in which we want the client to be a particular way or do a particular thing. It can be hard for us to tolerate someone wanting to do something other, especially if we perceive that it will not be in their own interests, that it will add to their suffering. It may be difficult to tolerate another's suffering, which can make us want to cheer someone up, to relieve our own discomfort, as we slip into one of the near enemies of compassion.

In order to act skilfully it is not enough to know what we should do or not do, we also need to have the necessary personal resources. Partly this comes from practice from exploring our mind states and actions from an ethical perspective and endeavouring to make our actions more skilful. Buddhism gives a number of lists of precepts which are guidelines for ethical behaviour. These are not lists of rules, but training principles to reflect on and use as a benchmark for what we do. One of the commonest lists is the five precepts which in their negative form consists of undertaking to abstain from killing beings, from taking the not given, from sexual misconduct, from harmful speech, and from intoxicants which cloud the mind. In their positive form they are the practice of loving kindness, of generosity, of contentment, of truthful speech and of mindfulness. The precepts describe how one who is inhabiting skilful mental states all the time would behave spontaneously (Sangharakshita, 1989).

In addition to examining our actions and their motives in relation to such a benchmark, we can aim to directly develop skilful qualities. The two most important qualities are mindfulness or awareness and *maitri*. *Maitri* may be translated as unconditional loving kindness or friendliness. It is a love which is disinterested in the sense of not wanting anything back, not sticky or expecting people to be a particular way in order to receive the 'love'. It goes beyond ties of family or lover and resonates with all beings. *Maitri* provides the emotionally positive basis which is needed to work with other people, particularly people in distress. It is the foundation for true compassion. But emotional positivity needs to be balanced by mindfulness. Mindfulness provides awareness of oneself and one's emotional states as well as of other people and the likely effects on them. Together, mindfulness and *maitri* can create the friendly space which is essential for therapeutic interaction. Developing these qualities enables us to see our patients as individual people. Craving is utilitarian and views the world for what it can obtain, people as objects to be manipulated and patients as so many bits of pathology to be treated. *Maitri* has eyes of appreciation and responds to the person, not just the schizophrenic or the addict. With *maitri* and mindfulness I have a chance of catching my irritation with patients who seem to refuse to use our work and of finding a more creative response. I am more able just to be with the man in his distress and allow change to take place.

Many things can help us to develop these qualities. Meditation is the traditional method, and the second step of the Threefold Way. It can be extremely useful as a way of learning simply to be with whatever is happening in us, without needing to act. As well as helping to develop mindfulness, it can also be a means to nurture into being the seeds of *maitri*. Friendship is also important to sustain us. In particular, friendships with those who share our values, who also see the importance of working on themselves. We also need inspiration to help give us a broader perspective, which may come from a wide variety of sources such as art, fine literature, other inspirational books or immersing ourselves in beautiful countryside.

Going about work there are plenty of opportunities to keep a practice of mindfulness going. When I am walking from one part of the institution to another I can bring attention to the soles of my feet and experience myself walking on the earth, rather than letting my mind be rushed off into the next event. Especially if I happen to be outside I can tune into the play of light, the trees, the sense of the season and the wider world. From time to time during the day I like to stop, just for a few moments, to allow me to catch up with myself. I might follow a few breaths, release accumulated tension in my shoulders from hunching in front of a computer screen or tune in to my feelings as they are right now. In this way we can keep a thread of awareness going through the day which helps to keep us resourced to engage with whatever is thrown at us.

When we then come into contact with our clients' suffering – or their intransigence – we will then be more equipped in our being to be with them. When it is difficult to be with them, or be with our own reactions, we can try breathing through (Macy, 1988). In this we follow our breath and let the pain or suffering enter our heart, our chest. We may feel some discomfort in our chest as we resonate with their pain. And then breathing out, we can let it go, but transformed somewhat. Using our breath our heart can act as a transformer, to transform the suffering that we meet. The breath is a great anchor which helps us simply to be with whatever is. It allows the development of true compassion.

In Buddhism the figure *par excellence* of compassion is the bodhisattva. The bodhisattva is a being who endeavours to alleviate the suffering of all beings. Yet the bodhisattva's activity is described as play. This is because the bodhisattva's compassionate activity is based on wisdom. The bodhisattva sees through craving and transcends it. He or she sees it for what it is. Many of us might choose not to inject heroin seeing the damage it causes, yet many addicts through craving will self-destructively inject heroin. By analogy, the bodhisattva has transcended *all* craving and the suffering to which it leads, and lives joyfully in freedom. The bodhisattva has a larger perspective. He or she sees the impermanence of all phenomena and sees the flux and play of all phenomena as a dance. Rather than obstructing the flow of the dance with craving and aversion the bodhisattva dances too, adding without interfering and allowing the natural changes to take place.

If we want to be a bodhisattva we need to be able to see what is going on without insisting on things being a particular way. This means we need to be able to tolerate others doing what we don't want them to do, and to be able to tolerate their suffering (including anger or hatred) and what it evokes in us. This requires work on ourself. In order to be able to just *be* with someone, we need to have developed our being. And in doing this we can be helped by trying to find a larger perspective. We can look for some lightness, a sense of play and not get bogged down in the seriousness of it all. However difficult it appears now, it will change. Sometimes we need to just be and get our own small selves out of the way to let real change take place.

REFERENCES

Macy, J. 1988: Taking heart: spiritual exercises for social activists. In Eppsteiner. F. (ed.) *Path of compassion: writings on socially engaged Buddhism.* Berkeley, CA: Parallax Press, pp. 203–13.
Sangharakshita 1989: *The Ten Pillars of Buddhism.* Glasgow: Windhorse.

15

THE PARADOX OF PSYCHIATRIC NURSING: MAKING A DIFFERENCE BY ATTEMPTING TO CHANGE NOTHING[1]

Ben Davidson

Ben Davidson introduces the third set of means by which one may develop an ethical practice, clinical supervision. The use of colleagues to provide feedback about your style of work and the form of your interaction with clients is invaluable in psychiatric nursing. It may take many forms, however, including individual supervision with a line manager, peer group supervision with colleagues, an external facilitator coming in to enable in-depth discussion of the work, and so on. If resources allow, however, it may be that there is no better form of supervision than from someone actually in the room watching your interaction with clients. Here a form of 'live supervision' is described where the supervisor, or 'support worker', makes comments on the process of the interaction during the session, in a way that allows the client, as well as the 'active' worker, the best chance to use any insights that emerge.

Recently I attended an interview for a senior clinical post in a nursing development unit. I had to choose an aspect of my practice to present in a ten-minute slot to the three interviewers and the group of six candidates for the post. I decided to use a case study. It was hard to find a piece of work that seemed exactly appropriate, harder still to condense it into that time, but there was one example that stood out. I worried that the life stories of the clients involved might distract attention from the particular aspect of my practice I wanted to convey, so I decided to highlight from the outset what aspect of my clinical practice the case study demonstrated.

---

[1] I should like to thank Ms Jackie Adeosun for her skilful use of the support-worker role in the following intervention. I wish also to acknowledge the training, encouragement, supervision and support given to me in the work described below by Mr Nicholas Watts CQSW, Project Manager, Cowley House Community Mental Health Day Centre, Directorate of Social Services, London Borough of Lambeth, UK. Cowley House has now closed due to cutbacks in the local government Social Services budget.

There were two main themes. The first theme related to the approach we take as psychiatric nurses. Do we join with psychiatrists in attributing mental pathology to events, processes and people, in working on someone's illness, in treating a problem? Or might our role be something different, to validate a person's experience, to facilitate a negotiated view of their situation as the natural upshot of their life history (Smail, 1984, pp. 12–13), to try simply to *be* with them in that situation? My second theme was essentially a practical application of the first. In the light of the tension between the two roles described, how should we view, and manage, a mental health crisis? This chapter is based on the presentation that I gave.

BACKGROUND

I work at a Mental Health Day Centre, which is a community resource owned and run by an inner city Social Services department. The central thrust of our work is large group facilitation and provision of a therapeutic milieu, in a homely building in Kennington, South London, with crisis intervention available for clients during periods of mental breakdown. This crisis intervention is conducted, as is other, preventative work undertaken at the Centre, through drop-ins and sessional therapeutic work, as well as through outreach support and practical help for people in their homes. We also undertake welfare work: getting people benefits, housing repairs, and so on. The approach taken to our clinical work is based on systems theory and group analysis. In practice this means we rely on the relationships within the group, client–client as well as client–staff relationships, to generate healing. Such relationships also provide the backdrop for our use of an innovative form of family therapy, employed to good effect even with people in psychotic states.

Ours is a group of clients who mostly don't like hospitals. Generally we manage to keep them out. They like, instead, our attempts to empower them to believe in their own strengths, our attempts to understand and validate their experience, our attempts to work with them analytically – but with a light touch – and as a large group. It is a cohesive large group.

The point of this chapter really is to show what it is like to work in this way with people in attending to their mental health needs. I hope to convey something of the experience of adopting a systems approach, seeing and relating to people and their problems always within a larger context. I hope also to show how psychotherapy is essentially, 'an obstinate attempt of two [or more] people to recover the wholeness of being human through the relationship between them' (Laing, 1967, p. 53). In preparing this chapter, however, it seemed it might be helpful to provide some basic themes about systemic family therapy, some of the techniques used. I have hesitated to do this as I am keen, first and foremost, to convey something of the experience of working in this way, rather than distracting the reader's attention by over-conceptualising it. Working therapeutically, after all, demands primarily an ability to be in tune with one's feelings and other aspects of one's own experience in relation to clients, as a way of beneficially accessing and bringing to light *their* experience and the way it influences their conduct. All too often we use ideas and theory as a crutch because we are daunted at the prospect of relying on our feelings, and then we censor and modify our experience in line with what we think we *ought* to be experiencing according to such ideas and theory. Nevertheless, a theoretical base from which to practise and a proper understanding of what the work involves are also important, so for a comprehensive text on family therapy and systems theory, I would recommend Skynner's *One flesh: separate persons* (1976) as a background to the following sketch of some basic techniques and concepts.

In the work described, two systemic concepts and techniques are pivotal – *homeostasis* and *paradox*. In relation to homeostasis, perhaps the simplest way to explain what lies at the heart of this concept is to say that 'nature balances automatically what we do not balance consciously' (ibid., p. 12). If a family has come to invest in the myth that 'in this family we never have arguments', it may be no surprise that conflict, hostility and jealousy, for example, get acted out unconsciously or expressed through other means. There may be a high prevalence of gastric or other somatic complaints in the family, as a means of concretising such feelings. Or conflict may come to be represented as occurring between the family (us) and some outside agency such as social workers, members of another race, grandparents (them), as a way of externalising rage and envy. Alternatively, one member of the family may come to *contain* the banished feelings on behalf of the whole group, and even be seen as abnormal, or formally diagnosed as having psychological problems or otherwise scapegoated as a result. An adolescent displaying a ferocious temper and sexual precociousness may be expressing the repressed sexuality and anger of some other, possibly more powerful individual(s), or possibly those repressed feelings of the whole family group. Viewed solely in the context of how a balanced individual might be expected to act, she may appear as though she is disturbed. However, in the context of the family system of communication and expression of affect, her conduct may be seen more appreciatively as representing (in exaggerated form) perfectly normal feelings which are otherwise denied throughout the group. And although their relatively repressive states of being will be less problematic for the other family members as individuals, the attention to manners and etiquette they display as a group, may more realistically be seen as equally exaggerated.

My suggestion, that families may simply 'come to' such an arrangement as this, ignores the operation of power within a group, as also it ignores the distress and pain experienced as such roles become increasingly polarised, entrenched and pathologised. In such circumstances, it may be that the services of a family therapist, operating from a model which takes into account the communication, or patterns of information exchange within the whole group is required, to restore equilibrium to the system. While polarisation of roles and feelings may be quite normal, there are occasions when the 'homeostatic' mechanisms which keep members of the system in balance cease to be effective, and some intervention is required to restore equilibrium.

In the following account, the role of paradox in such intervention is a central theme. A 'paradoxical injunction' is one where a message is given which promotes change by prescribing that things should stay the same (paradoxically). The reader will be familiar with some situation where, in exasperation at a defiant child, a parent tells it to do the opposite of what is required, having seen that the child's need to express defiance is greater than any other emotional consideration: 'OK, that's it, that was your last chance – you have taken so long to sit down to eat you are not going to get *any* dinner now.' Which, of course, is a risk – a sharp child (or one with no appetite) might see through this device and insist that such an arrangement suits him fine, he didn't want to eat anyway. However, if the intervention was well judged, the child's defiance wins over and the child insists that as he is now seated he is entitled to food immediately. Just so in marital or family therapy! 'Well it does seem as if the two of you are having the most awful time of it, and these problems certainly are very, very serious indeed – four different professionals is it, you said, you've seen now over the last year? – but I have to say that, from what I have gathered in this interview, there is really nothing I have to offer that you would be able to use to improve the situation. I really think you're just going to have to find a way of living with this thing. [Long pause; give some sign the interview is about to end, e.g. close the file, make as if to stand up.] Unless . . . No, it's hardly even worth wasting our time talking about it . . .'. Cue response from patient.

The form of paradox used in the following account is far more subtle than the above. In a form of intervention Skynner refers to as 'reactor analysis' (ibid., p. 188) the therapist lowers his emotional defences and allows the family attitudes to affect him, allows himself to be *sucked into* the communication system. As Skynner describes, such therapists

> operate rather like the fishermen of the Gilbert and Ellice islands . . . where one member of the team dives into the tentacles of the octopus while the second follows immediately behind and, by a sharp tug on the leg of his companion, raises them both swiftly to the surface where they can be disentangled. For equally cogent reasons the reactor-analysts also operate in pairs, one standing by to rescue his co-therapist as he is about to vanish into the 'dear octopus' of the family's pathology.

(1976, p. 188)

The therapist is a reactor in that he does not direct, so much as follow, or react to the emotional currents at play. He is an analyst in that he respects the potential of patients to discover their own way forward if only their motivation and insight can be harnessed. The means by which such harnessing occurs is the relationship between co-therapists (or active and support workers in the case of the model in operation at the Day Centre). The active worker dives in to the current of emotion and communication between the family members, specifically *not* censoring or having to think about his response – that is the job of the support worker, who 'tugs his leg' at appropriate junctures, and then initiates a conversation between the two of them as to his (the active worker's) emotional response, the roles the family participants are taking, the feelings that are getting expressed, those that are not getting expressed and so on, thereby eliciting insight in the clients. If the reader is able to recall a time in childhood when a parent discussed your conduct or character with another adult, in your presence, all the while excluding you from the conversation, that may give something of the flavour of such interactions. Although our experiences of such interactions are usually painful, as they were occasioned perhaps through a parent's feeling angry and rejecting, it is possible, I hope, to imagine how such a powerful form of relationship may be harnessed therapeutically in the patient's interests. In particular, where the active worker's emotional engagement with the family dynamics prompts him to want to intervene directively or prescriptively, the support worker is in a position to give that small tug (if they are working well together) and draw the former's attention to his mistake (subtly prescribing to the clients that they should not change – or at least should not *be made to* change), while at the same time drawing their attention to the way in which roles are being adopted and feelings shared.

I am Marjorie's key-worker at the Day Centre. Marjorie is a neatly dressed, 59-year-old, white woman, who has a 40-year psychiatric history, most of that time on high doses of neuroleptic medication, but without apparent side-effects. She presents as highly dependent on her carer, John, who, during the open door drop-ins we run twice weekly, will prepare her food, organise her medication and sort out the change she needs to pay for her tea. She is also, somewhat paradoxically it may seem, very intelligent, keenly aware of her environment and sometimes quite engaging. She was in psycho-analysis for a number of years in her twenties. John, who has been Marjorie's carer and partner for about thirty years, is a 74-year-old, small-framed, white man. He has led a colourful life, is widely travelled and looks intriguing with his long, silver-grey hair in a pony-tail, a meticulously shaped goatee and a perpetual look as if there is a party in his head. He used, in the years after the Second World War, to be a nurse at a mental hospital. He can be very patronising and controlling. He might greet us with a review of Marjorie's progress, talking to us about her as if she is not there: 'She's been very up and down this week, *haven't* you Marjorie?'

A crisis developed in the early autumn last year as Marjorie became more dependent, quite angrily so at times, insisting John get her things and complaining about the care he was giving her. The arguments ranged from a low-level bickering during drop-ins to quite heated outbursts and exchanges. Marjorie was violent on several occasions at home. A psychiatrist had intervened by changing and increasing the strength of Marjorie's medication. He had John's support in focusing his treatment this way. They both saw Marjorie as the problem, or at least as having the problems.

It was surely no coincidence, however, that in the summer it had emerged that John, or Janet, as he wanted from then on to be known, was becoming a transsexual. Janet began dressing in women's clothes and would talk candidly about the breasts she was developing as a result of her hormone treatment. At first we staff denied our anxiety about the couple and blamed our feelings of unease on the uncompromising way Janet asserted her transsexuality, interpreted by us as a need to shock. But this disabled us in responding to the wider situation and emerging crisis.

Things continued this way for some time until Janet accompanied Marjorie to a Women's Group at the Centre and asked to become a client in her own right so that they could attend the Women's Group together. Although it was presented as a strategic ploy to gain admission, this request seemed also significant as a statement from Janet regarding her status. We took the opportunity to respond creatively and decided our response should include Janet, even though she was technically too old to access our services.

Rather than give a full description of the sessions with Marjorie and Janet (or rather Beverley as she came finally to be known), I shall draw out some of the difficulties and highlights in the work, relating them back to my principal theme of the psychiatric nurse's role: Pathologisation versus validation.

THE WORK

Difficulties

From the time I first met this couple nearly two years ago, up to the point I just reached in my account, I resisted seeing Marjorie as 'the problem'. Increasingly, however, John/Janet/Beverley *was* the problem, so far as I was concerned. She was controlling, pathologising, shocking and in more or less complete denial of any need herself whilst evidently in the middle of probably the most traumatic event of her life, which she shared compulsively, in intricate detail and at length with anyone who would listen. All the while she would laugh off both Marjorie's and anyone else's difficulties about the gender reassignment as other people's over-sensibilities, not her problem. All sense of vulnerability, dependence and need in the relationship appeared to be vested in Marjorie. When I advised that they needed help to look *together* at the issues contributing to their current difficulties *as a couple*, Beverley expressed considerable ambivalence, insisting she was attending the sessions to help Marjorie with *her* problems. Although I offered, in the spirit of maximising client choice, to see Marjorie alone to give her support, I was glad that we all finally agreed they would be 'family' sessions. For some time though, despite this systemic emphasis, I retained my view that the problem was Beverley's, a response every bit as pathologising as the psychiatrist's.

We used the family therapy technique described above: I would engage directly with Marjorie and Beverley while a 'support worker', my colleague Jackie, was also in the room, sitting slightly to one side of me in a position where she could watch the interaction between the three of us and offer live supervision when necessary. This co-working relationship is difficult in many respects, not least of which is the fact that one's practice as active worker is under constant scrutiny and critique, in front of the client. It is of course also difficult to establish adequate trust with one's co-worker to allow the feedback to flow smoothly and to work with it.

I would often ask Beverley and Marjorie to review the session just before it ended. On one such occasion Marjorie had said what she thought we had covered in the session and how she felt about it. Beverley then took her turn. However, Beverley did not talk about how *she* felt, but about Marjorie. Despite several prompts from me, Beverley insisted on reviewing where Marjorie was at rather than presenting her own response. At a point of near exasperation with Beverley, where I had all but told her she was jeopardising progress by refusing to own her feelings, Jackie stepped in to remind me I had said the session would finish with Marjorie and Beverley's feedback, but now I was lecturing rather than listening to Beverley. I apologised and allowed the session to finish. On another occasion, in contrast, Beverley acknowledged not only how hard she was finding the gender reassignment and people's attitudes to her, but also how she felt nervous and unsure how to respond to Marjorie's anger. What an admission of vulnerability from Beverley, what a breakthrough!

'Marjorie, how do *you* feel the session has gone?'
'I don't think there'll ever be any change, he just mocks me all the time, Ben.'

I tried to coax some optimism out of Marjorie, angry at her fatalism, touched by Beverley's disclosure and scared that Marjorie was pushing them back again into their polarised positions. Again, Jackie intervened. She reminded me how Marjorie had said she was feeling; she suggested that difference was normal and healthy in any relationship and it was fine for Marjorie to be feeling pessimistic; she advised me to accept how Marjorie felt; and she told me that we now had to finish the session. Again, I apologised, echoed how Jackie had summarised Marjorie's position, and ended the session on that note. On both these occasions I had been drawn, by my own need to make things better, as well as by Beverley and Marjorie's fear of the confusion they faced, into trying to resolve things. I had on each occasion identified a problem: Beverley's denial of her needs; Marjorie's refusal to feel anything but helpless and fatalistic. On each occasion I had responded much as the partner in their relationship would characteristically respond – with anger towards Beverley and her denial in the first case (much as Marjorie felt), and with an attempt to control Marjorie's experience, to get her seeing things more positively in the second (acting much as Beverley would). Together, Jackie and I then produced an alternative response to these circumstances, which was in each case to highlight what was happening and, at the same time, *just to allow the situation to be*.

Highlights

The highlights of my work with Beverley and Marjorie were the occasions of positive change in their relationship. These seemed to occur just when my absorption in their relationship was at its greatest and when differences between them manifested in the relationship between Jackie and I (Skynner, 1976, p. 275), with me becoming more problem-oriented towards them and Jackie restoring a more neutral approach, as described above. Such breakthrough and change in the couple's attitude to themselves and to each other usually took the form of acknowledgement and acceptance by Marjorie and Beverley of the role reversal in their relationship. A good example was when Beverley eventually shaved off her goatee. I had mentioned some time before how much harder I found it to relate to her as a woman while she sported such an impressive beard, and both Jackie and I remarked on the change at the beginning of this session. Marjorie had not noticed though, until Jackie and I commented on Beverley's appearance, that the beard had gone, despite the fact that Beverley had shaved it off early that morning. Beverley tried to laugh this off and related how Marjorie had failed also over the previous three years to notice her developing breasts. She acknowledged, finally, in a rare outburst of emotion, how angry this lack of recognition had actually left her, and how her derisive laughter belied this. She also disclosed how rejected she felt by others and how awful her appearance now seemed to her, 'like an old hag'. Apparently as a result of expressing her own vulnerability, she managed to start taking Marjorie's more seriously. This included a willingness to hear Marjorie's expression of anger, outrage and hurt that she (Beverley) had kept her hormone therapy and gender reassignment secret for three years under the pretext of some sort of test to see if she (Marjorie) noticed. Marjorie also made breakthroughs. For example, she acknowledged how when she referred to Beverley as 'he' she wanted to hurt her because of her anger about the changes Beverley had imposed, without consultation, on their lives. Then, increasingly, she explored and learnt how she could be less dependent and how she could look after Beverley. Awkwardly and with rather closed questions at first, but with increasing confidence and skill, Marjorie would ask Beverley how she felt about things, whether she hadn't found aspects of her gender reassignment, interactions with people and aspects of their relationship together difficult to handle. And perhaps the most impressive example of her move from dependency to taking charge was in the role she took in recounting the history of their relationship together. Marjorie evidently felt proud at the increasing sense that theirs was a unique and impressive story of a life together. She asked whether I might write about the work I had done with them some day, and when I told her recently that I was writing this chapter, she asked (and then requested in writing) for her real name to be used.

COMMENTARY

It is easy to caricature psychiatrists as representing a force of pathologisation, while as nurses we do something much more creative. But this oversimplifies things to a ludicrous degree. This was the point about my practice that I wanted to convey, that it is much easier *for all of us* to find a problem in our clients and try to get rid of it. I, certainly, find it a constant struggle to act from the position I described earlier: Validating a person's experience, facilitating a negotiated view of their situation as the natural upshot of their life history, trying simply to *be* with them in that situation, attempting to change nothing (Laing, in Tongas *et al.* 1989). When I manage to do it though, often with supervisory help as described, it seems to me that, paradoxically, attempting to change nothing makes the most significant difference: in these circumstances even the most traumatised clients begin to accept their experience and begin to unfold as people (Davidson, 1992, pp. 202–3). In the case in point, it was when I was most absorbed in my relationships with Beverley and Marjorie, when I managed just to be there with them, attempting with Jackie's help to change nothing, that this sort of unfolding and growth took place; stagnation turned to breakthrough. It was possible for me to maintain this approach by using (live) supervision to help maintain an awareness of disequilibrium in our relationships, and using it also to help retain a focus on strengths and away from 'problems' in the couple's system.

Our plan had focused on validation, and validation is what we managed to offer. In particular, we validated Marjorie's experience of anger at the changes she was undergoing, anger at being kept in the dark and anger at not being taken seriously; we validated Beverley's experience of the difficulty of gender reassignment, her need to retain some semblance of psychic control in the face of these changes (which led to her difficulty in accepting she had needs) and her onerous responsibility of looking after a highly dependent, needy partner while she wanted to develop her own life for a change; and we validated their experience as a couple, especially as their relationship was, surely now more than ever in their 30-year history together, stigmatised and lacking in social validation: a psychiatric patient and her ex-nurse carer, living as man and wife; an elderly couple below the poverty line, facing death; two women, one a transsexual, in a relationship together.

We also managed to draw on strengths in Beverley and Marjorie's past experience together to help them through the current crisis. We helped them to see how this crisis emerged organically out of their life together and out of the roles they had adopted. We talked also about how the crisis might merge into their future together. If Beverley should die first, Marjorie might now manage independently and Beverley could go to her death more integrated a person, with needs as well as capabilities.

My individual approach failed to maintain a wholly systemic view of Beverley and Marjorie's situation, veering towards an idealisation of Marjorie's role and denigration of Beverley's. With the involvement of a support worker, however, a more truly systemic view was maintained, with much greater overall neutrality regarding the question of whose was the 'healthier' role. As a self-regulating, homeostatic system ourselves (helped in part by the supervision and the help with our relationship we received from our manager), Jackie and I together saw Marjorie and Beverley's ways of experiencing emotion, and their interpersonal functioning, much more as complementary and inter-dependent.

EPILOGUE

Shortly before giving the presentation I met with Beverley and Marjorie to make sure they were happy with my discussing them and to ask them for help with a review, three months on, of the work we had done together. They invited each other to respond, demonstrating the best of listening skills and respect, helping each other out as they talked. Characteristically now, according to colleagues, Marjorie took the lead, saying they listened to each other more, although sometimes needing reminders.

'Yes,' said Marjorie, 'Beverley listens to me more. But she does forget sometimes.'

'And *when* I forget, Marjorie, *you remind me*,' laughed Beverley.

Then, looking at me, Beverley added 'And *I* remind *her*, *too*, when *she* doesn't listen to *me*, you see.'

Beverley then again showed her vulnerability, asking me to tell the interview panel how much more difficult it is to go through a gender reassignment than people imagine. She lectured me in rather an abstract way about these difficulties though, as if they were not her own, and Marjorie raised her eyes to the heavens. Not everything had changed. But perhaps that was the most humbling aspect of this experience. By working consistently simply to *be with* Beverley and Marjorie, rather than trying to get something to change, certainly some things remained as they had always been. They will still no doubt both fall back on patterns of relating that they have each learnt early in their lives and practised for many more decades than I have been around. But at the same time Jackie and I had made it possible in some paradoxical way for quite a dramatic change to take place. The change was a restoration of balance and flexibility in their relationship. It felt very natural now for Marjorie to be taking something of a lead and for Beverley to be concentrating to some extent on her neediness.

Beverley's account of difficulties in relation to transsexuality was in full flow. But these were difficulties my interview panel should be informed about *for their education*. Beverley had stopped short of expressing them as problems she was finding it hard to manage, or could do with some support in talking through. She caught onto the irony of this and finally paused. Marjorie added, semi-automatically, 'I still have no idea how to help Beverley choose her dresses, she drives me mad, I don't know what to do. And I don't think my psychiatrist should decrease my medication, Ben.' Marjorie and Beverley glanced at each other, then at me, a self-parody of stuckness in their respective roles, and the three of us giggled.

REFERENCES

Davidson, B. 1992: What can be the relevance of the psychiatric nurse to the life of a person who is mentally ill? *Journal of Clinical Nursing*, **1**(4), 199–205.

Skynner, A.C.R. 1976: *One Flesh Separate Persons: principles of family and marital psychotherapy.* London: Constable.

Smail, D. 1984: *Illusion and reality: the meaning of anxiety.* London: J.M. Dent.

Tougas, K. Shandel, T. and **Feldmar, A.** 1989: *Did You Used to be R. D. Laing?* Channel Four, London and Third Mind Productions Inc., Vancouver, (TV documentary transcript).

16

TRYING TO TREAT THE SYSTEM: DOMINANCE AND NEGOTIATION IN FAMILY THERAPY

Chris Stevenson

Chris Stevenson concludes Part 2, highlighting the interplay of the two foregoing themes: there has to be a personal struggle to develop an ethical practice; and one may employ specific means in order so to develop.

A patient exists as part of a family or other social system, as well as manifesting a number of internal systems such as cognitive schema, object-relational structures, endocrinological processes, and so on. Clearly, a strong therapeutic prejudice by a clinician is likely to influence which part of the system is identified as well, which part is identified as ill. No doubt many of the clinician's more personal characteristics will also play a part in this ascription of health and illness. Here Chris Stevenson explores the ethical and practical difficulties in avoiding such prejudice and enabling truly informed choice of therapeutic approach and treatment plan by clients. Using a clinical vignette of some family work in which she has been involved, Chris explores the way systems theory can help in working with the group as a whole rather than one or another member. She discusses the advantages of this way of working. She also highlights the dilemma about whether this way of working itself allows free choice by individual members of the group, or an element of coercion. She reinforces the idea that a strong sense of openness to feedback from colleagues, in the context of a supervision group, offers some protection from ethical 'blind-spots' in this respect.

When I first became involved in family therapy I experienced something akin to what family members must undergo when convened to an initial family meeting. There was an alternative language, a strange structure to the sessions (including a live supervision team, one-way mirror and video) and, most importantly, a particular, formalised world view about how problems are generated and maintained. However, my induction over three years was smooth. In time I could 're-frame'[1] and 'paradox'[2] naturally. Once inducted, I behaved, like many colleagues, as if there was no other way in which to know, and change, the world of families. For a while I never questioned the necessity of convening the whole family. I never thought twice about the validity of the blueprint for healthy family functioning that I held.

> Somebody was saying to Picasso that he ought to make pictures of things the way they are – objective pictures. He mumbled that he wasn't quite sure what that would be. The person who was bullying him produced a photograph of his wife from his wallet and said, 'There, you see, that is a photograph of how she really is.' Picasso looked at it and said, 'She is rather small isn't she? And flat?'
>
> (Bateson, quoted in Keeney, 1983, p. 79)

The above is an example of individual variance in our interpretations of the world. We may see our own interpretation as both natural and exclusively valid. In the same way as Picasso's challenger assumes his photograph is the only genuine form of pictorial representation, so too may nurses come to encounters with people defined as having mental illness with certain assumptions about the *correct* way to view their problems. These assumptions may take the form of a particular type of picture, or an 'off the peg' story, about how people come to be ill and how they will be cured. For example, an individual's cognitive processing, their avoidance behaviour, the endocrinological systems of their brain or the ways they structure their experience can be the focus of therapy and seen as the basic 'treatment unit'. Similarly, the whole individual, a dyad (a pair), a family, a family and their network of professional carers, or even larger groupings, can all be seen as the source of the problem and the appropriate focus for therapeutic work. Within my own practice in community psychiatric nursing and family therapy, I have tended towards the latter views, finding it difficult to see the patient in isolation. For me, a person exists as part of a family, or part of some other family-like social system. Consequently I am tempted always to intervene at that level, trying to treat the family group, the system of relationships as a whole. My decisions about treatment plans for the people I see are thus not made from an ideologically neutral base.

It is natural that nurses adopt specific ideologies based on their interests, their training experiences and their professional socialisation. Such ideologies are likely to inform and influence nurses' decisions about what will be the focus of therapeutic attention. Working to a particular model can be helpful. It can provide structure to treatment, it can give the nurse a sense of conviction that gives hope to the patient, it offers some emotional security for the nurse and it is likely to enhance the nurse's interest in the work she does. However, a strong professional narrative will limit the options available to the person with problems. They may feel they have no choice but to acquiesce in the professional's view of their problem and particular form of treatment. If so, are they giving fully informed consent to treatment?

This chapter is concerned with informed consent and choice in treatment generally. In particular, I shall explore my own experience of trying to use my chosen model of therapy with clients at the same time as 'negotiat[ing] a view of what the patient's predicament is about which both the patient and therapist can agree' (Smail, 1988, p.4).

---

[1] Offer a different, usually positive, interpretation of an event.
[2] Give a message which promotes change by prescribing that things should stay the same.

Stated simply, any practitioner will, as part of their assessment, adopt a particular outlook regarding which part of the system is ill and which is well. This is true whether the system in question is an individual's biological system, his psycho-physical organism as a whole, his family network or the whole social system he finds himself in. The critical ethical dilemma concerns how any disagreement amongst the various parties involved in the therapy is resolved: whether the professional tries to convert the individuals (or other treatment unit) to a view which matches his own, or whether the disagreement is resolved more democratically. I shall offer two case studies which illustrate this issue. These are linked by my continuing interest in systemic explanations for mental health problems. They are distinct in that they set out quite different ways of negotiating the diagnosis and treatment of an individual and his family.

INFORMED CONSENT: THE MEETING OF IDEOLOGIES

Coulter (1973) argued that long before any contact with professional agencies there will have been 'lay labelling' of any mental health problem. Wynne *et al.* (1992) suggested that, when illness is perceived by the 'key players', a retrospective search to undertaken for relevant antecedent causes. Four main classes of causes have been identified. These are: (a) supernatural events; (b) physical/biological agents; (c) unconscious (psycho dynamic) processes; (d) societal processes, e.g., poverty, community disorganisation, etc. I have concluded from my own research (Stevenson, 1995) that, when a psychological problem is detected, the majority of family members favour explanations of the problem which are concerned with how internal or external forces have acted on the individual. The person is labelled as an innocent victim, mad or bad. For example, the person who 'drops out' of her/his studies is the unfortunate victim of examination stress, or is mad because of biological changes/unresolved developmental phases, or is behaving wilfully because of a failure in socialisation. These labels all involve a negative connotation.

When family members see an individual as problematic, and the professional holds a similar view, the potential for conflict with the labelled individual arises. The person being defined as problematic may not experience their distress as illness (Wynne *et al.*, 1992). Walrond-Skinner (1976) noted that the person defined as having the problem may hold a radically different view of the situation compared to other family members. In my own practice, the people defined as problematic have sometimes stated that it would be helpful to *someone else* in the family if another session was arranged. Taking a case example, Luke is a 19-year old black youth, adopted into a white family as a baby. He had been diagnosed as having a psychotic illness and had been hospitalised, during which time he was established on a medication regime. He was subsequently, following his discharge home, monitored by out-patient follow-up. Luke was invited to attend a family session with the family members he thought it would be helpful to include. During the first session, to which his adoptive parents and one sister came, Luke noted that his adoptive parents had never discussed the implications of his adoption between themselves. He suggested that his adoptive parents might like a session to themselves in the future, to allow them the opportunity to converse around the adoption issues.

Hoffman (1985) argued that the politics of family life can involve scapegoating through powerful collective attribution. The person defined as problematic may experience a sense of betrayal as she/he is channelled into an 'illness' role (Goffman, 1961). In these circumstances, for the person defined as problematic, an explanation outside the usual lay framework of explanation is helpful (Stevenson, 1995). Systemic explanations widen the focus to include the patterns of information exchange between family members. Such explanations are a means for the person defined as problematic to free her/himself from negative labels. However, when the person defined as problematic by the family explains the problem in a way that both challenges the family's view and matches the professional's, the larger network can feel alienated from the decision-making process. Teisman (1980) noted that the introduction of systemic family therapy conflicts with family members' favoured explanations of the problem and their expectations about intervention. Such systemic explanations are not well understood at a 'lay level'. Wynne *et al.* (1992) claim that there is a strong social and historical tradition of labelling the individual as sick and no equivalent concept that can be applied to families as a whole.

Systemic explanations do not consist in linear cause and effect relationships, e.g., that Sally's poor relationship with her mother causes her to behave in a psychotic way. It is the interlocking patterns of information exchange, involving *all* family members which sustain the problem. Causality is circular. For example, Sally's idea that she is being persecuted by a teacher in relation to her academic work, leads Tom and Jane to try to reassure her by constructing a story about how professional the teacher's attitude is, in order to 'correct' Sally's misconception. But the story serves to make Sally even more distrustful, now not only of the teacher but also of Tom and Jane, as *any* response the teacher makes to Sally is simply interpreted by her as a professional veneer concealing something more sinister. Sally's increased suspiciousness prompts Tom and Jane to embellish their story further, leading to a further increase in Sally's paranoia. The cycle continues *ad infinitum*. However, whilst circular explanation is a well-rehearsed explanation within systemic practice, most family members simply do not see the world in circular terms.

Different kinds of causal explanation entail differing amounts of responsibility by the 'non problematic' family members. While family members may be willing to identify their contribution to past events which have had a negative effect on the person defined as problematic, such past actions are easily and often rationalised as 'water under the bridge', or 'doing what seemed best at the time'. If the individual is seen as mad due to biological disturbance, no responsibility is entailed for anyone. Conversely, a systemic explanation entails more responsibility on the part of family members other than the person defined as problematic, and more blame for them than that associated with individualistic explanations. A systemic definition, which sees the family as *a problematic unit*, may make family members, other than the person defined as problematic, feel betrayed. For example, a systemic explanation of Sally's aggression towards her mother would involve an account of the pattern of communication between the two. Consequently, a systemic explanation might be perceived by Sally's mother as entailing responsibility for her. In this circumstance, her mother and other family members may complain vociferously that they have been inducted into therapy without informed consent. Although they have come to the therapy session, they have done so to help the person defined as having the problem with her/his difficulty. So whilst the person defined as having the problem is freed from negative labels and responsibility by a systemic explanation, it may be a liberation at the expense of other family members' rights to be free from responsibility.

When the person defined as problematic perceives that other family members are keen to maintain an individual focus, she/he has a dilemma. The individual focus is not satisfactory, in that it leaves the person defined as problematic in a negatively labelled position. A systemic focus is unsatisfactory if it creates a split between the person defined as problematic and the family network. If the tension is not managed, the person defined as problematic is likely to make a forced decision to retreat to an individualistic definition and take on an explanation offered by another family member. However, if a context of respect for different perspectives on the problem is set, as argued below, the person defined as problematic is spared the dilemma of choosing between explanations.

In summary, whenever priority is given to the accounts of one part of the system over another, a subjective sense of betrayal, blame and responsibility can occur. It is into this arena that the therapist steps. Her/his challenge is to manage the presentation of explanations in such a way that each participant feels respected.

INFORMED CONSENT: PERCEIVED PROFESSIONAL POWER

The issue of professional power, in relation to informed consent, is problematic. Foucault (1975) argued that knowledge/power creates an hierarchy. For Foucault, power relations are embedded in social discourse. Professional jargon, based on 'superior knowledge', is a form of discourse which functions to maintain the hierarchy. The very language of therapy may be pejorative to the client's position if, as Foucault argues, dominance and submission are embedded in social discourse. In particular, the language which has developed in relation to structural/strategic family therapy apparently serves to uphold the dominance claimed by the therapist. The language, e.g., the problematic child is a *distance regulator* between parents, is not accessible to non-trained people and is used in the private domain of therapy. The therapist's implicit power is further endorsed, because society provides well rehearsed scripts which help legitimate professionals' power position.

In reviewing the practice of therapists taking different approaches to family meetings, I proposed that systemic family therapists have implicit power in the context of being expert helpers approached for help by the family in distress (Stevenson, 1995). Some try to exercise their perceived power by dictating the paradigmatic constraints of 'good' therapy. The family members' explanations were seen as inferior to those of the therapy team, who were ideologically driven to promote their own systemic world view.

Building boundaries between clients and professional means that knowledge is privatised within the domains of specific therapy approaches. A specific ideology constrains the therapist's perspective and discourse, and devalues the experience of the family. Furthermore, ideology as dogma may encourage the therapist to engage in a battle with family members. Referring to structural/strategic family therapy, Napier and Whitaker (1978) have asserted that there is a battle for the structure of sessions, between the therapist and family members, concerning who will attend sessions, with power and control at stake. When a battle is anticipated, therapists who claim power adopt a therapeutic vocabulary based on war and adversarial games. Intolerance is implicit within the vocabulary.

However, power relations are more complex than implied above. People can refuse to acknowledge professional power, leaving the way open for negotiation between parties. Bateson (1979) suggested that power is a myth. Although professional and client may perceive the professional to be powerful, the power is illusory. Through looking at the accounts of family members I found that clients will sanction a thera-pist's claim to power if, and only if, their own views are respected (Stevenson, 1995). If they are not shown an adequate amount of respect, family members will participate conditionally in the therapy process. The power relation is an agreed story constructed in partnership by the therapist and family members. Family members behave *as if* the therapist's power is real, so long as their own explanations for the problem are respected.

The proposition that power is contractual fits with social constructionism. From this position there are no incontrovertible truths about problems, owned by therapists. The only 'reality' is the co-constructed story which players create. For example, the therapist and family co-author new accounts of the family's situation from which new behaviours can emerge. Producing shared narratives simply does not require a thera-pist outside the system in a position of absolute power.

INFORMED CONSENT:
TREATING THE SYSTEM WITH CONVERSION OR RESPECT

Two positions on power are outlined above which have implications for the approaches professionals take to people who are seeking help. The implications are outlined below, as I reflect on the different forms of family therapy practice which I have undertaken.

Conversion

According to family therapy theory, contextual factors bear on the process of reaching an agreement about a problem explanation and work in favour of the therapist. Pearce and Cronen (1980) predicted that the context will exert a strong force on the emergent meaning of a situation. Conversely, the substance of communication, e.g., the prof-fered explanations of family members will offer only a weak force towards defining meaning. When I researched therapists in action during sessions I found that some family therapists had difficulty in hearing the individualistic problem explanations given by family members (Stevenson, 1995). In the past, I have experienced similar difficulty because I was convinced that the 'truth' about families was systemic. The therapists' reluctance to hear family members' views was consistent with the advice within the family therapy literature, where the superior interpretation of the therapist is touted. For example, Minuchin (1974) asserted that the family need to be *educated by the therapist* about the family structure and dynamics through which the problem is maintained. To accept the accounts of family members involved the therapists 'putting on hold' what they considered to be 'good' therapy. Thinking back to my own strategic practice, the team philosophy was that the family must be compelled to change. The therapy team knew best about what was good for the family because they could divine the true problem. The team issued injunctions to bring about the 'necessary' change to convert the family to the therapist's blueprint of a healthy family.

When therapists seek conversion to their world view, or to a 'correct' family form, family members who do not subscribe to the therapist's 'correct' explanation are simply seen as resistant. Therapists use this construction of 'resistance' as a justification for exerting covert pressure on the family, in order to develop a systemic focus, for example, through paradoxical intervention. In the latter scenario, informed consent is compromised by the imposition of the therapist's view through techniques whose purpose is not discernible by the clients. An example from my own strategic practice illustrates the use of paradoxical intervention. The team had been dealing with a family in which a 23-year-old son had failed his university entrance examinations and had since been living at home unable or unwilling to leave the house except on rare occasions. During one session the team carefully constructed a long metaphorical story, loosely based on the *Pilgrim's Progress* by John Bunyan, which the team thought would implicitly convey a message that the parents would be forever burdened by a child who was problematic, as Pilgrim was burdened. We thought that the message would be resisted by the family, and that they would be forced to change in order to defeat the therapists. The family members may have been amused, bemused or confused, although they were probably constrained by politeness from saying so.

From reflecting on my practice, I now doubt whether overt or covert attempts to force families to change either work, or are acceptable ethically. Through the process of researching the beginning of therapy I recognised that structural/strategic therapists find themselves in a therapeutic position when they 'put on hold' the strong socialisation (Stevenson, 1995), which Rogers *et al.* (1993) pointed out is part of a therapist's career. In this context, therapeutic does not refer to an outcome, but the preconditions under which therapy can begin. The preconditions are met when respect is shown by each party for the views of others. The professional is not a 'knight therapist' who arrogantly struggles against family dragons in order to convene and convert family members to her/his systemic ideology. In the latter scenario, there can be no informed consent. Dogma about what constitutes good therapy is disrespectful to the family members and simply narrows the opportunities for therapeutic work. An example of restricted practice is found in Carpenter and Treacher's (1983) recommendation to limit therapy to one initial assessment session unless *all* family members are present.

Respect

My current practice is 'reflecting team process'. It is based on the work of Andersen (1987), and is consistent with social constructionist ideas. Our group strives to reduce the hierarchy between the family and therapy team, and work collaboratively towards creating new ideas about the problem by setting up opportunities for 're-reading' existing stories. For example, some of the team listen carefully to the conversation between the therapist and family members. At a mutually agreed point in the session, the family members are offered the opportunity to swap places with the listening team members. The family members, and the therapist who has been engaged in conversation with them, can listen to the speculative reflections of the rest of the team. The process frees up conversation and so encourages informed choice. The family members and therapist then have a chance to comment on what they have heard.

Within such social constructionist family therapy, the family members' explanations are legitimated. The therapists are much less likely to work covertly towards a problem redefinition, or use strategy to convene absent family members. In acknowledging the client's contribution, the therapist asks questions of a different form to those adopted by structural/strategic therapist which are geared towards discovering some underlying pattern of family dysfunction. For example, Andersen (1992, p. 61) suggested that, early in the session, questions of the type, 'How would you like to use this meeting?' are helpful, in that they immediately acknowledge the collaborative nature of the therapy process.

The diverse explanations that family members give for the problem that has encouraged them to seek help are respected by our team. Atkinson and Heath (1990) assert that therapists should not try to know everything about a problem or impose their view on the family. To do so leads to a premature explanation of the problem which, once arrived at, negates and devalues alternative explanations. If one version of the problem dominates, and/or the owner of that definition is seen to have won in the negotiation, there is likely to be the perception by other participants that they have lost. For example, White (1989) related the case on an encopretic child. As White described it, 'The poo was making a mess of Nick's life' (p.6), and that of his parents. White labelled the problem as 'sneaky poo'. In doing so, he offered a problem definition and explanation which lay outside the individual and the family system. However, the externalised definition, which transcends the different explanations of family members, necessarily subjugates their views.

When therapists respect alternative explanations of the problem, even though they conflict with their own systemic ideology, resistance becomes a redundant concept. Resistance is a valid, rational reaction to a power relation in which the therapist attempts ideological conversion. Resistance arises in response to a perceived lack of respect from others. As Epstein (1993) asserted, the *validity* of client 'resistance' should be acknowledged by professionals.

When I practise within a reflecting team, I feel that the family members are empowered in interaction with the therapist. There are many explanatory 'truths'. The position is beyond that of Rogers' (1942) liberal humanism, where the therapist's neutral stance involves a conscious suppression of her/his own value judgement, or singular truth, in favour of the person finding their own solution. In reflecting team process, as I perceive it, the team expose their prejudices in order that the family members can judge the ideas the team express in the context of the framework of those prejudices.

Speculative information is provided by the team for the family to assess in terms of its usefulness. As French (1985) advocated, the therapist may exercise a non-coercive authority. The potential for therapy entering into the conversational domain is identified by Anderson and Goolishian (1990). The family may have beliefs about exercising their own expertise. Their perception of expertise is related to their conviction about the 'goodness' of their own explanations of the problem.

Hoffman (1992) asserted that therapist and family can co-author, co-evolve and co-construct explanations within therapy. When mutuality and collaboration are present, it is possible for people to share ideas, and receive the other's view of 'reality' in a non-exploitative relationship. The result is an enriched ecology of ideas, which will facilitate change. I experience less angst than previously when I tried to cure the family by implementing 'smart' interventions which, I realised on some level, were based on my personal and professional prejudices.

A case example taken from my recent practice illustrates the preceding points. A couple were invited to a series of meetings as the husband, Tom, had been recently discharged from in-patient treatment for depression and there were marital difficulties identified by both himself and his wife. At the first interview, Tom was suggesting that the marriage was unrewarding but that it must continue for the sake of the children. He was expressing, very forcibly, his belief that therapists as a breed were likely to advise marital separation because of their mistaken, liberal, social science-based education. His wife, Margaret, was offering a very different perspective, saying that as Tom had withdrawn from the relationship with her, there seemed to be little point in continuing the marriage.

It would have been easy for me to draw on well-rehearsed systemic explanations from my previous professional socialisation to help me account for the function of Tom's depression in maintaining the marriage and the family system, and to inform our thought about the best way to intervene. Initially, I heard Tom's concern about therapists as an affront to much of what has constituted my professional education or even as evidence of 'closedness' or resistance to therapy sessions. However, the family team and Tom and Margaret, perhaps because of the way sessions tend to allow space for reflective conversation at different levels, began to explore in more depth the reasons why Tom was concerned about separation. As I listened and spoke I found myself less outraged about Tom's prejudices about social science and more aware of the extent to which my own values are embedded in limited ideas about children and families. I was able to express this within a team reflection. I think because I tried to listen in spite of my initial reading of Tom, I was able to recognise the special concern he had about disunited families, his overwhelming love and consideration for the welfare of his sons and his fears driven by his own experience of parental loss. One part of the conversation explored how estranged parents can find ways to relate to their children even though the difficulties were recognised and spoken about.

The couple eventually decided, some time after the final family meeting, that their marriage should end. I cannot say how far the family meetings were instrumental in their reaching this decision, or whether this outcome should be deemed as successful. However, Tom said of reflecting team process, 'It's much more humane than I imagined it would be' and wrote a letter expressing his gratitude that the meetings had taken place. Margaret expressed her view that she had had the opportunity both to express and be listened to in a different way than had occurred before. I like to think that, because there was not a therapist view imposed on Tom, he was able to think about different possibilities for family life.

Summary

The chapter has focused on informed consent in trying to treat the system. The professional and the lay person differ in the narratives they tell about mental health problems. With systemic family therapy, professional and lay ideologies meet in the family session. A strong professional narrative may limit the array of choice for the person defined as problematic and their social network. It reduces the opportunity for informed choice to take place. If therapy participants reject the professional narrative, they are often labelled as resistant, and in need of conversion to the superior perspective of the therapist.

When conflicting explanations for 'illness' exist, there is potential for betrayal, blame and responsibility to be experienced at different intensities by family members, according to which narrative dominates. The ethical therapist is well advised to manage the presentation of explanations so as to ensure that each participant feels respected. Without sensitive handling, family members who are made to feel responsible may be left with many feelings, including resentment, that they have been inducted into therapy without informed consent.

Some systemic family therapists try to exercise their perceived power. Power wielding does not set a respectful context in which alternative views about problems are allowed. Rather, therapist and family members engage in a battle for power and control. When therapists behave as if their power is real, they are likely to have fixed ideas about problems and their solutions which are the basis for active intervention. 'Failure' of the family members to change is interpreted as resistance, and the therapist responds by using techniques of change which are veiled from the recipients.

Therapists who believe their power is real are naïve. Therapist power is contractually agreed on the basis of the family members feeling respected. When power is contractually agreed, covert attempts at converting others to a specific world view are unnecessary. Such attempts deny informed consent. Therapeutic encounters are more likely to arise when therapists 'put on hold' definite ideas about what constitutes 'good' therapy.

Practice which accepts the collaboratively, co-created nature of explanations necessarily entails an increased client voice. It opens up a range of alternatives for defining, and re-defining, problems and their treatment. The available choices are expanded. Family members are empowered in giving informed consent to a way forward in therapy.

REFERENCES

Andersen, T. 1987: The reflecting team: dialogue and meta-dialogue in clinical work. *Family Process* 26: 415–28.

Anderson, T. 1992: Reflections on reflecting with families. In McNamee, S. and Gergen, K.J. (eds), *Therapy as social construction*. London: Sage, pp. 54–68.

Anderson, H. and Goolishian, H.A. 1990: Beyond cybernetics: comments on Atkinson and Heath's 'Further Thoughts on Second Order Family Therapy'. *Family Process* 19, 157–63.

Atkinson, B.J. and Heath, A.W. 1990: Further thoughts on second order family therapy – this time it's personal. *Family Process* 29, 145–55.

Bateson, G. 1979: *Mind and nature*. New York: Dutton.

Carpenter, J. and Treacher, A. 1983: On the neglected art of convening and engaging families and their wider systems. *Journal of Family Therapy* 5, 337–58.

Coulter, J. 1973: *Approaches to insanity*. London: Martin Robinson.

Epstein, E.K. 1993: From irreverence to irrelevance? The growing disjuncture of family therapy theories from social realities. *Journal of Systemic Therapies* 12, 15–27.

Foucault, M. 1975: *The archaeology of knowledge*. London: Tavistock.

French, M. 1985: *Beyond Power*. New York: Summit Books.

Goffman, I. 1961: *Asylums*. Harmondsworth: Penguin.

Hoffman, L. 1985: Beyond power and control: toward a second order family systems therapy. *Family Systems Medicine* **3**, 381–96.

Hoffman, L. 1992: A reflexive stance for family therapy. In McNamee, S. and Gergen, K.J. (eds), *Therapy as social construction*. London: Sage, pp. 7–24.

Keeney, B.P. 1983: *Aesthetics of change*. New York: Guilford.

Minuchin, S. 1974: *Families and family therapy*. London: Tavistock.

Napier, A. and **Whitaker, C.** 1978: *The Family Crucible*. New York: Harper and Row.

Pearce, W.B. and **Cronen, V.E.** 1980: *Communication, action and meaning: The creation of social realities*. New York: Praeger.

Rogers, A., Pilgrim, D. and **Lacey, R.** 1993: *Experiencing psychiatry: users' views of services*. London: Macmillan in association with MIND Publications.

Rogers, C.R. 1942: *Counselling and psychotherapy*. Boston: Houghton Mifflin.

Smail, D. 1988: Taking care: an alternative to therapy, London: J.M. Dent.

Stevenson, C. 1995: *Negotiating a therapeutic context in family therapy*. Unpublished PhD thesis. University of Northumbria at Newcastle.

Walrond-Skinner, S. 1976: *Family therapy: the treatment of natural systems*. London: Routledge.

White, M. 1989: Introduction. In White, M. and Epston, D. (eds), *Literate means to therapeutic ends*. Adelaide: Dulwich Centre Publications, p. XV.

Wynne, L.C., Shields, C.G. and **Sirkin, M.I.** 1992: Illness, family theory and family therapy: I conceptual issues. *Family Process* **31**, 3–18.

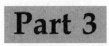

Part 3

Ideology

We slide relentlessly towards the millennium, that symbolic watershed between our past and our future. What are the ethical issues which concern us in the dying days of this century? If popular politics and media attention are anything to go by, one would have to include animal rights; abortion; sexual exploitation of children; euthanasia; embryo research. And yet, to what extent *should* these questions form such points of focus for our ethical scrutiny? Are there not certain interests at play in setting the contemporary ethical agenda? What of the claims on our ethical attention that might be made by issues such as (political) asylum; employment; the welfare state; racism; free market capitalism?

It may be that the reader has been hard pressed to construe the 'professionalisation of care' itself as an *ethical* issue demanding priority attention, when at work tomorrow morning there will be weightier matters to attend to and practical choices to make: Patients will require restraint, and in the press some *exposé* of diplomats importing child pornography will unavoidably impinge on one's ethical sensibilities. Who says that the professionalisation of mental health care is a pressing problem? The editors? Who are they? Who, for that matter, says that the exploitation of children in the overseas manufacture of sports footwear should demand one's attention? And if the exploitation of children by multinational sports footwear manufacturers is, self-evidently, an ethical concern, then how come it is only *now* that this concern is being presented, for one's immediate attention? Who sets any of these agenda?

The questions which might stimulate any kind of science of ethics in psychiatric nursing might appear simple, if not simplistic. 'Who decides what may or may not be done to us?' 'What can or cannot be done to us when we are in a state of mental (or perhaps physical) collapse?' 'How should we treat one another when we are helpless?' And indeed, answers to many questions along these lines have been attempted in the foregoing pages. But the reader may recall our assertion earlier in the text that 'there are . . . powerful interests exerting an influence on current ideology as to what is "right" and "wrong", to some extent quite independently of what ethicists might say and to an extent ominously lurking behind their views'.

Despite being self-styled 'everyday moral philosophers' and ethicists, we, the editors, have to admit that our views, hard come by through many hours of lonely battle with our consciences though they may be, are also influenced by ideology. We believe that it is possible to battle through the influence of ideology to develop one's own views of right and wrong to some extent. But never can our conduct or thinking be entirely impartial to the influence of partisan bias and narrow interests, including our own self-interest. Of even more concern, perhaps, is the fact that some such interests, ominously lurking behind our moral views, are, as yet, hidden, and may well remain so.

Some may argue that morality has no basis except in the expression of people's (self-interested) opinions. According to Nietzsche (1969) it was a fiction which mankind couldn't possibly live without. Ayer (1982) argued that ethics involved nothing other than a confusion in the meaning of certain words. As editors, we certainly subscribe to the view that morality does not so much exist as *is created*. But the very fact that we continue to argue about the rights and wrongs of various patterns of human conduct suggests that moral discussion and argument must make some kind of sense, beyond what the positivists would argue was a mere prescription-in-disguise.[1] We take it as an article of faith that there *is* a realm of our psycho-physical being, an ethical realm which is both the moment-by-moment reverberation within our psyche of the choices we make and their resonance with other living beings, and which has also somehow a sort of momentum, something like an aggregate thrust of all the choices we have made, particularly momentous choices, for good and evil. In which case, it is surely crucial that we discern, as far as we are able, the way in which ideological forces impinge on the direction our conduct is taking, whether or not we are induced to believe and argue that such direction is right and fitting. In this way we may sort out unexamined prejudice and partiality from the genuine article of ethical choice.

Part 3 addresses that very issue: how are ideological forces impinging on the direction our conduct is taking? Whose interests are being served? Was it really right to close that day centre? Who decided how the statistics for client usage of the centre should be prepared? Might we have looked at it another way, paying more regard to the quality of work carried out there, and less to the quantity of client contacts per week? By sending that memo to management declaring that the union's refusal to co-operate with plans for the transition was putting clients at risk, were we really helping clients? Or have we merely allowed ourselves and our interests to become a tool for a right-wing political agenda to undermine the union's negotiating position and let clients go to the wall? Did the possibility of winning favour with management and enhancing our promotion prospects temporarily blind us? Was not our attempt to publicise this turn of events in the media simply a hopeless non-starter, too little, too late? What does it mean that we now have a case management system and contracts with clients for short-term, focused interventions based on inevitably problem-centred (and thus pathologising) need-assessments? OK, so now we are building bridges in the community between health and social service teams, ensuring that the clients we see are those most in need. But in these circumstances, should we not pause also to wonder what happened to our former clients' spirit of self-reliance and community? What happened to our empowering, preventative, *health*-focused work, capitalising on and validating client's strengths? What happened to the client sit-ins at the centre of yesteryear, when last the council attempted to close the place down to save money? And is it any longer possible to facilitate discussions as a group conductor through which clients can see how so many of their problems are ordinary social, political and emotional problems of living in this society, which all of us (including the conductor and other staff) have to negotiate, rather than the result of some stigmatising 'mental illness' that leaves them feeling inadequate and bad?

Citizens' charters are in fashion. When we set up user groups, who, exactly, do we encourage to participate? To what extent do we facilitate and enable such groups? Do we do so with money or with staff time? What hand do we retain in their business? And if they have developed a degree of autonomy, what objections do we raise to taking their demands seriously? The rhetoric and reality of user empowerment is the subject of Chapters 17 and 18.

In Chapters 19 and 20, the possibility of approaching our work from an angle that takes seriously the political and social aetiology of mental illness is examined. Can anything realistically be done to politicise psychology? And whatever has become of collectivist and

---

[1] The 'emotivist' view is that any moral statement can be reduced to two components: preference and prescription – 'I like things this way; comply with my preferences!'. For example, take the statement: 'We should operate the principle *from each according to his ability; to each according to his need'.* The translation and more intelligible rendition of this is, for the emotivist: 'I want some of your resources; give them to me!'.

interpersonal approaches to mental health care? Has the rhetoric of democracy and the free market masked something much more evil going down in the way individualistic approaches have taken over in the treatment of the mentally ill?

Of course, there has to be accommodation of principles of quality assurance in mental health care, as in all public services. And why should there not be development of some means by which the quality of the work we do is audited? Chapter 21 seeks to find a way of advancing such principles at the same time as assuring that it is quality that is being measured in such circumstances, and not simply an arbitrary collection of data that can be used to bolster policy and resource decisions originating in partisan ideology. In a similar vein, perhaps it is right that short-term, focused and scientifically proved interventions, brief therapies are being purchased by the state for those most in need, in place of long-term and costly treatment modalities. But to what extent is this ideology, to what extent the moral high ground? Chapter 22 attempts to offer a structure and context for such judgements by setting out at some length the philosophical, cultural, political and ideological contexts in which the three main therapeutic modalities emerged, developed and took root. In this way, by high-lighting the ideological context of the current situation, we may be able to develop greater clarity as to what is genuinely right and fitting, however hard it is to extricate oneself from the web of ideology and interest in making any final ethical judgement as to the state's current choice.

In Chapter 23 one such form of 'brief therapy' is exemplified through the experience of a practitioner attempting to use a form of cognitive reconstruction to come to terms with his own experience of terminal illness. The chapter is offered by way of an example of the creative use of such principles in practice, in contrast with the shallow rhetoric with which perhaps any therapeutic ideology may be purveyed by practitioners who are not willing themselves to experience its effect. In Chapter 24, developing the theme of mental health carers with their own forms of distress and disturbance, an appeal is made to the experience of practitioners generally in developing the concept of the wounded healer. One thought behind this is that by dissolving artificial social barriers between *us* (the sane) and *them* (the insane), we reduce the likelihood that such distance can be exploited ideologically and enhance our ability to respond authentically and empathically to the experience of others. The improbability of such an idea gaining ground against the ideological forces that keep our own madness safely hidden, however, is emphasised

For many people a major problem with ethics – if not with philosophy in general – is its abstract nature. But we all have values. Most of us are sensitive to what those values mean to us and where, perhaps, we acquired them. No matter how difficult and abstract ethics might be, could we imagine living any kind of life without a moral philosophy of some description? If we abandoned our ethical philosophy today, by tomorrow we would probably have established a new moral order, based either on an ethics of personal conscience, or on ideological rhetoric, or based on some mixture of the two. Our only problem would be the age-old one of deciding if it was the *right* moral order.

REFERENCES

Ayer, A.J. 1982 *Language, truth and logic.* Harmondsworth: Penguin.
Nietzsche, F. 1969 *The genealogy of morals.* trans W. Kaufmann, New York: Random House.

17

LISTENING TO CLIENTS

Peter Campbell

There is supposed to have been a laudable move towards listening to clients, and this has ostensibly been supported by the recent government. A patients' charter would be an impressive innovation if it achieved its aim of empowering users of mental health services in making their opinions heard and effecting the changes they want in care provision. The rhetoric of citizens' rights and the notion that, at the time of writing, the Conservative government wants to make a charter with psychiatric patients (among others), to give them what they want, belies the fact that mental health service users' opinions and preferences have been freely available for years. They have, however, been ignored, simply because they are not overly valued by those who have the power to make a difference. Here Peter Campbell details the development and contribution of the user movement. He addresses the central ethical issues of power and its abuse, powerlessness and protest in people's experience of society and psychiatric treatment. Peter explores how realistic the prospect of a user-led service is. He discusses the possibility of advocacy work and of facilitating self-advocacy by users of psychiatric services. He questions the nature of expertise on mental illness and mental health care and argues that the special insight into the nature of madness accessible to service users puts them in a unique position of expertise. Such expertise remains largely untapped by psychiatric nurses and other mental health carers. Peter endorses the case for more collaboration between service users and providers as a moral, also a practical imperative, but questions whether powerful and to an extent hidden ideology will allow it.

WHERE ARE WE, WHO ARE WE – CONSUMERS, CITIZENS OR MAD PERSONS?

The position of mental health service recipients in the United Kingdom has changed significantly in the last ten years. When discussions about the design and delivery of mental health services occur, it is now increasingly likely that recipients, individually and collectively, will be near centre-stage rather than in the wings. In the House of Commons Social Services Committee report on Community Care published in January 1985, the members wrote: 'As a Committee, we have had difficulty in hearing the authentic voice of the ultimate consumers of community care . . . Services are still mainly designed by providers and not users, whether families or clients, and in response to blue-prints rather than in answer to demand'. In November 1994, as the NHS Executive's Mental Health Task Force approached the end of its two-year programme of work, a conference of 200 service users and 100 managers from all over England was held in Derby. Organised by the Task Force User Group, it presented the written products of the 'user movement's' collaboration with the Mental Health Task Force initiative: *Guidelines for a Local Charter for Users of Mental Health Services;* and *A Code of Practice for Advocacy.* While it is still possible to question what is and is not authentic, it is no longer credible to propose the difficulty of hearing the voices of recipients within mental health services.

In the last decade there has not only been a rapid growth in the number of recipient-led projects at a local level but recipients have won a place on the management councils of national voluntary organisations and contributed to Department of Health reviews and to the House of Commons Select Committee on Health. In certain respects it could be argued that the consumer of mental health services has not only stepped behind the counter but has also got a sight at the doors of the candy cupboard itself.

Yet the triumph of mental health service consumers should not be overstated. In the first place, persons with a diagnosis of mental illness are now and always have been a good deal less than consumers. No-one who has queued for medication in a psychiatric admission ward can be unaware that they are using a delivery system backed up by compulsion. This is not a setting for nice decisions on economy or styling, for delicate or impulsive choice, or for leaving with nothing but a polite nod towards the assistant. An informal novice will soon discover that, courtesy of Section 5.4 of the 1983 Mental Health Act, you are always less than three minutes away from a transformation to formal status. Furthermore, diversity has never been a conspicuous feature of mental health services. Despite far-reaching changes in the location and mechanics of service delivery in many places, the menu itself has remained substantially the same. In some instances it could be argued that choices have become more restricted. Drugs, electroconvulsive therapy and long periods of enforced idleness were the staple diet of psychiatric inpatients in the 1970s. They remain the core of the psychiatric approach in the 1990s. Outside observers will not need long conversations with anyone diagnosed as mentally ill to reveal that their relationship to services is hardly that of the empowered consumer in the open market place.

And, of course, the diagnosed mentally ill have always been a good deal more than mental health service consumers. Particularly in this decade, the majority of us live in the streets of British towns and cities and not within the walls of Victorian asylums. Our neighbours are more likely to be ordinary citizens than fellow psychiatric patients. Despite official rhetoric which focuses on our capacity or reluctance to consume or be consumed in the welfare markets, we are usually concentrating on our capacity to be human beings, to be citizens and equal members of everyday society. We are worrying about how to tell future partners that we are lunatics. We are recovering from patronising rejections for jobs for which we are already overqualified. Consuming mental health services is frequently the least of our concerns.

Unfortunately, there is no way that the progress of the diagnosed mentally ill towards full citizenship in the United Kingdom can be suffused with the same glow that some apologists would apply to the advance of the welfare consumer. At the time of writing and even in the light of opinion polls suggesting public support for the government's community care policies, it is an open question whether society really wants 'loonies' on its pavements. Nothing that has happened in the last decade has had a significant impact on the Not In My Back-Yard philosophy that has always oppressed people with a suspected history of madness. Indeed, the last two years – years that have coincided with and immediately followed the final stages of implementing the government's community care changes – have seen a notable renaissance of the stereotype of the mentally ill person as violent maniac or tragic victim. At a recent conference on media images of mental health (London School of Economics, December 1994), Sashi Sashidharan, a consultant psychiatrist, spoke of the public perception of 'madness seeping out of the institutions' and the threat that carries. In the current climate of opinion it would be difficult to deny that fears of this kind are a prime element in public responses to the mentally ill.

At the same time, we have witnessed not only the persistent blocking by government of all attempts to introduce comprehensive legislation to prevent discrimination against disabled people but also sustained action to extend the power of mental health workers to control and threaten their clients beyond the hospital and into the community itself. The government has now amended the 1983 Mental Health Act to create a power of aftercare under supervision. Whatever type of citizenship remains open to people with a history of mental illness, it seems likely to be citizenship with a difference.

One key to improving the status of those who use mental health services is to enable change in their relationships to the world around them: relationships to mental health services, to service providers and mental health workers, to society as a whole. This has certainly been recognised in the rhetoric of the last decade with repeated exhortations to 'listen to clients', 'work together' and 'create new partnerships'. The Report of the Mental Health Nursing Review Team (1994), whose executive summary includes the statement 'The work of mental health nurses rests upon the relationship they have with people who use services. Our recommendations start and finish with this relationship' is one example of this new vision. Unfortunately, in this and other investigations into the condition of mental health services, the extent of re-thinking about relationships between professional and client remains uncertain. The suspicion persists that the agenda for action is well outlined before professionals ever invite clients to the threshold of their new partnership.

The Mental Health Nursing Review is by no means a betrayal of people with a diagnosis of mental illness. On the contrary, it goes further than might be expected towards an accommodation with the concept of the mental patient as consumer of mental health services. Genuine efforts were made to involve service users during the course of the review, both by the inclusion of representatives on the review team and by individuals giving evidence at regional conferences and in private session. The report itself enshrines the idea of an individualised, needs-led service, recommends the participation of people who use services on service planning, education and research groups and recognises the impact that limited services, uncertain solutions and the compulsory element in care can have on creative relationships. There is much that activists in the British 'user movement' can welcome. Yet there are also fundamental questions that the review and, more importantly, the mental health nursing profession do not address clearly. What kind of relationship do the diagnosed mentally ill want to have with mental health nurses? What nursing interventions do recipients find most helpful and unhelpful? Do mental patients really want or need mental health nurses? At a time when the future role of mental health nursing is regularly considered in the press and some researchers are finding significant differences between what nurses and patients think is helpful, the absence from the debate of users' views is instructive and ominous. Perhaps there are still some areas where consultation is too hot to handle.

Clear focus on the possible relationships between givers and receivers of care is obscured by confusion about the true and potential identities of the parties to that relationship. As the relationship alters, so will the identities of the participants begin to change. But who are the participants? What parts of them are touched by the relationship? Who is it possible for them to become? To some extent this question is relevant to both parties, for by changing the relationship mental health workers presumably seek to change themselves to become more effective, more fulfilled, more caring, more human. But it has overriding significance for recipients of care.

I have already used a variety of words to characterise people who would popularly be described as 'mental patients' or 'the mentally ill'. Other definitions, including 'mental health system survivor' – the one I would soonest choose for myself – have not yet featured. This diversity can partly be explained in terms of political correctness or circumlocution. It is partly due to legitimate arguments about the causation of problems or the desire of people to avoid being encapsulated in terms of an illness even when illness is not disputed as a cause of the problem. But, while it is true that increasing numbers of people with a diagnosis of mental illness, particularly those connected with user-led organisations, no longer wish to see themselves as 'mental patients' or as 'one of the mentally ill' and are making efforts to avoid use of these terms, it is also clear that most of us are struggling to discover exactly who we have and may become. Barham and Haywood's study of the lives of long-term service users in a North of England town (1991) confirms the centrality of questions of identity to anyone who has received a psychiatric diagnosis. To enter the mental health system is not only to lose one identity but to acquire an unsolicited and irrevocably tarnished replacement. Challenging this exchange is the underlying agenda both of organisations of service users and survivors that currently form the 'user movement' and of every individual with a diagnosis of mental illness regardless of whether they are currently consuming services or not. This scrutiny of language is not a sterile exercise. Some 28 years after becoming a 'mental patient' I am still wondering what hit me.

It is doubtful whether current enthusiasm for involving service users can in itself adequately address these questions. Although the transformation from 'victim of a brain disease called madness' to 'mental health service user' that may occur within a Mental Health Strategy Working Group is not to be dismissed, it is unclear how much significance it retains in the long corridors of the asylum, let alone in the parks and highways of this land. Service providers, while inviting users into positions of influence, control the nature of the relationship and offer identities that merely exalt a client status. They prefer the diagnosed mentally ill to talk about their use of services rather than their madness. Too much of the latter interferes with the business in hand.

Despite the all-pervasive approbation of empowerment, the dilemma for the diagnosed mentally ill remains acute. As welfare consumers, we will always remain inferior, however nicely the care is packaged. As citizens, we are caught in confusion in the face of a society that is not reconciled to disabled citizens and is quite uncertain if community mental patients really can be citizens. And, of course, remaining a madperson is not a possibility. Mary O'Hagan who explored the psychiatric survivor movement in the USA, Britain and the Netherlands (1993) comments on the degree to which people only saw themselves in relationship to psychiatry and quotes one survivor from Holland:

> We should explore a total other direction. My fancy is that it could be a cultural movement where we defend the right to be mad and give some positive attribution to it instead of nurturing the idea that somebody should actually get well again. People have the right to be who they are; they have the right to be mad.

This may appear a romantic vision and far beyond the remit of collaboration between service users and mental health workers. Perhaps it is time to question whether mental health workers contribute more to society than the mad.

LISTENING TO CLIENTS

Consultation is a primary mechanism for changing the relationship of service users within services. Whatever else providers may be committed to in the pursuit of working together with service users, they seem to be unanimous in their desire to talk and listen to clients. This desire is partly a necessary reaction to new legislative requirements: Section 10 of the Disabled Persons (Services, Consultation and Repre sentation) Act 1986 relating to the co-option to relevant committees of persons repre senting the interests of disabled people, the need for local authorities to involve disabled people in the preparation of local community care plans. But it is also a result of a genuine realisation, engendered by the consumerist approach to welfare, that evidence from direct recipients of services is central to securing improvements in services. Consultation has become the *sine qua non* of good practice in mental health service provision.

This turn of events contains a major irony for many people with a diagnosis of mental illness. Our most persistent complaint has always been and still remains that no-one really talks or listens to us. Statements of this kind are so ubiquitous that it would be reasonable to claim that not being listened to is a defining characteristic of mental patient status. While providers and users continue to assemble around the convenient and attractive banner of collective consultation, we must recognise that the individual reality is one of the continual devaluation, discounting and denial of personal experience.

Esso Leete (1989), a woman diagnosed and treated for schizophrenia and an active member of the user/survivor movement in the USA says:

> I can talk, but I may not be heard. I can make suggestions, but they may not be taken seriously. I can voice my thoughts, but they may be seen as delusions. I can recite experiences, but they may be interpreted as fantasies. To be a patient or even an ex-client is to be discounted.

This statement certainly encapsulates my own experience. I have been discounted both as an agent in my own life and in the life of others. During an admission in the mid-1980s, I recall being ignored and subsequently severely reprimanded when I entered the nursing office to correctly warn staff that a fight was likely unless they intervened between two fellow in-patients. More recently, I was told 'Just remember who you are. You're only a patient' when I tried to advocate for a friend on my ward. Until the last few years, mental health workers have routinely shown no interest in aspects of my life I consider important – my spirituality, my creativity, what it means to live with a diagnosis of mental illness for decades. In crisis I have had to shrink my distress to fit a 'mental health state examination' approach.

Any attempt to improve the care people receive in the mental health system must consider in depth the anger and resentment being expressed by so many individuals world-wide. Where does this originate? Why are so many demanding to be treated with respect and dignity? Is this just the illness talking? Is it a massive failure of the caring imagination? While it is possible that some of the causes will lie largely outside the province of services, those that lie within are not likely to be answered through consultation and mental health consumerism alone.

Nor should the eagerness to consult with consumers obscure misgivings about the effectiveness of consultative processes in securing change. David Brandon (1991) shows how 'consultation can, however, be a way of marginalising those who are beng consulted if their suggestions and advice are simply discarded'. Even if service users' advice is not discarded, the impact of the process on public perceptions of our status is open to question. There are profound and long-standing reasons why the House of Commons Select Committee could claim they were unable to 'hear the authentic voice of the ultimate consumers'. It was not because we were not there. People have been recipients of institutional psychiatry for over 150 years. Nor was it because we were not speaking out, although the authenticity of our voices may have been affected by a lack of organisation and by the fact that, until recently, they were broadcast largely through the agency of charitable and voluntary organisations. But literature is well stocked with accounts of mad persons protesting their case. The voice of the diagnosed mentally ill has not been listened to because it has not been considered worth listening to.

Whatever has happened in the last decade in respect of our credibility as welfare consumers, our credibility as persons remains debatable. It is only a little more than 50 years since the concept of 'life unworthy of life', first advocated by a psychiatrist, Alfred Hoche, in 1920 was used to justify the murder of 100,000 to 200,000 mental patients in Nazi Germany. It is less than a year since a court case regarding mistreatment in mental health services was dismissed because mental patients were judged incapable of being credible witnesses. It is easy for the majority of society to ignore mad people. They are way out on the margins, beyond the clearing and into the woods. Consulting with us as clients is a notable improvement but it is a peculiarly indirect way of attacking the prejudice that blights us.

The generalised lack of credibility attached to the role of mental health service user, the feeling that because you are using these services you must automatically 'be in the wrong' in a variety of ways, is one major obstacle to successful consultation. But there are more specific concerns about credibility in consultations. One of these revolves around the mechanics and desire for representativeness – from the service providers' viewpoint, the question: 'OK, we're talking and listening to users, but are they the right users for our purposes?'.

Representativeness has become important, both for user action groups and for outsiders, including service providers, who seek to work with them. Beresford and Campbell (1994) suggest there is an underlying difficulty here, arising from the collision of different models of democracy: 'While movements of disabled people and other service users have placed an emphasis on a participatory model of democracy, the service model is firmly located on a representative system of democracy and bases its efforts to involve service users on a representative model of democracy'. They also point to anger within user organisations that: 'people's representativeness assumes importance if what they say threatens or challenges the status quo'. Conflicts around representation are far from being resolved, indeed, they are rarely openly addressed. While national networking organisations such as Survivors Speak Out repeatedly disclaim their representative role, they are constantly being drawn into positions where their capacity to speak on behalf of the user movement is assumed. At the same time, their ability to fully involve even their own membership may be limited. On the other hand, service providers suit themselves on what criteria to adopt regarding representativeness and when to declare them. They may snipe at user groups' representativeness but they rarely give them the money to do anything about it. Every so often leading figures from the mental health professions will make veiled public statements about the dangers of working with 'professional users' as if they still cannot accept that users can get organised and join in the game too. Even within services, our status as partners remains precarious.

Many of the problems concerning consultation with service users are to do with mechanisms. We are a long way from making planning systems accessible to non-experts. It is also well past the time when those with the power should make clear what the rules really are, so that they can be openly scrutinised. For example, when and how does representativeness affect the validity and weight of evidence, does representativeness affect all groups equally or is it more important for groups of radical survivors than traditional psychiatrists? But successful consultation also depends significantly on attitudes and intentions and, for an increasing number of service users, on results. And here misgivings at the collective level are nicely reflected by questions at the individual level. Are they really listening? And why do I still feel so bad?

THE CONTRIBUTION OF THE USER MOVEMENT

Despite the close and extensive relationship between the user movement and the mental health service system, it is important to remember that the user movement encompasses a wide range of activities, many of which are not directly related to services. Creative activities – art, theatre and poetry – are increasingly becoming features of the movement. People come together to discuss new understandings of their interior experiences. Public education, in particular through attempts to influence the media, has become a major concern for national networking groups. One of the user movement's outstanding features in the last ten years (and it may not always have been a strength) has been its willingness to do almost anything it was invited or encouraged to do. Diversity rather than coherence has been one of the results.

Pragmatism has been dominant in much user action in the UK over the recent years. This distinguishes the current movement from the activity of the 1970s and may help explain its greater initial success. Ideological debates have not been a primary concern and user groups at national, regional and local level have usually avoided contentious issues that might create splits within the movement. Total opposition to compulsion, for example, has not become a defining point in the same way it did in action within the USA. The anger of individuals at the personal damage mental health professionals have caused is still a 'strong and common motivating factor and activists may be united more by this feeling of a common wrong rather than by any agreement on an analysis of its causes or priorities for a solution. Consciousness-raising, the process through which users talk together about their personal experiences and seek out new understandings of their situation, has been central to much action in other countries. In the UK, the warmth and rapidity of the consumerist welcome for the user movement may have gone some way to diminishing the importance of this activity.

The links between anti-psychiatry and user action are frequently cited. Indeed, blanket references to such links have become an easy way for mainstream psychiatry to dismiss the contribution of the user movement. As we approach the end of the 1990s, references to anti-psychiatry seem to have lost specificity and it is often unclear what citing anti-psychiatry really means, except that in many quarters it is usually about a shadowy grouping of discredited ideas whose influence can be both feared and casually abused. In fact, references to the classic anti-psychiatry texts are relatively uncommon within the user movement and there is some evidence now of a preference for a post-psychiatric approach or a search for approaches that relegate the need for reference to a psychiatric lodestar. While it is certainly true that the ideas of R.D. Laing and David Cooper and contact with people who knew them personally were influential on members of the British Network for Alternatives to Psychiatry (BNAP) which was a seedbed for the earliest independent user groups in the 1980s, such thinking has had a diminishing impact and is not crucial now. The user movement may have shown Laing and Cooper greater respect than most of the psychiatric professions (and that could be because they showed mad persons more respect than is usual amongst the professions), but it has never accepted or used their ideas wholeheartedly. If the user movement in the UK does develop a coherent ideology, it may owe a debt to anti-psychiatry but is likely to be based on a model more rooted in the social model of disability developed by the wider movement of disabled people.

One of the most profound impulses behind the formation of the first independent user groups in the early 1980s was the desire to speak for oneself. Individual lives where relatives and doctors and nurses judged our best interests and spoke on our behalf were mirrored at a collective level by voluntary organisations like National MIND that marginalised our participation but still claimed to be advocating for patients. This desire to promote individual viewpoints and to avoid at all costs substituting one kind of paternalism for another has had important implications for the way the user movement has developed. It was a major factor in deciding that the first user networking organisation, Survivors Speak Out, should support the creation of local action groups almost regardless of what they were campaigning for, rather than develop a consistent and agreed platform of demands. It remains one of the reasons that there is still reluctance and suspicion within the movement about proposals to develop a unifying analysis or a united user voice. For those with direct experience of madness who seek its proper valuation, the idea of conformity may be particularly problematic.

Whatever its origins, we must currently acknowledge the diversity of intention and ideology within the user movement. It still contains people who believe their problems are caused by illness and seek an improvement in psychiatry alongside those who see the medical model as the root of their oppression and alternatives to mental health services as the only viable way forward. The movement has also appropriated aspects of relevant contemporary thinking, including lessons from consumerism, civil rights campaigning, disability politics. Some of this material it has taken as its own, some it is still digesting and some it seems to have laid aside for later. It is interesting that user organisations have done relatively little work to support campaigns for civil rights for disabled people, yet are starting to consider whether their problems may fit into the individual impairment and social disability model so significant in the work of organisations of disabled people.

A commitment to empowerment is one unifying factor among user organisations. Although characteristically under-defined, the desire for empowerment usually includes some implicit criticism of both consumerism and the medical model. The medical approach is seen as reinforcing the individual's loss of control in crisis and creating long-term powerlessness through disinterest and disrespect for the totality of individual experience. Consumerist approaches, while valuable in many respects, are revealed as unlikely to involve people in a way that gives them a meaningful say, either in their own care and treatment or in the wider shaping of services. On a scale of empowerment, user satisfaction questionnaires and consultative forums are inferior to user-controlled budgets or user-run services. Empowerment also implies a wider vision of individuals as citizens whose lives extend beyond the boundaries of welfare systems.

In twenty years time it may well appear that the greatest contribution of the user movement in the last decade has not been to criticise the psychiatric approach to distress but to assert and demonstrate the capacities and competencies of people with a diagnosis of mental illness. Although we are still closely attached in the public mind to the twin stereotypes of violent threat and hopeless victim, the ropes may be starting to loosen. Mad people have been successfully running user action groups (voluntary organisations) for ten years. Service users have made television programmes that have been broadcast nationally. Loonies have been earning a living educating mental health workers. Deflecting the impact of these events through circumlocutions like 'the worried well', 'the professional user' and 'the misdiagnosed' cannot hide the underlying reality. The mad are not who they are conceived to be – not because of what they claim to be but because of what they do.

POWER AND THE NURSE–PATIENT RELATIONSHIP

Empowerment and disempowerment must be central practical concerns for mental health nurses. Nurses have a unique capacity to influence service users' day-to-day experience of living through and living with their distress. The great majority of people who enter psychiatric units are making genuine attempts to come to terms with their problems and to gain greater control of their lives. The extent to which nurses are prepared to exercise power over them or to share power with them is critical in a practical and a moral sense. Rosenhan (1973) states: 'Neither anecdotal nor "hard" data can convey the overwhelming sense of powerlessness which invades the individual as he is continually exposed to the depersonalization of the psychiatric hospital.' Unless mental health nurses are persuaded to comprehensively examine how their caring practice maintains the powerlessness of service users, it is inevitable that the long-term damaging of individuals will continue.

My own impressions of nursing care over the last ten years, based on five periods as an in-patient and numerous visits to friends in various hospitals, suggest that mental health nurses may spend less time relating to in-patients than in the two previous decades. Certainly the nurses' attachment to the nursing office is a constant feature of users' accounts of current life on admission wards. At the same time the possibility of nursing staff and in-patients collaborating as a caring force within the ward seems almost more remote than it was in the 1970s. Whatever good intentions trainee nurses are taught in classroom settings, the prevalent atmosphere in many day rooms is not of cooperation and involvement but of discouraging 'interference'.

I believe there is a strong common-sense argument that giving and taking are central elements in a creative human relationship. It should not be assumed that this no longer applies when one of the parties is diagnosed as mentally ill. Furthermore, many in-patients are likely to be looking for a wider range of interactions with those charged with their care. If this is so, the comparative absence of mental health nurses except on the bank shift and the tendency for dialogue to only take place in, or on the fringes of, the nursing station may be movements in the wrong direction. Some service users also complain that the introduction of the key nurse has encouraged a move towards 'nursing by appointment' or 'sessional caring'.

In whatever locations caring may be taking place, it seems essential that nurses are sensitive to the barriers that obstruct reciprocal communication and the difference between having power, even benificent power, over a subordinate and sharing power with a partner. When the caring is haunted by compulsion, this sensitivity is at a premium. It is far from clear how seriously the implications of compulsion for person to person transactions are currently investigated by mental health nursing experts. If recipients of compulsion or people who have lived with the possibility of compulsory interventions have been coherently consulted on the repercussions – positive or otherwise – the findings do not appear to have been widely cited. Perhaps it is now time to stop canvassing abstractions in the classroom and open a concrete and specific debate on the wards themselves.

But the subordinate position of people diagnosed as mentally ill is not simply a matter of our actual or potential legal status. That merely reflects a wider and more profound inferiority relating to the particular character of our supposed incapacity. What type of person is a disabled person? What type of disabled persons are those with impairments of reasoning and insight? Is it possible to restore these people to full humanity when we actually fear their difference so much and when they themselves secretly feel less than human? How can you validate the mad when you are ignorant of their experience and ignore what they tell you about it? These are some of the conundrums facing professional care-givers who want to share their power. It would seem almost impossible to give positive value to mad people when you will not give positive value to their madness. If you do not recognise a central part of an individual except in terms of disease, it will be difficult for that person to be anything but of a different order to you, and of a lower order to you. Particularly if they are asking you for help.

I have recently trained mental health nurses at one of the most prestigious psychiatric hospitals in Britain who both told me that they were taught not to talk to people about their madness and that R.D. Laing and Carl Jung ended up with mental illnesses because they talked to their patients in this way. This seems to me to be a gloomy reflection on the prospects for empowering people with a diagnosis of mental illness, either within their periods of crisis in psychiatric units or in the rest of their lives in the outside world. It may also begin to give some clues to the reasons why service users are so insistent that no-one is listening to them. Edward Podvoll (1990) has identified what he calls 'the asylum mentality' and writes:

> The most subtle form of asylum mind has been called the 'silence that humiliates', a studied interpersonal rift between doctor and patient. The professional separation between them creates a loneliness and silence for the patient in which to reflect on madness – to intensify it, so that it might mock itself.

Asylum mentality is not confined to doctors. The greatest power that mental health nurses hold is the power of denial.

Any re-evaluation of the status of the recipient within the caring relationship should include an extensive investigation of the nature and source of desirable expertise in mental health care. Such an investigation has not yet gone far enough. There is little research comparing the needs and wants of service users with professional skills and attitudes. While there is some recognition of the expertise of service users as direct consumers, this expertise has only been partially exploited. Service users' expertise in madness has barely been explored. As Jan Foudraine (1974) wrote: 'What concerns me most is why we do not see that those who are called psychotic or schizophrenic can teach us most about the human condition; why we have been so unprepared and unwilling to listen especially to them'. Giving a new value to our madness has been a persistent covert activity for many people involved in the user movement and there are now signs that concerns of this kind may become more overt. The dynamics of the mental health nursing relationship could benefit from further demystification of professional expertise in the face of madness. Greater respect for the insights of mad persons would not only be courteous, it would be useful.

Rogers et al. (1993) have described the increasing incompatability of professional and lay discourse about mental health issues. The concern of some service users that nurses are being taught the wrong skills and are becoming less rather than more conversant with the day-to-day practical and spiritual concerns of their clients is one aspect of this split. At the same time, the potential role of service users in new collaborations is quite narrowly circumscribed. Although self-help among those with a diagnosis of mental illness is demonstrably effective, the use of people with direct experience as a therapeutic resource within services is extremely inconsistent. The debate about the nature of madness, a debate that could still be central to the quality of life of most service users in the long term and an area where they have the most powerful contribution to make, remains peripheral. It is clear that mental health workers and mental health service users are talking and listening together more. What is open to question is both the quality of discussion and the boundaries of debate.

Improvements in mental health services, however desirable in themselves, will not transform the position of the diagnosed mentally ill in our society. Nor will the change from mental patient to mental health service consumer ultimately amount to very much. Consumer rights do not necessarily ensure respect or understanding. As such a consumer, I can still be locked up for hours alone in a police station cell at my greatest time of crisis while awaiting expert assessment – a practice with no justification at all save in terms of logistics or punishment. Furthermore, I know almost nobody, and certainly nobody with a diagnosis of mental illness, who seeks a destiny of consumer. The role of mental health service consumer may be a step out from under the stairs but to suggest it is where most of us will be happy to stop is unrealistic. This is not to deny that there may be important differences between the diagnosed mentally ill and the majority of society or that our difficulties are not substantial. But the nature of those differences and the identities left open to us by society must now be available for equal debate. It is time that madness and mad persons were evaluated outside the cages of medicine. It is no longer acceptable that we should be presumed to have so little of value to say about madness or about living with madness. The crucial debate is about social understandings not service systems. Mental health workers, including nurses, should put aside their notes and badges and work alongside us.

REFERENCES

Barham, P. and **Hayward, R.** 1991 *From the mental patient to the person.* London: Routledge.

Beresford, P. and **Campbell, J.** 1994 Disabled people, service users, user involvement and representation. *Disability and Society,* **9**(3); 315–25.

Brandon, D. 1991 *Innovation without change?* London: Macmillan.

Foudrane, J. 1974 *Not made of wood.* London: Quartet.

Leete, E. 1989 The role of the consumer movement and persons with mental illness. Presentation at the Twelfth Mary Switzer Memorial Seminar in Rehabilitation, Washington, DC, 15–16 June.

Mental Health Nursing Review Team 1994: *Working in partnership: a collaborative approach to care.* London: HMSO.

O'Hagan, M. 1993 *Stopovers on my way home from Mars.* London: Survivors Speak Out.

Podvell, E. 1990 *The seduction of madness: a compassionate approach to recovery at home.* London: Century.

Rogers, A., Pilgrim, D. and **Lacey, R.** 1993 *Experiencing psychiatry.* London: Macmillan/ MIND.

Rosenhan, D. 1973 On being sane in insane places. *Science* **178**, 250–8.

18

CLINICAL SOCIOLOGY AND EMPOWERMENT

Peter Morrall

Here Peter Morrall considers some further issues in relation to empowerment, starting from the point that the empowerment of users and consumers of health services has been on the policy agenda for a number of years, while health service administrators and personnel are now specifically required to consult with users and carers. The rhetoric and reality of empowerment for people with enduring mental disorder are, however, clearly distinct. Much of the interpersonal communication and therapy practices of mental health workers can be experienced as disempowering. Can clinical sociology provide users with avenues through which real power may be gained by addressing the origins rather than the symptoms of disempowerment? Or is there simply nowhere to start in the face of issues such as homelessness, the removal of mentally ill from GPs' waiting lists and other structurally disempowering situations? Is the provision of training and awareness-heightening initiatives for mental health practitioners from the realm of academic sociology, the traditional bastion of radical critique of societal institutions, an important initiative? Or is it just another example of the sort of crude territorial acquisitiveness and professional imperialism (*clinical* sociology) that academic sociology sets out to critique?

> The history of madness is the history of power . . . It requires power to control it. Threatening the normal structures of authority, insanity is engaged in an endless dialogue . . . about power.
>
> (Porter, 1987)

Gibson (1991) has noted that a general interest in the concept of empowerment was stimulated by the World Health Organisation's approach to health promotion in the 1980s, which focused on helping people to take control over their own lives. The involvement of users and carers in the delivery of mental health services has been recommended in a number of recent reports (Audit Commission, 1994; House of Commons Health Committee, 1994). The Audit Commission noted:

The past few years have seen an increasing recognition of the need to take account of the views of the people who use mental health services and their families. Listening to users is important if professionals and service managers are to avoid falling into the trap of making assumptions on other people's behalf, since their views often differ widely from those of users.

(Audit Commission, 1994)

The English National Board for Nursing, Midwifery and Health Visiting (ENB), along with many voluntary organisations involved in mental health, has endorsed this policy. The ENB has encouraged nurse teachers to include people with enduring mental disorder (PEMD) and their representatives in the development and implementation of educational programmes (ENB, 1996). A significant part of the ENB's 1995 annual mental health nursing conference was committed to the issue of user and carer participation in the delivery of care. This trend complements the recent government's initiatives directed towards empowering individuals in their interaction with both public and private institutions. The ordinary citizen now has a 'charter', and the passive customer has been reconstructed in contemporary society into the 'active consumer'. It has thus become professionally and politically correct for nurses to seek and act on the opinions of service users and carers.

However, it can be viewed as politically naïve to believe that this will empower users of the health services and in particular those suffering from chronic mental illness. The impression that PEMD are being offered an opportunity to participate in the organisation of their care and treatment may well serve to give a token illusion of empowerment, which is in itself disempowering. It can be said that it is not in the interests of the state or professionals to dilute their influence by investing power in PEMD (or any other service user or carer group).

More fundamentally, empowering service users and their carers will have enormous – and hence prohibitive – cost implications. Scull (1983, 1984) has suggested that, with the development of the welfare state, institutional segregation of the mentally ill as a mechanism of social control became too expensive, and thus the policy of community care was determined by economic considerations. The resourcing of care in the community remains a topical political issue. With reference to mental health, there continues to be the claim that there is insufficient funding for an effective community care policy. For example, the Audit Commission (1994) has reported that a serious under-resourcing of community care is occurring because most of the funding for adult mental health care in England and Wales (£1.8 billion a year) is spent on hospitals.

Scull's view is that the consequence of under-resourcing community care is the creation of a 'nightmare existence' of neglect and homelessness for discharged mentally ill people (Scull, 1983). In fact, very few homeless people in this country are former psychiatric in-patients (Audit Commission, 1994), but the plight of mentally ill people living in the community, even if they have not been 'decarcerated' from a hospital, is still stark:

> Surveys have shown that the proportions of mentally disturbed people in single homeless hostel populations have grown . . . In the 1980s most surveys found that 30–40 per cent had overt psychiatric disorder . . . The number of destitute people with serious mental disorder now living more or less permanently in this way is reckoned to be 60–90,000.

(Murphy, 1991, p. 211)

The Audit Commission (1994) recognised that poverty and inadequate accommodation are common among the mentally ill in the community. But how can mentally ill people living in severe and perpetual poverty or homelessness be empowered in reality?

The report of the Mental Health Initiative into homelessness among the mentally ill (Craig *et al.*, 1995) recognises many examples of good practice, and concludes that the aims of the four teams in the study (to identify homeless people with mental health problems, and ensure they were in contact with the relevant agencies) were, in the main, achieved. However, the authors also note resource constraints that preclude effective empowerment:

> The idea that statutory services would be willing and able to take on large numbers of clients with long-term, high support needs has proved somewhat idealistic . . . Statutory services were not adequately prepared for taking on such cases, which simply add to demand on their already limited and over-stretched resources.
>
> (Craig *et al.*, 1995, p. 142)

Furthermore, how can people with enduring mental disorder be empowered when health care professionals have the authority to refuse to offer treatment? The Association of Community Health Councils for England and Wales' survey of over 200 community health councils (Brindle, 1994) found that, in one year, general practitioners removed from their lists approximately 30,000 patients. Many of these patients were elderly, chronically ill, or mentally disordered, who are time-consuming and costly to treat.

What 'empowering' intervention can the mental health services offer in these structurally disempowering situations? Psychosocial therapy? Psychoanalysis? Supervision registers? Community treatment orders? Alternatively, should not the efforts of the therapist be directed towards helping PEMD gain a home, employment, a living wage and genuine control over her or his life? That is, therapeutic interventions should be addressing the origins, not the symptoms, of disempowerment.

ACTIVE CONSUMER

How empowered in general is the consumer of health services? Has there been a shift in power between the service user and the professional, to the benefit of the former? In the last 20 years there has been an explosion in information, and in increased access to information. Clinical knowledge has become more codified and less indeterminate. As Nettleton (1995) records, computerised expert systems (used, for example, in the diagnosis of illness) allow members of non-professional and quasi-professional groups entry into bodies of knowledge that were formerly esoteric. Furthermore, the perceived existence of a more active and knowledgeable service user may also threaten the social distance between the patient and the medical practitioner.

From the 1980s onwards in the UK, the structural and bureaucratic limitations on the clinical autonomy of the medical profession would include the restructuring of the health service and the rise of 'new managerialism'. New managerialism replaced what Harrison *et al.* (1990) describe as the 'diplomacy model', which had operated since the 1960s. Managers under the earlier system were not leaders or agents of change; their role was primarily to help the professionals in their clinical work by solving organisational problems as they occurred. In contrast, the new managers are expected to be much more pro-active, innovative, and consumer-oriented. This management style also involves the comprehensive auditing of clinical work; this, it can be argued, erodes further the autonomy of the professionals.

Freidson (1988) recognises the development of consumer movements, and the 'active' and knowledgeable service user. However, he questions the effect these developments have had on the power of the professional:

> While the traditional arrangement in which the physician is active or guiding and the patient passive or co-operative has been tempered somewhat, there is little evidence that it has changed so markedly as to have become routinely egalitarian, involving truly mutual participation.
>
> (Freidson, 1988, p. 388)

However, the explosion of information is entering into a new and dramatic phase. Computer-based technology is now operating in a realm that has been described as 'cyberspace' and has the potential to offer consumers immense and immediate access to knowledge on a global scale. But, although access will be available to all, these information systems will be susceptible to expropriation by both established and new breeds of experts, who have (or will have) the techniques and resources to analyse and synthesise data on this scale. Given the imperialistic and market-oriented tendencies associated with medicine in the past, and its success in promoting a techno-scientific base in modern health care, future strategies are likely to include expeditions into and colonisation of cyberspace. As Freidson observes (1994), the better informed consumer is competing with medicine's continued technological and knowledge expansion. Service users simply cannot keep up with medicine's progressively sophisticated knowledge base and technical competence.

Furthermore, the formulation of a Citizen's and a Patient's Charter may not be achieving the projected goals of empowering the individual in her or his encounter with the health care industry. For example, a survey for the Royal College of Nursing concluded that respondents knew little of their rights under the Patient's Charter, with less than a third being able to identify any of its components (Brindle, 1994).

Illman (1991) also questions the reality of the active consumer. He argues that many consumers are not 'active', because they may not know what they need in the first place, do not have the skills or motivation to assess the quality of the service they have received, and still believe that 'doctor knows best'.

If it is doubtful that service users overall are as knowledgeable, active and empowered as government policy implies they should be, it is highly improbable that the severely mentally ill are in a stronger position. Freidson points out that it is the very nature of the service users' contact with the health industry which creates inequality in terms of control over treatment:

> owing to . . . the emotional and physical incapacitation that often accompanies illness, patients are not in a position to be adequately informed and fully rational customers who are capable of looking after their own interests in the medical market place.
>
> (Freidson, 1994, p. 190)

PEMD are by definition not 'fully rational', or 'capable of looking after their own interests'. Consequently, they have a disadvantage in their relationship with the health services. Moreover, the way in which the use of psychopharmacology contributes to the social control of PEMD is obvious. However, it can be argued that psychotherapy (in the broadest sense of the term) is at best inadequate with respect to empowering its users, and/or unsubstantiated empirically. At worst, psychotherapy is deceptive, disabling, and an abuse of power. In particular, the talking treatments, as Masson observes, implicitly (and often explicitly) encourage the individual to accept responsibility for what are, at root, social problems:

> Every therapy I have examined . . . displays a lack of interest in social justice . . . Each shows an implicit acceptance of the political status quo . . . It is easier to make the assumptions necessary to remain a member of the profession of psychotherapy, for example, that everybody is responsible for his or her own situation in life . . . I believe that therapy is never honest.
>
> (Masson, 1992, p. 285)

For Masson, therefore, therapy is dishonest because it accentuates individual accountability in situations where the state, a section of society, or society as a whole, is ultimately responsible. It is the social system that is dysfunctional in these circumstances, not the individual.

CLINICAL SOCIOLOGY

Central to this process of individualising social problems is the issue of power. In all social relationships, including those designated therapeutic, power exists as a potent factor. Power is distributed unequally in society. Consequently, equality is rarely established in social and interpersonal communicative processes.

Frequently, the powerful in society, and in interpersonal relationships, achieve their goals through manipulating or 'distorting' communication (Malhotra, 1987). Habermas (1970, 1972) comments that what is being communicated has the appearance of being understood, equitable and acceptable to all participants, but below the surface there is virtually always an 'hidden agenda'; a sub-text which is orchestrated by the person or group with power. Systems of communication (language, the media) are organised so as to ensure an outcome which is in the interest of the powerful. It is indicative of the power of the individual or group that communication processes can be fabricated in this way.

Hugman provides the following example of power-distorted communication from the health care setting:

> a caring professional asks a service user to comply with an intervention (to take medicine, do the exercises, take part in family therapy), but the request is directed to accomplishing the professional goals, and not to reaching an agreement with the service user which gives the service user's goals an equal status in the relationship.
>
> (Hugman, 1991, p. 35)

Domination by the powerful in society is operationalised through the selection of the content and character of what is being communicated. The formulation of communicative processes on the basis of power is described as 'discourse'. Foucault (1970, 1972, 1973) argues that powerful factions in society, including health care professions, produce their own discourse. Foucault (1980) examined how medical knowledge has been constructed to form an ostensibly authentic and socially sanctioned way of viewing the world. He suggests, however, that there cannot be one 'legitimate' way of viewing the world. Different societies (both historically and cross-culturally) have alternative, and possibly competing, realities. The manner in which service users perceive and refer to their bodies is controlled by the concepts, theories and symbols that have been supplied by health care professionals. The medical discourse in turn is a reflection of what those with power in society have deemed to be of significance at that point in time.

Sociology, with its range of theoretical perspectives, when applied to the clinical arena, can highlight the power configurations that manipulate and distort communication:

> Sociology, because of its concern with social structure, draws attention to aspects of life such as occupation which are relatively ignored by existing treatment professions, and through concepts such as social class stresses the interconnection between advantage and disadvantage in the various spheres of life.

> (Blane, 1993, p. 64)

At the University of Teesside, a skills-based module in clinical sociology has been introduced to the undergraduate programme. This programme is offered to health care professionals and students of the social sciences. Egan's (1993) multi-stage and eclectic model of counselling has been adapted to include theoretical insights from a variety of sociological approaches. These insights are used at each part of the counselling process. The aims of the module are:

- to develop the participants' communication and counselling skills, and
- to raise the consciousness of the individual seeking help with respect to the root cause of her or his problems, and to help her or him to act on this awareness.

The latter may include engaging in collective action (through self-help or pressure groups) with the express purpose of instigating social change.

Conclusion

Empowerment is frequently available to individuals. However, without acknowledging the social, political, and economic conditions which shape our existence, the potential to alter our personal circumstances is minimal.

Clinical sociology empowers by helping clients (for example, PEMD and/or their carers) to realise their 'true discourse' (Malhotra, 1987). That is, the individual becomes aware of what her or his authentic interests are, and this forms the foundation for future action towards achieving her or his 'demystified' needs. There is, therefore, at this critical juncture in the development of mental health care policy, the opportunity for practitioners (psychiatric nurses, medical sociologists) to participate in a therapeutic *perestroika*.

REFERENCES

Audit Commission 1994: *Finding a place: a review of mental health services for adults.* London: HMSO.

Blane, D. 1993: Clinical sociology: what might it be? In Payne, G. and Cross, M. (eds) *Sociology in action.* Basingstoke: Macmillan/British Sociological Association, pp. 57–68.

Blom-Cooper, L., Hally, H. and **Murphy, E.** 1995: *The falling shadow: one patient's mental health care 1978–1993.* London: Duckworth.

Brindle, D. 1994a: GPs rid lists of difficult patients. *The Guardian,* 11 July.

Brindle, D. 1994b: Named nurse scheme fails publicity test. *The Guardian,* 25 April.

Craig, T., Bayliss, E., Klein, O., Manning, P. and **Reader, L.** 1995: *The homeless mentally ill initiative.* London: Department of Health/Mental Health Foundation.

Egan, G. 1993: *The skilled helper.* Fifth edition. California: Brooks-Cole.

English National Board 1996: *Regulations and guidelines for the approval of institutions and programmes.* London: ENB.

Foucault, M. 1970: *The order of things: an archaeology of the human sciences.* New York: Pantheon.

Foucault, M. 1972: *The archaeology of knowledge.* New York: Pantheon.

Foucault, M. 1973: *The birth of the clinic: an archaeology of medical perception.* New York: Pantheon.

Foucault, M. 1980: *Power/knowledge: selected interviews and other writings 1972–1977.* New York: Pantheon.

Freidson, E. 1988: *The profession of medicine: a study of the sociology of applied knowledge.* Chicago: University of Chicago Press.

Freidson, E. 1994: *Professionalism reborn: theory prophecy and policy.* Cambridge: Polity Press.

Gibson, C.H. 1991: A concept analysis of empowerment. *Journal of Advanced Nursing* **16** 354–61.

Giddens, A. 1991: *Modernity and self-identity.* Cambridge: Polity Press.

Habermas, J. 1970: *Towards a rational society.* London: Heinemann.

Habermas, J. 1972: *Knowledge and human interests.* London: Heinemann.

Harrison, S., Hunter, D. and **Pollitt, C.** 1990: *The dynamics of British health policy.* London: Unwin Hyman.

Hugman, R. 1991: *Power in caring professions.* London: Macmillan.

Illman, J. 1991: Not enough patient power in the waiting rooms. *The Guardian,* 29 March.

Malhotra, V.A. 1987: Teaching of clinical sociology: Habermas' sociological theory as a basis for clinical practice with small groups. *Clinical Sociology Review* **5,** 181–92.

Masson, J. 1992: *Against therapy.* London: Collins.

Murphy, E. 1991: *After the asylums.* London: Faber and Faber.

Nettleton, S. 1995: *The sociology of health and illness.* London: Sage.

Porter, R.A. 1987: A social history of madness: stories of the insane. London: Weidenfeld & Nicolson.

Scull, A.T. 1983: The asylum as community or the community as asylum: paradoxes and contradictions of mental health care. In Bean, P. (ed). *Mental illness: changes and trends.* Chichester: Wiley.

Scull, A.T. 1984: *Decarceration: community treatment and the deviant: a radical view.* Cambridge: Polity Press.

19

COMMUNITY PSYCHOLOGY: A SOCIAL ACTION APPROACH TO PSYCHOLOGICAL DISTRESS

Steve Melluish

Amid expectations that we should form power-sharing relationships with clients in which we have the humility to look to them for expertise, and while experiencing pressure from management to ration care and prove cost-efficient performance, as mental health professionals we also often have to operate within reorganisation and dramatic local disruption to our services. Just as crises within families and individuals may be opportunities for development and growth, so too within a profession. Here Steve Melluish describes how both as an individual and as a member of a team, it has been possible to capitalise on such changes. In developing a departmental approach based on 'community psychology', however, certain questions arise. What is the interface between psychology and politics? Is it right (or, indeed, really possible) for mental health care to move into the sphere of political action? Steve considers the extent to which primary prevention in mental health work and social action to target at-risk groups can effect change. Steve challenges the notion of *empowerment* and questions whether it is possible to effect any real change even within the context of the most 'empowering' client–professional relationship. He suggests that social action, professionally facilitated or led, may lead only to more confusion. It may be that the most that can be expected of professionals in this field is for them to attempt to demystify psychological problems. That is, they can help to refocus both clients' and society's attention on the origins of these problems within people's social environments.

> Man must get rid of illusions that enslave and paralyse him . . . he must become aware of the reality inside and outside of him in order to create a world which needs no illusions. Freedom and independence can be achieved only when the chains of illusion are broken.
>
> (Erich Fromm 1980, p. 172)

Freeing ourselves from illusions and confronting the reality of our existence is, according to Fromm, common both to the enterprises of psychoanalysis and Marxism. He argues that both the psychotherapist and the political activist are involved in forms of 'consciousness raising' or demystification: the psychotherapist seeking to help the individual obtain some degree of freedom from the 'inner' forces to which his/her life is a reaction and the political activist seeking to enable community or social groups to act collectively upon 'outer' or public forces. Fromm's work is part of a wider critical literature within psychology, psychiatry and psychotherapy that has sought to bridge the separation between therapeutic and political forms of intervention and provide a framework for understanding the link between the private and public domains.

Community psychology is part of this critical tradition. It has evolved over the past 30 years as a reaction to the prevailing ideas and practices within traditional clinical psychology with its emphasis on the individual. Community psychology aims to develop an understanding of people in their social worlds and to use this to improve people's psychological health through social action. As an approach it is a relatively undefined field in terms of any 'coherent theory, methodological preferences or substantive issues' (Fryer, 1994, p.13) and has evolved both as an area of theoretical study and as a basis on which to build psychological practice.

My interest in community psychology has developed through my training and work as a clinical psychologist where I have often felt frustrated at the tendency of clinical psychology (along with other mental health professions) to ignore and deny the link between social inequalities and psychological distress and to offer individually based solutions to problems of social origin. Community psychology seemed to me to be an approach that rather than simply accepting the social backdrop actually spoke of improving it and advocated the need for social rather than just psychic change.

As I have become more familiar with the writing and practice of community psychology I have become increasingly aware of the complexity, at a conceptual and ethical level, of broadening the focus of one's practice to consider the social realm. In this chapter I consider some of the practical, ethical and conceptual issues involved in trying to develop a more community psychology approach. I begin by tracing the origins and development of community psychology, placing particular emphasis on the influence of ideas drawn from Public Health and Community Development models. I then discuss how these ideas have been adapted in the work conducted by Sue Holland in the White City Project and in the work of myself and colleagues in Nottingham which has attempted to develop a community approach as part of our work as NHS clinical psychologists. I then examine whether it is possible or right for psychologists or other mental health practitioners to become involved in the wider concerns of a community and to engage in political and social action.

THE GROWTH OF COMMUNITY PSYCHOLOGY

It is difficult to attribute the origins of any particular social movement or social change to an exact time and place in history. However, in the literature on community psychology, it is stated that a conference held in Swampscott, Massachusetts, in the Spring of 1965 was the official birthplace of 'community psychology'. A number of background factors are regarded as influential in this development. First, during the

1960s there was criticism of institutional forms of care following the work of Goffman (1963) and other social critics who documented the detrimental effects of incarcerating people in overcrowded psychiatric hospitals. Second, there was growing concern about the efficacy and limitations of individual psychotherapy. Eysenck's study (1952) was influential and, although itself subject to much criticism, provided evidence for practitioners' dissatisfaction with individual psychotherapy and acknowledged the importance of the environment, if only at a micro level. Third, awareness developed as to how social and environmental factors affect people's health and how stress underlies many illnesses. Within mental health services this led to a recognition that 'mental disorder' could not be viewed in isolation from its social context. Lastly, the influence of feminism and the women's movement led to a shift in the traditional class-based analysis of society with factors such as sex, race, disability and age seen also as contributing to structural social inequalities.

The confluence of these factors led to a recognition of the need for a new approach. The term 'community psychology' was conceived to indicate that the role of the psychologist in the community was to be broader than that of community mental health teams and would encompass prevention and the need to examine the wider social context.

The emergence of community psychology in America was paralleled by a less formalised development in Britain. Although during the late 1960s and early 1970s, there were many British psychologists who expressed dissatisfaction with a purely individualistic approach, in terms of practice it was the setting up in 1973 of the Battersea Action and Counselling Centre that perhaps marked the beginning of community psychology in Britain. This project operated from a shop front in South London and aimed to provide a psychotherapy service along with other forms of material aid such as welfare advice, a crèche and a food co-op. The project lasted five years before its funding was withdrawn in 1978. A few of those involved went on to set up a similar initiative in Lambeth (The Lambeth Community Mental Health Group) and Sue Holland went on to develop 'The White City Project' on a housing estate in West London which continues today as 'Women's Action for Mental Health'.

These innovative projects in the 1970s did not significantly influence the provision of most mainstream mental health services but they did provide the inspiration for a few clinical psychologists, in the late 1980s, to revive interest in community psychology as an approach. A few individuals such as Janet Bostock and Gill Edwards began to integrate community approaches into their work as clinical psychologists in primary care and began to explore and write about the need for psychologists to attend to the social aetiology of much emotional distress (Bostock, 1991; Edwards, 1989). This was supported by the work of Jim Orford (1992), David Smail (1993) and David Fryer (1990), whose writings challenged the individual determinism of much conventional psychology. More recently, in 1994, a meeting was held in Newark, which formally marked the establishment of a national network of psychologists in Britain who were interested or involved in community psychology.

The small but growing interest in community psychology in Britain over this period can perhaps be attributed to the disillusionment of psychologists working within community mental health teams (C.M.H.T.s), which many saw as failing to fulfil their promise of reforming psychiatric practice. In many C.M.H.T.s the medical model persisted and psychiatry continued to dominate. This led to the retention of an individualistic focus and a preoccupation with relieving the symptoms rather than addressing the causes of distress. Sue Holland (1988) in commenting on the arrival of the C.M.H.T. on the White City estate said:

> The problem is that the old mental illness teams have hijacked the concept of health but are still applying the old remedies. The move from hospital to community has not grown out of a real sense of community with its residents, their histories, their struggles, their anger and desire, but merely extends the walls of the hospital into the community.
>
> (p. 126)

THE PRINCIPLES OF COMMUNITY PSYCHOLOGY

The recent interest in community psychology has coincided with the decentralisation of the NHS towards more local services and the rediscovery of 'community' as a central concept in discussions of social policy. The move to a less centrist approach to health has come, in part, from a re-examination of 'third world' models of primary health care and from the ideas drawn from the public health movement and community development. These two approaches have in common a number of principles that include aiming at public participation; valuing 'lay' knowledge; and being directed towards action and often involved in popular struggles for social change. Community psychology has attempted to apply these principles to mental health provision.

Public health

Central to community psychology has been the fundamental tenet of public health that 'no condition is ever prevented by treating the victims of the condition itself'. The American psychologist, George Albee has published a number of articles (Albee 1982, 1985, 1988) stressing how traditional mental health services cannot respond practically to the enormous prevalence of psychological distress and arguing for existing resources to be channelled into primary prevention. He calculated that less than 20 per cent of 'seriously disturbed' individuals and an extremely small proportion of 'the larger group of people with problems' are actually seen by mental health services in the U.S.A. (Albee, 1982). Community psychologists in Britain (Bostock, 1991; Edwards, 1989) have restated this argument, advocating that psychologists and other mental health workers should direct their energy and expertise towards working with communities to support them in gaining greater influence and control over their environments.

Community development

In proposing social change, community psychology has drawn on ideas from community development in thinking about how to 'empower communities'. Community development has its origins in the work and writings of Paulo Freire, a Brazilian educationalist, who helped initiate a number of successful literacy campaigns in Brazil and other countries during the early 1970s. Although his focus was literacy, his method termed 'conscientisation' set the field of literacy within a wider discourse about oppression and he argued that to become literate was congruent with becoming conscious of the effects of injustice and oppression.

When community development projects were first set up in economically deprived areas throughout Britain they were often run by activists who aimed to foster solidarity and engage people in the political process. In these community development projects the everyday concerns of people such as housing, childcare and family relationships were seen as political issues and part of a wider struggle against an oppressive system. This was a departure from earlier ideas of how to organise politically, which had primarily focused on trade unionism within the workplace and was predominantly the preserve of men. Community politics, instead, principally involved women organising on a local level to address the issues that affected their communities. In advocating social action, community psychologists argued that psychologists should act as catalysts for change by taking up such struggles and by helping to articulate the way in which people's private troubles are connected with an exploitative social structure and an inequitable distribution of resources.

Sue Holland in The White City project adapted Freire's model of conscientisation to provide a framework in which to link individual psychotherapy and community action. In this framework individuals are seen as moving from a position in which they view their private troubles in terms of symptoms, through a stage where they question the origins of their psychological difficulties, to a further stage at which they ask what changes they desire for themselves and others, and finally to a position in which they are able to engage in social action to alter the conditions that make them vulnerable to psychological distress. In practice the project combines, 'intensive focal psychotherapy, group work, mental health education and the stimulation of mutual-help initiatives within the neighbourhood' (Holland, 1988 p. 131).

THE NOTTINGHAM EXPERIENCE

In Nottingham, the ideas of community psychology have influenced the thinking and practice of the adult clinical psychology service. I began my current post in July 1993 working as a clinical psychologist in primary care, which entails responsibility for offering a psychological therapy service to GP's in the west area of Nottingham. I also have as part of my job a community psychology remit.

Community initiatives

Due to the large size of the west area of the city I decided to concentrate any community psychology activity on one defined geographical area. This area includes a number of estates built in the post-war period as part of slum clearance programmes and now termed 'outer city estates'. The one particular estate where I first attempted to apply the principles of community psychology comprised low-level, repetitive housing with a road layout based on some planner's utopian vision of 'community' with three concentric road loops intersected by numerous radial roads all leading to a central roundabout, on which stood the community centre. While on a map the design looks neat, on the ground it is disorientating and confusing.

There were a number of reasons why this estate appeared to be an area in which to consider applying a community psychology approach. Geographically it was on the edge of the city far away from any commercial district and with very few local facilities, the nearest shops being located on the perimeter road. Census information revealed there to be high rates of unemployment, many people dependent on some form of state benefit and a significant number of households with a member regarded as having a chronic illness. Furthermore, amongst residents on the estate there had been growing concern about joy-riding, burglary and violence and in the summer before I took up my post there had been riots.

These riots, along with the joyriding, led to an initiative set up by the city council to try and address the problems of the estate. Initially, debates about the estate raised the spectre of the 'problem family' and the city council carried out a number of evictions of certain 'problem families' who were thought to be the source of the trouble. This breach of tenancy rules to counter wider problems of crime and disruption within the community had previously been applied in Hackney in what was regarded as a successful approach to reducing crime levels. I found the idea of the evictions very disturbing and was confused at the apparent consensus amongst local people, as reported in the local media, for such action. It seemed in fact that no systematic attempt had been made to gather the opinions of local people, neither had any opportunities been created for them to discuss the policy. Furthermore, it seemed that in spite of the policy's reported success in reducing crime, its underlying message was that the problems of the estate were to be found within individuals. The policy thus perpetuated 'victim-blaming' and prevented any exploration of people's experiences of their community or alternative ideas that took account of their positions within an oppressive social structure.

I was interested to understand more about the community on the estate and along with two community workers and four local residents became involved in what was variously termed the 'community survey' or 'quality of life' group. The aim of this group was to ascertain how local residents felt about the estate and to use the survey as a means of encouraging local participation and of opening up a debate about issues affecting the estate.

A questionnaire was devised which included open and closed questions asking how people felt about the estate, what they saw as the main issues of concern and what they thought needed to be done. Questions were also included enquiring how residents felt the estate was viewed by outsiders and what was the nature of their own involvement in the community. Members of the group conducted individual and group interviews in a number of settings such as the community centre, outside the local post office, and in people's homes.

As a result of the survey, a number of accounts about the community emerged, reflecting differing degrees of optimism about the future of the estate and what needed to be done. The findings from the survey group were presented at a meeting of residents, local workers and city council officials. The findings were accepted by this audience as constituting a local voice, representative of residents. However, the hope that this would be seen as the start of an ongoing dialogue has not been realised.

For me, being involved in the survey group allowed me to become familiar with the needs and concerns of people living on the estate and to participate in a shared endeavour. It revealed the difficulty for local people in having a say in local policy-making, and how hard it was to influence decisions about resources in the area in which they lived. Although the community research did not have tangible results in terms of resources for the estate, it provided a space for critical discussion and reflection about how people experience their community.

Community research as described is just one example of an attempt to apply the principles of community psychology. For me it has also involved attending community meetings, being part of a group to look at health issues on the estate, running seminars for local health visitors offering non-medical understandings of psychological distress and setting up and running community support/study groups for people experiencing psychological distress. Other work in the Nottingham department has involved a wide range of initiatives including a survey of local people's views of their general practitioners and a preventative health project that aims to employ lay health workers.

Although such initiatives are minimal in terms of the enormity of the problems affecting people living in such areas, they can perhaps be seen as part of a wider struggle within such communities to break the silence about the injustices of an economic system that leaves so many people feeling excluded and marginalised.

Clinical practice

On a practical level, community initiatives, such as those described above, have enabled me to become more aware of local resources and also better informed about the issues affecting people living in the local area. They have also provided a context for working clinically with individuals.

At a conceptual level, the principles of community psychology offer a perspective on an individual's experience and suffering that is different from traditional clinical psychology or psychotherapeutic approaches. Instead of viewing an individual's difficulties as signs of their dysfunctional adaptation, community psychology aspires to focus on a person's strengths and competencies in a world that is not functional for them. Psychological distress is thus seen as arising from environmental causes rather than intrapsychic ones and it is seen also in the context of the increasingly inequitable distribution of resources in our society. Community psychology also explicitly recognises that low social status defined by class, gender, race and age creates social injustices that have psychological consequences. This perspective is perhaps best illustrated by a case vignette.

Case study

Mr C. was referred by his GP for panic attacks. He was in his mid-forties and had been a resident on the estate for most of his life. Up until 6 years ago he had worked in a factory but was made redundant and since then he had devoted his time to a number of community projects aimed at providing activities for young people.

At our first meeting, Mr C. was markedly distressed and tearful and spoke about the disabling effects of his anxiety. He explained how he was fearful to go out and that he had great difficulty relaxing and sleeping. He described how he felt useless and a failure and uncomfortable when around people, even his family who held him in high regard.

On further discussion, it transpired that Mr C.'s panic attacks began shortly after the riots on the estate. Following the riots, it was rumoured that through his involvement in his voluntary work, he had been helping the police identify those involved in the riots. Although this was untrue, this view gained acceptance and he and his family were subjected to threats and intimidation. He felt trapped and asked to be rehoused but was informed that he would have to wait. After several weeks of waiting his frustration reached a point where he went to the housing office and threatened to set fire to his house unless he was moved. On the basis of this threat he was offered new accommodation.

In our sessions together we explored the parallels between his sense of impotence in trying to be rehoused and the young people's impotence to change their circumstances. In both cases these feelings of despair and frustration had led to destructiveness (or threats of destructiveness) and, as a result of this, action had been taken. In Mr C.'s case he was rehoused, whilst the riots brought the estate to the attention of the authorities and plans for improvement were developed.

My being in a position to place Mr C.'s distress in the context of the wider concerns and issues on the estate helped us to elaborate an understanding of his experience that did not mistakenly locate blame either within him or in others such as the 'rioters', but sought connections between his suffering and the problems facing the wider community.

ETHICAL CONSIDERATIONS AND CRITICISMS OF COMMUNITY PSYCHOLOGY

Community psychology, in its attempt to become engaged in social change, raises a number of ethical as well as theoretical issues. Any attempt to intervene in a system, such as a particular community, is likely to have a number of effects, some of them difficult to predict and perhaps unintended and some even harmful. Below I discuss some of these ethical and theoretical issues such as the risk of pathologising communities, the tension between being involved and also being an outsider, the importance of language, the danger of inadvertently contributing to community passivity and, lastly, the concept of empowerment.

The risk of pathologising communities

Community psychologists have mostly tended to work within economically deprived communities. Although at one level this represents good common sense as such areas are in most need, it can also lead to an inadvertent psychologising of social problems. For example, by responding to a community's concern over joy-riding there is a danger that this problem becomes viewed as individual or group pathology rather than primarily as the result of the economic circumstances of a community that deny its youth any hope of stable employment or vision of a productive future.

Being an outsider

Working within economically deprived communities can also create a tension between being an outsider and striving to belong. Although as an outsider one is able to think and construct an understanding about a community, this position is often uncomfortable as it is a privileged position often denied those living in the deprived areas in which one may work. At the same time, becoming involved in a community raises other issues such as the blurring of one's professional role and also the inevitable development of allegiances and alliances that can distort one's objective stance and lead to a partisan view of the problems within a community.

Language

Community psychology's attempts to gain closer proximity to the 'community' creates possible conflicts over forms of discourse and there is a real danger of ordinary language and values being taken over by technical jargon. For example, commonly used terms such as 'unhappiness' become changed to 'psychological or emotional distress'.

There is a danger that community psychology may serve to make people express their concerns in a more manageable fashion, one which is no longer clamorous, insisting or disruptive. In some ways the community survey discussed earlier can perhaps be seen in this light as it attempted to present the concerns of local people in a form acceptable to the council officials, as a result of which people's passion, urgency and anger were no longer conveyed with such force. Although I think there is a huge gulf between community psychology and psychiatry in this respect, it is perhaps still important for community psychologists to be careful to avoid redefining the experiences of people or a community and to avoid undermining the capacity of people to retain and express knowledge of their own lives.

Passivity

Psychologists or other mental health professionals becoming involved in the concerns of a community can lead to a passivity and resignation from local people in tackling their own issues, fostering further dependence on professionals and the state. This point is made by Nocum Chomsky (1987): 'proliferating numbers of experts and specialists to not breed greater insight into the innermost workings of society, but obfuscate it, making people feel passive and less able to effectively participate'. Professionals becoming involved in a community may actually undermine existing community initiatives and reduce the confidence of local people to trust their own feelings and judgment. It is interesting how a recurrent issue for local professionals is 'how to involve local people' in the projects, schemes etc. that they (the professionals) are running. Rarely is there discussion about *who should be* running these projects or how to shift the balance of power from people and agencies who make decisions to the people who are on the receiving end of those policies.

Empowerment

Central to the rhetoric of community psychology is the desire to empower others to effect social change. The notion of empowerment is seen as coming through a process of raising people's awareness about their oppression so that they can then become engaged in social and political action. Such a notion of empowerment has, however, been the subject of much debate.

Critical perspectives such as those of Smail contest the view that through a superior form of consciousness people can escape the system of power and be liberated. Smail (1994) argues that this notion is based on a misunderstanding of the nature of power. He suggests that power is not solely a psychological phenomenon, based on the strength of a person's individual will or insight, but is linked to 'coercive, economic and ideological factors'. This conceptualisation of power implies that 'empowerment' can only take place when there is a shift in such resources towards those in less powerful positions. Psychologists, or other mental health workers, bring little in the way of material resources to the communities in which they work and are perhaps, regardless of their good intentions, at risk of contributing to an obfuscation of reality through inadvertently advocating psychologised notions of empowerment. Chomsky (1987) argues that the academic social sciences actually function within society to 'deflect people's attention away from things that matter, so that those in power can do what matters without public interference' (p. 36).

Community psychologists such as Bostock (1991) acknowledge the limited scope of community psychology to empower and express concern at how the onus for social change is placed on those with least resources. She points out how community psychology fails to address the 'disempowering of the powerful and instead tends to focus on facilitating the empowerment of those who are powerless'. These criticisms pose fundamental challenges to the idea of community psychologists actually empowering communities to effect social change and raise questions about the possibility for psychologists or other mental health workers to act politically.

CONCLUSION

I have discussed the emergence of community psychology as a framework for thinking about the social origins of psychological distress and as a means for combining therapeutic and political forms of intervention. Whilst I believe the ideas of community psychology can lead to a fundamental revision of current mental health practice, I do not believe that it can or should attempt to be a substitute for political action. Community psychologists and other mental health workers must be wary of misguidedly appropriating politics in searching for means to address the social inequalities underlying much psychological distress. I believe they can, however, offer both support and also frameworks for understanding the experience of personal distress to those engaged in struggles for personal meaning and for a more equitable and just social order.

C.P.N.s, by virtue of their presence in the community and the relative autonomy with which they practise, are in a good position, both individually and as teams, to adopt a more environmental approach and to become involved in the struggles and the wider concerns facing residents. This will involve thinking beyond the narrow confines of the medical model, however, and will require a willingness to recognise the salience of social and economic forces on people's psychological health. This reorientation in both thought and practice is well put in this quote from (Heller, 1989) cited in Orford (1992, p.5):

> Our professional traditions tell us to attend to symptoms of depressed affect, such as the number of days when it is hard to get up in the morning, and to ignore signs of political apathy, such as number of years of not registering to vote. We ask about queasy stomachs, sleepless nights, and family conflicts, but not about feeling safe in the streets, the number of persons in our block that we know by first name, or the availability of recreational centres for teens. We ask our teenagers about their experiences with drugs, alcohol, and sex, but do not ask them about their hopes

for the future, the community attributes they value, or whether they believe that they can make a personal impact upon the way they, or others, will live 10 years from now.

(p. 12)

As psychologists, community psychiatric nurses or other mental health workers, we are very limited in our ability to bring about material change within a community. Nevertheless, I believe we can try to resist and subvert what Chomsky termed our ideological function, that is our unwitting role of obfuscating the origins of people's distress. We can do this by drawing attention to how people are psychologically harmed by the injustices of our inequitable society. On a practical level, this involves challenging the individualistic models of understanding so often used within mental health services, which obscure or deny the wider social context. It also involves helping to facilitate and amplify the voices of those who are most oppressed.

Our task is, in short, to free ourselves and others from the illusions that mystify our understanding of how our society works. With an undertaking of such proportions, we have to be on our guard against losing our humility and our ability to be personally reflective, for as much as we can see others as enslaved by ideology and chained by illusion, it is often hard to envision ourselves in this way.

REFERENCES

Albee, G. 1980: Towards a just society: lessons and observations on the primary prevention of psychopathology. *American Psychologist* **41**(8), 891–8.

Albee, G. 1982: Preventing psychopathology and promoting human potential. *American Psychologist* **37**(9), 1043–50.

Albee, G. 1985: The answer is prevention. *Psychology Today,* Feb., 60–4.

Albee, G. 1988: Prevention is the answer. *Open Mind* **35**, 14–16.

Bostock, J. 1991: Developing a radical approach: the contributions and dangers of community psychology. *Clinical Psychology Forum* **33**, 2–6.

Chomsky, N. 1987: *The Chomsky reader.* London: Serpents Tail.

Edwards, G. 1989: Finding that Broad Street Pump. *Changes,* April, **7**, 61–4.

Eysenck, H. 1952: The effects of psychotherapy: an evaluation. *Journal of Consulting Psychology* **10**, 319–24.

Fromm, E. 1980: *Beyond the chains of illusion.* London: Abacus.

Fryer, D. 1994: Commentary on 'Community psychology and politics'. *Journal of Community and Applied Social Psychology* **42**, 11–14.

Fryer, D. and Ulah, P. (eds) 1987: *Unemployed people: social and psychological perspectives.* Milton Keynes: Open University Press.

Goffman, E. 1963: *Asylums.* London: Penguin.

Holland, S. 1988: Defining and experimenting with prevention. In: Ramon, S. and Giannichedda M. (eds) *Psychiatry in Transition: The British and Italian Experiences.* London: Pluto, Chapter 11.

Orford, J. 1992: *Community psychology: theory and practice.* Chichester: Wiley.

Smail, D. 1993: *The origins of unhappiness: a new understanding of personal distress.* London: HarperCollins.

Smail, D. 1994: Community psychology and politics. *Journal of Community and Applied Social Psychology* **42**, 3–10.

20

DEMOCRACY IN PSYCHIATRIC SETTINGS: COLLECTIVISM VS. INDIVIDUALISM

Gary Winship

While the NHS has opted to purchase forms of treatment generally known as 'brief' therapies, there are powerful moral and practical arguments in favour of alternative approaches to 'illness' and care. Here Gary Winship charts the progress of democracy in psychiatric settings, relating this to cultural and political changes in society over recent decades. He begins by making a distinction between collectivist approaches to therapy (*therapeutic collectivism*) and approaches derived from a philosophy of individualism. He describes how a small, maturing therapeutic community under his management aspired to a system of democratic functioning, detailing the scope and the limitations of the work as well as the practicalities of working in such an environment. Gary sets the material he presents in the context of a broader discussion of political ideology and the nature of democracy.

The politics of pluralism, the deconstruction of the Soviet Union, the dismantling of the Berlin wall, are emblemic events exemplifying the blurring of many of the old (cold war) frontiers of geographical and political constitution. The distinction between left and right in politics has, arguably, become less visible and the debate about democratic ideals in this (post-)modern era is bristling as we approach the end of the millennium. According to Dunn (1992), the pre-dominance of democracy as the exclusive claimant of legitimate political power, is 'in some respects remarkably recent' (p.239). Dunn's view of the 'completeness of democratic triumph' (p.240) within a *trusted* system of capitalism ensuring prosperity and 'long-term overall advantage to it's participants' (p.254), needs to be contrasted with Chomsky's (1991) formidable study of democracy in the modern world and in particular in the US. Chomsky is more troubled about the current perception of democracy, feeling that it has become a rhetorical and propagandist political facade that disguises the brute authoritarianism of so-called democratic administrations.

The debate about democracy and the legacy of the systems of capitalism from which democracy emerges 'cannot be reduced to a one dimensional formula' (Rustin and Rustin, 1983). For example, the divergence of views between Dunn and Chomsky, above, cannot be resolved by appeal to historical 'facts'. Such issues are fundamentally emotive and their debate is inevitably polemical, as personal and cultural interest are inextricable from political theory. It seems that currently our efforts to understand the operation of political power and organisation on our personal experiences are especially obscured. For any illumination we need to account for a far wider web of influence than in previous eras, perhaps with some sort of concept of inter-cultural globality such as Habermas (1989) has developed. The task of assessing how the political culture of 'democracy' and individualism impact upon the development of interpersonal theory and practice in psychiatry is therefore a complex one.

Democracy in health care treatment settings might be described as the introduction to therapeutic encounters of consensual decision-making procedures, derived and adapted from political theory. Democracy, from this perspective, might be viewed as an algorithm of patient empowerment. The interest in genuine (rather than tokenistic) democracy in therapeutic settings rests most explicitly with the application of the principles of the Therapeutic Community (TC). However, beyond the work of Rappoport (1960) and Crozier (1979), the discourse is rather limited. Of course the notion of emancipation of the mentally ill is a project founded long before Rappaport, dating back to Tuke, but the focus of this chapter is the indisputable radical changes in the second half of the twentieth century. These more immediate developments merit discussion, and I shall examine how the changes in the theory of the therapeutic milieu have been interwoven with the co-existing political changes. The delivery of health care moves in tandem with the governmental politics of the day where there is a reciprocity of action, ideas and public influence through the various strata of social organisation – an ebb and flow of influence between social bureaucracy and cultural forces. According to Habermas (1989), the structuring of the Welfare State and its relationship to the administrative strata, influencing organisations such as pressure and lobbying groups, and the public sphere, is not well understood. There is a kind of trickle-down/up effect where political ideologies, like moral and cultural values, move back and forth between societal strata. If we begin from the premise that no milieu is an island, then cultural and political forces will penetrate milieux such as welfare care systems and therefore be implicated in the development of ideas in treatment settings.

The impact of national crisis and political upheaval on therapeutic processes was examined recently in the journal *Group Analysis* (1993). Papers from Mexico, Russia and Croatia showed how political and social crises impact directly upon the material that patients bring to therapy. Hailsham (1978) likewise posits that there is a link between an unstable political climate and its social implications, citing that a breakdown in family values, increased crime and violence, unemployment, sexual permissiveness and general unhappiness are all symptoms of political unrest. He goes as far to suggest that the cause of this 'whole syndrome starts with political insecurity' (p.79). Whether we agree that the trickle-down effect is the primary or secondary cause of psychiatric illness (nurture versus nature causation), we can be sure that fundamentally the subsequent therapy necessary to alleviate distress cannot be extricated from the sociopolitical climate of the day. Family conflict, school experiences, unemployment, divorce, poverty, racism and other social phenomena are determinants both of distress (illness) and its alleviation. Are there ways in which we can see how the tandem between psychiatry and the over-arching political infra-structure has evolved?

THERAPEUTIC COLLECTIVISM

The cognisable growth in interest in group therapy following the Second World War was a concomitant of the political and social climate of the day where there was a generally perceived need for a more socially inspired societal construction. In 1945 in his manifesto, Clement Atlee, the incumbent prime minister, promised a programme of public ownership and a new social order. The devastation of the war had made some redefinition of human and moral values urgent. Health and life itself were the central focus of popular aspiration and there was a consensus in favour of sharing resources. This can be seen in the context of people's experience of food-rationing, also of communal shelter after the experience of the Blitz in London, the Midlands and the North East. Neither such basics as food or shelter could then be taken for granted. In this desire to share resources can also be seen a need for a reparative form of inter-relations, a will towards an integrative union of different people, pulling and pooling together. The concept of equality during the war had reached new heights as women shaped events with their commitment to tasks normally left to men.

The pioneering work of the therapeutic community movement has its roots in this atmosphere and its early development coincided with the need to have a collective sense of re-building, the need for affiliation, for community support and co-operation. The backbone to the TC approach arose from the discourse of group analytical psychotherapy. The early experiments with group therapy (in the UK) had began during the latter years of the war and the work of Bion and Foulkes at Northfield in Birmingham is notable here. Notable also is the work of Maxwell Jones at Mill Hill with the evacuated patients from the Maudsley Hospital. Bion and Foulkes, like Jones, found that a group therapeutic approach was an extraordinarily powerful tool in their work with soldiers who were suffering the painful psychological after-effects of the war. Self-help and mutually led group support challenged the generally held belief that the therapist knew best (basic assumption leader dependence, Bion, 1961). It was a shift from the authoritarian version of the doctor–patient relationships, to one where the patients became co-physicians.

Thus the foundations for group therapy took place at a time when there was a need for a new vision of living with others. However, after the celebrations of victory had subsided, the nation faced years of rationing and the dream of houses fit for heroes floundered as a world recession took hold of the economy. Nevertheless, the plan for a fair and equitable system of health care was finally instituted in 1948 with the birth of the National Health Service. In the context of this nationalised and publicly owned health service, a social vision of therapy enjoyed such solid foundations that it thrived through subsequent Conservative governments in the 1950s. Likewise, group therapy flourished. TC practice in psychiatric institutions also became exemplars of radical and progressive practice. In the 1960s, again in tandem with a new era of socialist government, a social model of therapy became firmly grounded in the philosophy of health care with the growth of *social psychiatry* (Jones, 1968). Here the traditional role and function of the doctor were superseded by the concept of a treatment community able to look after itself (Rappoport, 1960).

It may be useful to delineate the type of socially inspired therapy so far described. These modes of therapy, namely TC and group therapy, might be described as *therapeutic collectivism*. Although TC and group therapy are clearly encounters that involve a collection of people, the term therapeutic collectivism is not intended to preclude the orientation of individual therapies which are *inter-subjectively* constructed, i.e., therapies which consider the interpersonal interaction between the patient and the therapist as primary. These dynamically orientated interpersonal therapies do in fact pay close attention to the familial mental constructions that are within the patient, the collective inside, so to speak. Richards (1987) says that our understanding of society and the world around arises from an experience of 'others inside' (p. 46).

The notion that our inner world is *many peopled* is the foundation of object relations theory. Many psychotherapists talk about the family being under the couch when they see a patient individually. I have noticed on many occasions how a patient will gesture to an empty chair or space and speak as if the person they are thinking about is there. The term *therapeutic collectivism*, therefore, is one that envelops a conception of the therapeutic dyad as a social space. Here we are working from Rustin's (1991) notion that 'social relationships are always primary' (pp. 20–1) and that individuality arises from an intricate experience of dependence on others. In this way we may consider that group dynamic understanding has its roots in our inherent social disposition, the very beginning of life being a group experience of sorts. The therapeutic dyad, considered in this way, becomes a question of group dynamics which Freud noted when he referred to psychoanalysis as a *group of two*.

I am suggesting here that psychoanalytic theories of intersubjectivity, whether applied to individual, group or milieu therapies, begin from a premise that individuals do not exist and cannot recover health, in isolation. This psychoanalytic axiom begins with Foulkes (1938) who, in reviewing the work of Norbert Ellias, said that psychoanalysts should consider the patient's whole network of social inter-relations, there being 'no sharp line of demarcation between what we are accustomed to describe as inside and outside' (cited in Pines, 1983, pp. 265–85). I now contrast this socially derived concept of therapy, which I have called therapeutic collectivism, with its political counter-part, that of *therapeutic individualism*.

THERAPEUTIC INDIVIDUALISM

Popper (1966) describes individualism as the 'basis of Western Civilization', interpreting a central doctrine of Christianity as a prescription which falls short of an all-encompassing sense of community: 'Love thy neighbour say the scriptures, not love thy tribe' (p.102). Popper tells us that it is also Kant's central doctrine that we should 'always recognize that human individuals are ends and not means to your ends' (p.102) although this sounds rather more like a defence of the individual against the oppressive power of a group, rather than a denigration of the collective *per se*.

The concept of individualism arises from the political philosophies of the eighteenth century. John Stuart Mill's (1859) notion of liberty was a philosophy that viewed the collective of society as a 'tyranny of the majority' (p.63), advocating instead a notion of *personal sovereignty*. The concept of individualism also runs through the ideas of Marx and Durkheim where it is conceived as a phenomena associated with the growth of labour where there is a development of occupational specialism which fosters talents, capacities and attitudes which are not shared by everyone. The concept of maintaining an *elitist* structure endorsed by Hailsham (1978), where certain individuals are seen to have the capacity to lead and govern, also derives from this source.

Therapeutic individualism has ridden in tandem with the influencing political climate and can be framed particularly within the last 15 years in Britain, which has been dominated by the politics of free market individualism. Individualism has come to represent a philosophy and psychology of 'self', although it is important to note that the concept is distinguishable from *individuality*, which pertains to the uniqueness of experience, and *individuation*, which has a rich psychoanalytic discourse relating to the differentiation between the infant and its mother. The modern notion of individualism has redefined who may be seen as a worthy member of society. Individualism may be characterised by the belief that one should stand independently (look after number one) and take responsibility for yourself and your immediate family. The monetarist vision of individualism focused on putting money back into people's pockets so as to give them individual choice about how to spend their money. With the philosophy of privatisation and private ownership, and the capture of large markets by businesses selling private health care, private pensions and private insurance, the thrust towards a radical individualism has resulted in the deconstruction of collectives where the concept of public has been vilified and degraded.

During the last 15 years of individualism we have witnessed the denigration of not only collective organisations such as trade unions, but also the destruction of a large number of industrial production communities. In the wake of the dismantling of these communities is large-scale unemployment and an increased gap between poverty and wealth. But the price of running down these large-scale industries – steel, coal, shipping – should not be measured only in terms of the loss of manufacturing output, nor only in terms of the economic and emotional strain of massive unemployment. The attack on the National Health Service is a measure of how damaged the social perception of joint ownership is. Habermas (1989) has gone so far as to say that true conservatism would aim to maintain public and welfare services in their current state, but in Britain the process of their de-construction is well under way. On the surface perhaps we can see how organisations and communities have been assaulted, but less visibly, probably unconsciously, our ideology has also been violated. It is the concept of 'collective' (and associated concepts such as group, union, movement, gathering, community, society) that have been the real casualties of the last 15 years. This attack has inevitably filtered through the social matrix and therefore exerts an influence over treatment settings.

In the health service there has been a conflict between the philosophy of individualism and the process of patient empowerment. This is apparent in the reduced social orientation of the therapies of individualism. Approaches such as cognitive and behavioural therapy have been the predominant mode of therapy during the 1980s and 1990s. Individualistic approaches conceive of the patient in an insular way, viewing the patient in isolation from their historical, interpersonal network. Taking no account of the dynamic of transference, the therapist is often in the role of teacher or educator. For instance, in behaviour therapy the patient may be shown how to do thought-stopping exercises or is set 'homework', emphasising the role of the therapist as director, where treatment is prescribed and therapist interventions are mainly authoritative. In my experience of the behavioural therapies, and notwithstanding efforts made on more progressive courses to address the need for a 'negotiation' of the pace and goals of treatment with the patient, disempowerment is contingent to the therapy and rather than being examined, it is in fact at some level always a pre-requisite to treatment.

CLINICAL NARRATIVE

It was against this backdrop of individualism that a small treatment community (Witley Two) attempted to develop a more collectively orientated approach to treating drug users. The process of empowerment was considered as basic to the work of the community in the treatment of patients whose drug addiction was symptomatic of their powerlessness over the course of their lives. The ward had a well-established hierarchical structure with a ward manager, a charge nurse, several staff nurses and a care assistant. In 1988 the ward was not operating as a therapeutic community. The new ward manager was keen to develop a psychodynamic approach reminiscent of the work of Ward Six at the Maudsley Hospital, which explicitly derived its approach from other psychotherapeutic treatment miliëux (Jackson and Cawley, 1992; Jackson and Williams, 1994). The approach on Witley Two therefore followed an approach where the transference dynamics in the nurse/patient relationship were observed and gently challenged, addressing the imbalance of power in the staff/patient relations on the ward. Gradually a culture emerged where the analysis of the nurse/patient dyad and the staff/patient group dynamics were extended to examining the total ward milieu from a psychoanalytic perspective.

Sharing food (for thought)

In 1988 the system for ordering and storing dry stores was entirely the responsibility of the staff. The staff would assess how much food the residents needed and then fill in the appropriate forms. When the dry food stores were delivered on a Tuesday morning the staff would check that the food was correct and then store the food in different places. Some of the food would go into the patients' kitchen and some would be stored in the nursing office, unaccessible to the patients and then rationed out during the week. The ward manager suggested that the system for storing food in the nursing office should be changed, suggesting that the patients could take responsibility for their own food. Some of the staff thought this was a good idea but others thought it would be disastrous because the patients would eat all of the food at once. The staff were concerned that all the food would be eaten too quickly. At a staff business meeting it was apparent that some staff felt most strongly that the system should not change. However, at the end of the meeting there was a general agreement in favour of an experimental phase of two months with a system which involved the patients rationing and storing the food themselves. When the idea was discussed with the patients, they too were worried that there would be a greedy consumption of the food. Some favoured continued control by the staff. However, there was again a general concensus in favour of a trial period.

The first week was a disaster. The orange juice and biscuits were gone within two days of the food arriving on the ward. Other foodstuffs, such as cereals, were consumed almost as quickly. The second week was not much better. However, by the third week the food was beginning to last. In the ward therapy groups there was much discussion about greed and fair sharing, and an atmosphere of peer pressure and feedback. After two months there was much progress, the food was lasting through to the weekend and so it was decided to continue the trial. The advantages of the system were noted in so far as the patients did not have to keep asking the staff when they needed something like jam or sugar. The 'ward rep' (a patient who acted as a representative of their peers, usually someone who was in the latter stages of their programme) was identified as the person who would liaise with the staff when ordering the food, assessing which food stuffs needed to be topped up and which items were already adequately supplied. The ward rep would also be jointly responsible for checking the food coming into the ward. After several months there was much less wastage as the amount of over-ordering decreased. Staff of the hospital kitchen stores department were impressed and noted that the previous wastage of milk and other stuff diminished. Eventually the patients found that the system allowed them to vary the type of food stuffs they ordered and so they were able to ensure that their favourite foods could be procured and less popular stuffs could be deleted from the order.

The ward rep role therefore took on the added responsibility of ordering food and dry stores. Over the following two years the ward rep role began to assume further responsibilities. Eventually the ward rep's responsibilities included ensuring everyone was up in time for the morning programme and co-facilitating the weekly introductory group for new residents with a member of staff. The ward rep also became responsible for ordering and distributing the linen (this included holding the key to the linen cupboard), ensuring the bedrooms were prepared for the new residents, attending the staff business meeting and organising the morning cleaning group. Because of the increased sharing of administration it was felt necessary to institute an evening business meeting, which the ward rep would chair, in order to air issues and discuss organisational matters. These business meetings were held every evening at 18:30 hours, lasting up to half an hour. One could say that these developments simply served to ease the load of the staff. However, in reality these developments presented a tremendous challenge to the staff team.

The business meeting became a place where grievances were aired, but also a place where plans for events and outings would be made. During one meeting there was a dispute about which videos would be hired for the weekend. The discussion did not lead to an agreement and at the end of the meeting it was still not apparent which video would be most agreeable. A show of hands was suggested and as a consequence the most popular video was selected. This was the genesis of a system of voting which became increasingly pivotal to the community.

Atmosphere of democracy

As the culture of the community matured the number of matters that came under the scrutiny of a democratic process increased. It was rarely necessary to have a formal show of hands, indeed, this was used as a last resort if a consensus was not arrived at otherwise, but there was a growing awareness that a democratic vote was a tool for resolution. However, there were occasions when the staff found themselves in a position of suggesting that the discussions be extended rather than resorting to holding a vote. At these times it seemed necessary to promote the spirit of discussion, persuading the residents that even though a vote would resolve a dispute or summon up at a decision quickly, that it was the value of the discussion that was still uppermost and fundamentally therapeutic. So, although voting was occasionally used, it was more emblemic of an *atmosphere of democracy* rather than being the all-pervasive system of decision-making.

Three years into the period I am describing the culture took a final turn towards democratic functioning. There were often occasions when a resident *stretched* one of the house rules. Although there was a clearly defined list of house rules which the residents agreed to prior to coming to into the unit, that basically stipulated that violence and drug use were grounds for discharge, the rules were fluid enough to allow for a number of grey areas. Although the ambiguities in the rules proved to be continually problematic, it was the working through of the finer points that often carried the greatest therapeutic currency. For instance, residents repeatedly stretching the boundaries by coming back late from passes aroused conflicts which often repeated, in the transference, the patient's root family conflict. Deliberating over the conflicts in the here and now was, on the one hand, a diagnostic tool and, on the other, an opportunity for a reparative experience, allowing an opportunity for the resident to negotiate the developmental task at hand rather more successfully than previously.

But on the occasions when the boundaries were overstretched beyond tolerance, the staff would take the decision to discharge the client. These banishments would always cause consternation. In the atmosphere of the growing empowerment of the clients it seemed wholly inappropriate for the staff to decide about these grey areas alone. The ward manager began to air doubts in the community about the autocratic way that some discharge decisions were made. Over a period of several months the ward manager and soon other staff began *consulting* the residents about decisions regarding discharging clients. The process was described as a consultative one because the nursing staff took the final responsibility for discharge. These consultations gradually became more formalised until a system evolved whereby the resident who had transgressed the boundaries would have his or her transgression discussed in a formal group. The resident would then be asked to leave the group and the rest of the group would vote on whether or not they felt the person should be discharged or not. At first this was done by a crude show of hands but was superseded by a system of balloting using slips of paper with each resident and staff member voting. The votes would then be counted by a member of staff and the ward rep.

This balloting system on major issues occurred on less than ten occasions in the following 18 months. Sometimes the community voted for sanctions, for instance, for a resident to be grounded for a period. On two occasions the resident was voted out. Subjectively, it appeared that, on most occasions, the decision reached by the community as a whole was the one that the staff would have arrived at independently, and certainly the decision the ward manager would have made.

Therapeutic impact

What was the impact of these developments where the living learning experience increasingly embraced a democratic ideology? One important outcome to these developments was noted in the results of audits on the ward. In 1988, at the beginning of the phase described, an audit showed that the average programme completion rate was only 1:8 and the bed occupancy was only 55 per cent. Four years later the completion rate was 1:3 and the bed occupancy rate was averaging over 80 per cent. This data is important on its own. However, the most important offshoot of this cultural shift was the improvement in communication between the residents and the staff. There was a much more harmonious atmosphere on the unit where conflicts could be aired. The milieu became one of a greater level of containment. A deeper understanding of the dynamics of the nurse/patient relationships from a sociocultural perspective went hand in hand with a psychodynamic conceptualisation of the process.

It was crucial that the residents found that what they felt and what they said were listened to. The residents began to realise they had power and authority to influence the world around them. Authority was not so much of a dirty word and it was not something that was alien to them in so far as one of their peers was invested with authority. Being in the role of authority was a new experience for most of the residents. Authority for most of them resonated with an experience of punishment from police, school teachers and, commonly, abuse from parents. The aggregate experience of authority that the clients brought to the community was therefore essentially a negative one. The ward rep system served to confront this conception of a punishing and retributional type of authority. The community's therapeutic task was to create, nurture and maintain a system where authority was disciplining but also caring and 'holding' too.

DISCUSSION

Democracy emerged as part of the endeavour to harness and quell the destructive power of primitive urges that caused disequilibrium in the community. The impulses and primitive drives towards self-destruction – the forces at the root of the pathological addiction to drugs – were confounded by the community will towards a more benign and reparative constitution of relations. The process was an evolutionary one where democracy occurred as a result of piecemeal social architecture as Popper (1966) described, rather than through a radical upheaval and overturning of established structures. The principle of a therapeutic community emerged from the general development of the milieu rather than being stipulated by the staff. For the most part, the changes happened rather quietly. Had the changes that were taking place come under the scrutiny of hospital policy-making bodies or ethical committees, some of the developments may have been thwarted. Ethical dilemmas were apparent throughout. The change in the food system in effect meant that the patients were without their full quota of rationed food for a short period (Bion was sacked for far less at Northfield). Allowing patients to co-facilitate introductory groups and chair business meetings might be said to impose too high expectations on them, compromising their right to therapy. Indeed, many patients often said that they wanted to be treated like a patient and not like a resident with responsibilities. A system wherein patients in hospital make their own beds would still seem to be a radical notion, and one which may be quite disagreeable to many nurses. And from a therapeutic perspective, certainly from an analytical perspective, it might be said that the high expectations of community living deprived the patients of an opportunity to regress. This, in point of fact, was not the case. The patients were still able to reconnect with those parts of themselves which struggled to be adult, though this work was contained with the all-important therapeutic sessions. Once the formal therapy was over, the business of getting on with the daily living began. The task for the staff, like the residents, was that of wearing different hats, moving between levels of therapy.

The capacity of the group to work between these levels of therapy is perhaps best illustrated with an example. The residents had written to the hospital's catering manager to raise some points of concern about the uncooked food that was sent to the unit, and had invited him down to a business meeting. The catering manager, on receiving the letter, had been very angry and wrote to the ward manager saying that he did not think that it was correct for the patients to be writing to him directly. The ward manager diplomatically pointed out that the residents were encouraged to take such action and that this was part of the therapeutic experience. The catering manager eventually agreed to come to the ward for the meeting with the residents. This was the first meeting of what was to become a regular fixture in the administration of the ward. The meeting was a mutual opportunity for discussion about how to make the most efficient use of the resources, e.g. there was often an unecessary wastage of milk on the unit. The residents were also able to plan to make better use of the funds allocated for food by the hospital. Following the meeting, the catering manager congratulated the ward manager and said he was most impressed with the residents who had behaved with great maturity. The ward manager was, too, 'impressed' by the residents' maturity which was a source of some frustration as he found them in the small psychotherapy groups as rather truculent and badly behaved adolescents. This type of split may be criticised. However, the feeling of the staff was that the difficulties and conflicts were being increasingly contained within the all-important formal therapeutic sessions. The concomitant outcome indicators, such as the eradication of drug use on the ward, were a measure of the effectiveness of developing such a seemingly 'split' approach.

The approach to developing this partnership cum group democratic process, a type of collectivism, was based on a belief in the common integrity of the community members, an idea that resonates with Foulkes' (1948) notion that a group has a propensity towards a healthy wholeness. Foulkes (1948) found that the process of free associative discussion enabled an interplay of opinion where 'disruptive forces are consumed in mutual analysis, constructive ones utilized for the synthesis of the individual and the integration of the group as a whole' (p. 31). The notion that human nature is underpinned by innate capacity towards goodness, as in Foulkes' philosophy, bears close resemblance to the philosophy outlined by Rustin (1991, 1995) in his work conjoining traditional sociological enquiry with psychoanalysis.

The atmosphere of democracy that emerged served to offer a containing structure where the clients were empowered to take adult responsibility for many day-to-day organisational tasks. This experience of empowerment for the clients became a workbench for exploration, although this living/learning experience was not divorced from the formal psychotherapeutic work that took place individually and in group sessions.

Each client received at least two individual sessions per week, often more, and attended three formal small psychotherapy groups. The relationship between the adult experience of dealing with the not-always-welcome expectations of the community, arising from the process of empowerment, were counterbalanced by the opportunity to be supported through the experience in the individual and group therapy sessions.

Fear of the collective approach

Psychoanalytical group therapy, allied to the principles of the TC, applied to the organisation of a ward community, proved to be a most useful approach to adopt. However, it is apparent that there is a great fear of groups in psychiatric practice. It is often said that, 'groups do more damage than good'. And yet, in 15 years of working in acute psychiatry with at times very disturbed and violent patients, I have only ever witnessed one violent incident taking place in the formal setting of a group therapy session (one incident of violence in some 4,000+ hours of formal group therapy). In several years of supervising nurses' group work, I cannot recall hearing about a violent incident happening in a group therapy session, even on wards where proportionate to the overall incidence of violence one would expect a random violent incident to occur in a group. I have always been struck by the effectiveness of the simple containing structure of placing chairs in a circle and asking very angry people to sit down with each other. And yet many nurses and doctors feel a good deal of antipathy towards group work. I would suggest that the antipathy towards group work rests in a more ubiquitous fear of collectivism.

It is not just in psychiatry that there is a fear of collectives or people gathering together. The UK's Criminal Justice Bill (clauses 63–66 especially) appears to be the latest vivid emblem of how a fear of the collective can lead to political manipulation. To say that the Criminal Justice Bill is likely to make it difficult to organise peaceful collective protests and gatherings in the future, while undoubtedly true, trivialises the magnitude of the social and cultural forces that have brought this Bill about. This Bill did not emerge from the Home Secretary, Michael Howard's mind alone, and was perhaps to some extent even a response to public will. The Bill suggests that by incarcerating more people, the streets will be a safer place, appearing to offer a sort of social containment by dissolution.

I would like to discuss some of the false assumption about collectives which I believe are at the root of the fear of the collectivism, and in order to examine the origins of such assumptions I shall re-visit the cultural climate that was the backdrop for the early experiments in milieu and group therapy during the Second World War.

Sprinklings of the fear of mass mentality germinated in Freud's writing long before the rise of fascism in Germany. In some ways it could be said that Freud and others had predicted the very worst of mass mentality that emerged, mid-century, in the masses' fanatical allegiance to despotic rulers. In *Group psychology and the analysis of the ego* (Freud, 1921) Freud quoted extensively from Gustave Le Bon's (1895) study of group mentality. Le Bon believed that when people assembled in a mass they became less individually identifiable and more subject to a contagion of racially inherited behaviour – an instinctive driving force that caused a herd mentality. According to Reicher (1991), Le Bon's wish to understand crowds was subsumed by his desire to tame them. Le Bon was not alone in his rather disparaging theory of the mass. In

Germany Friederich Nietzsche (1892) concluded that 'Once spirit was god, then it was man, now it is even becoming mob'. This was a culmination of his ideas about the herd mentality of the human condition first outlined in *Beyond good and evil* (1886). Nietzsche philosophised about the human condition against the backdrop of an ever more industrialised Europe. He saw the new democratic European as being a useful, highly serviceable, industrious herd-animal. However, he warned that this emerging mentality would result in the involuntary breeding of new tyrants to lead the herd slave race. These tyrants, he said, would be men of a dangerous and enticing quality. Nietzsche was prophetic in his pessimism. Unfortunately his ideas were hijacked by Hitler as Hitler hailed Nietzsche as the founding father of the Third Reich philosophy.

Whilst Freud agreed with the basic thesis of Le Bon's and Nietzsche's concept of the crowd and its propensity towards a herd mentality, he added that it was necessary to distinguish between unseen forces dictating group behaviour emerging from an ancestral racial inheritance, as Le Bon described, and the unconscious behaviour of 'social anxiety' (1921 p.7) that emerged as a result of the mechanism of repression. Freud attempted to distinguish between that which was natural group behaviour and those aspects which could be understood as a pathological attachment to an idealised leader. Schematically, from this point, Freud developed his argument about transference (object love) in the group, the group reverie which he applied to his study of the church and the army.

The extreme transferential, infantile attachment to a leader that Freud noted, was clearly manifest in the relationship between Hitler and the masses in Germany. Freud's negative view about mass mentality, following Nietzsche, was an intuit about the winds of change in Europe in the early twentieth century, that proved to be well founded. But not even Freud's worst fears of the herd mentality could have predicted the eventual outcome of the rise of fascism. In 1938 when Freud was evacuated from Vienna with his family it was a close call, in particular for Anna. Had she stayed in Vienna for another 24 hours, which she very nearly did, she would have been arrested and sent to a concentration camp. In a resigned letter at the time Freud wrote that the human race had progressed because now they were only burning his books. In the Middle Ages, he quipped sardonically, they would have burned him. He did not live to see how wrong he was. Freud's misreading of the world around him is interesting because he has always been considered as a champion of pessimism about the failings of the human condition. Yet even in his most distressing moment of fleeing from his home to freedom, we can see that he maintained a kernel of benignness about the world around.

The twentieth century has seen the very worst of collective persecution. That is undeniable and something which will perhaps haunt the memory of our epoch for-ever. There is something, however, that we might learn from these atrocities. Philosophically, Hitler's vision of social organisation might be described as the *omnipotence of individualism*, where 'the strong man is mightiest alone' (Hitler, 1924, p.462). Hitler believed that the masses were ripe for leading and that it was the revolutionary intent of individual figures that had shaped the course of history. He believed that the elite should take their rightful place at the willing sacrifice of fundamental moral values. For instance he compared the workers' collectives as a bunch of cripples that were held together by a 'belief that eight cripples joining arms are sure to produce one gladiator' (ibid., p.469). Hitler went on to say that 'one healthy man among the cripples . . . used his strength just to keep the others on their feet, and this way he was himself crippled' (ibid., p.469). Hitler's belief that the strong individual should be supreme and the weak should be sacrificed was apparent throughout his political, cultural and social engineering. To say this philosophy was misguided and narrow would be to greatly understate the desperate legacy of his influence. Hitler's conception of social change, fuelled and led by the ambition of an individual, or elite, with a devalued and dispensable collective, influences us still. The symmetrically alternate view, argued above, is of leadership emerging through a more gradual evolutionary process that is born out of, and is congruent with, the collective.

The suppression of the collective is the fount of social stagnation. Even Freud (1921) said that 'in certain circumstances the morals of a group can be higher than those of the individuals that compose it, and that sometimes only collectives are capable of a high degree of unselfishness and devotion'. He postulated that there was a powerful force holding the group together. He couldn't disagree that there was something child-like in the adhesive processes Le Bon described, but for Freud it was not solely an unruly child, more importantly, it was a manifestation of the capacity for love that held the group together 'and to what power could this feat be best ascribed other than to Eros, which holds everything together in the world' (1921, p. 24). So for Freud, it was love which, at best, underpinned the group's unity.

To summarise, I have suggested that a belief in the healthy wholeness of the group and society, where the forces of goodness and love are primary, is the basis for a vision of democracy, where there is an explicit and effective trust in the judgement of the people. I have shown also how this political philosophy can manifest in a treatment milieu, where the atmosphere of democracy in an evolving therapeutic community became an algorithm of patient empowerment, a process of working which I have called therapeutic collectivism.

It remains to be seen if it is possible to rescue the notion of the collective as something other than a negative force that wreaks havoc upon civilisation. If the notion of collectivism is to be seen more positively then it will be necessary to re-appraise the predominance of individualism and move towards a more optimistic view of human nature constructed on a mutual trust of each other.

REFERENCES

Bion, W.R. 1961: *Experiences in groups.* London: Tavistock.

Chomsky, N. 1991: *Deterring democracy.* London: Verso.

Crozier, A. 1979: Attempts at democracy. In: Hinshelwood, R.D. and Manning, N. (eds), *Therapeutic communities: Reflections and Progress.* London: Routledge, 263–71.

Dunn, J. (ed.) 1992: *Democracy: the unfinished journey 508 BC to 1993 AD.* Oxford: Oxford University Press.

Foulkes, S.H. 1938: Review of *Uber den Prozess der Zivilization* by Norbert Elias. *International Journal of Psychoanalysis* **19**; 263.

Foulkes, S. 1948: *Introduction to group analytic psychotherapy.* London: Heinemann.

Freud, S. 1921: *Group psychology and the analysis of the ego.* Standard Edition, vol. 18. Harmondsworth: Penguin.

Habermas, J. 1989: *The new conservatism.* Cambridge: Polity Press.

Hailsham, Lord 1978: *The dilemma of democracy.* London: Collins.

Jackson, M. and Cawley, R. 1992: Psychodynamics and psychotherapy on an acute psychiatric ward: the story of an experimental unit. *British Journal of Psychiatry,* **160**, 41–50.

Jackson, M. and Williams, P. 1994: *Unimaginable storms: a search for meaning in psychosis.* London: Karnac.

Jones, M. 1968: *Social psychiatry.* London: Tavistock.

Le Bon, G. 1895: *La psychologie des foules.* trans. 1947. Paris: Alcan.

Mill, J.S. 1859: *On liberty.* Harmondsworth: Penguin.

Nietzsche, F. 1886: *Beyond good and evil.* trans. R.J. Hollingdale (1973), Harmondsworth: Penguin Books.

Nietzsche, F. 1892: *Thus spake Zarathustra.* trans. R.J. Hollingdale (1961), Harmondsworth: Penguin Books.

Pines, M. 1983: The influence of S.H. Foulkes. In Pines, M. (ed.) *The evolution of Group Analysis.* London: Routledge, pp. 265–85.

Pines, M. (ed.) 1993: Special section: *Group Analysis* in times of national upheaval. *Group Analysis* **26**(1), 81–119.

Plato 1955: *The republic.* London: Penguin.

Popper, K.R. 1966: *The open society. vol. I.* London: Routledge.

Rappoport, N. 1960: *Community as doctor.* London: Routledge.

Reicher, S. 1991: Politics of crowd psychology. *The Psychologist* **14**(11), 487–91.

Richards, B. 1987: *Images of Freud.* London: J.M. Dent & Sons.

Rustin, M. 1991: *The good society and the inner world.* London: Verso.

Rustin, M. 1995: Lacan, Klein and politics: the positive and negative in psychoanalytic thought. In Elliot, A. and Frosch, S. (eds), *Psychoanalysis in contexts.* London: Routledge, pp. 223–45.

Rustin, M. and Rustin, M. 1983: Relational preconditions of socialism. In Richards, B. (ed.) *Capitalism and infancy.* London: Free Association Books, pp. 207–25.

21

QUALITY ASSURANCE: THE ETHICAL DIMENSION OF MEASURING WORK

Hugh McKenna and James Brown

Here Hugh McKenna and James Brown review the prevailing ideology of the market-place as it influences psychiatric nursing care. They examine the intrusion of the business ethos with its unsophisticated ideas of financial accountability and audit. They consider the implications of this on the running of the NHS and provision of health services. In particular, they consider the effect of measuring clinical outcome using primitive methods and its dehumanising effect on staff and the resulting deterioration of quality in their relationships (and therefore also their clinical work) with clients. Hugh and James highlight the morally dubious ways that data from such *quality audits* can be used and the interests its use can serve. They look particularly at how ethical standards, confidentiality for example, as well as standards of care, can, paradoxically, be compromised. They then look at ethical problems in research generally with those who are mentally ill. Finally, they highlight various ethical difficulties in artificially soliciting and using clients' opinions on care provision. In conclusion, Hugh and James stress the importance of developing ways of assessing clinical standards which are genuine, rather than ideological manoeuvres, and which also protect both clients and staff from abuse.

This chapter examines the ethical dimension of the currently popular market ideology and one of the ways in which that ideology has influenced mental health nursing: Quality Assurance. We consider the background and the ethical commitments of quality assurance, the practical issues raised by the implementation of quality assurance schemes, and the ethical costs of quality assurance. The appropriateness of a radically individualistic understanding of accountability for the quality of patient care is called in question.

We will introduce the subject by examining the political and ideological background to the heightened profile of evaluation and audit in clinical practice and service provision. Then we will look at quality assurance from seven perspectives: basic principles; current forms of implementation; implications for the shift to community nursing;

conflicts between quality assurance and cost containment; staff and management ownership of quality assurance; the appropriateness of the consumerist metaphor; and the ethical costs of quality assurance itself. What is the way forward? We discuss initiatives in which we have been involved where some of these problems were addressed. In particular, we seek to show how quality assurance, far from being at odds with the practice of psychiatric nursing is integral to it. And we highlight some of the ways in which soft measures of clinical excellence can be incorporated into joint management and staff quality initiatives, to the benefit of team morale, patient empowerment and care, and budget control, both in hospital and in the community.

BACKGROUND: IDEOLOGY, MORALS, MARKETS AND QUALITY

In 1979 the Thatcher Government came to power and a new broom approach was adopted, both to private enterprise and to public service, with an emphasis on scrutinising comfortable orthodoxies, rooting out bad practices, removing over-manning, and reducing restrictive practices and inefficiency. There was also a move towards individualism, a market-place ethos and more open and smaller government.

Individual recipients of public welfare were to be restored to the dignity of standing on their own two feet and taking responsibility, as far as possible, for their own lives. They were to be liberated from servile dependency on a nanny state. In this spirit, recipients of health care were to be seen more as users who actively make choices and do things; they were to be seen less as patients who are passive while things are done to them or for them.

More generally, what had previously been perceived as public goods came increasingly to be viewed as private ones. Assets passed from public ownership into private ownership. Public sector institutions, which many had thought of as a shared birthright, began to be fenced off for private enterprise. Interpersonal relations and transactions began to be seen more in terms of individuals each pursuing their private interests and less in terms of shared projects, group values and common goods.

In short, government sought to roll back the state, to let individuals choose and be responsible for the consequences, and to free market forces to do their work (work that is sometimes harsh in the short term but is, they believe, ultimately benign), to restore the economy and our culture to a healthy state.

From this perspective collectivities came to be looked upon with suspicion. This was in part because responsibility for the actions of a collectivity can become so dispersed and diluted that for practical purposes it disappears. Similarly, within collectivities, quality being viewed as everybody's business may lead to it becoming nobody's business. Morality in the public arena would therefore be better seen, it was claimed, as a matter of the actions, rights, responsibilities and duties of individuals. Individualism as a moral and economic imperative was thus central to the government agenda in the 1980s, both in relation to individual citizens and to public servants. In this way, Thatcher's radically individualistic market ideology claimed the moral high ground.

According to market ideology, compliance in private enterprise with certain ethical norms is crucial for the fair and effective functioning of markets: non-coercion, truthfulness and fulfilling bargain–commitments, for example. Parallel ethical imperatives arise in public service, it was claimed. For example, the duty to offer value for money. Organisations which were using the public's money had to be able to show that they were using it well. Officers were not only to act in ways they judged to be correct; they had also to be able to present their reasoning to the public and, if necessary, to defend their actions.

In the 1980s government reports highlighted the importance of improving the quality of health services. The Griffith Report (1983) stated that the NHS lacked any real continuous evaluation of performance against explicit standards. It called for all services within the NHS to examine what they do. The resultant, radically restructured NHS management arrangements placed great emphasis on the need to specify and assure the quality of health care. This trend of putting quality assurance on the health care agenda continued with the World Health Organisation's Target 31 (1985) which stated 'By 1990 member states should have built an effective mechanism for ensuring quality for patient care within all health care systems'. Most western countries set their sights on this target. In Britain this target was made manifest with the White Paper *Working for Patients* (DHSS, 1989) which specified a need to improve the quality of services to users whilst at the same time making best use of the resources available.

QUALITY ASSURANCE

Assuring quality: the basics

Mental health professionals have a moral obligation, enshrined within traditional professional codes, to give good care. In medicine there is the centuries old 'Hippocratic Oath', while in nursing there is the 'Nightingale Pledge'. Both lay down ethical guidelines specifying that practitioners give the best treatment and care possible. Modern professional codes also share this focus. The United Kingdom Central Council's Code of Professional Conduct (1992) made explicit that 'the practitioner seeks to achieve and maintain high standards'.

Although market thinking has stimulated increased interest in quality assurance in health care, the case for quality assurance in health care is not dependent on market thinking, as evidenced above. Indeed, the sort of exclusively individualistic understanding of moral responsibility endorsed by the Conservative ideology described earlier may even interfere with quality assurance. As Onora O'Neill observes, 'Unless we find ways of deliberating that can guide action and can speak not only to the individuals but to the . . . collectivities which might make a difference, . . . there is no chance of applied ethics which converges with "uplifted" politics' (O'Neill, 1986, pp.6–7).

Let us review some basic and, hopefully, uncontroversial principles of quality assurance which may equally apply to private enterprise and public service. First, if something is worth doing, then it is worth doing well. And, if you wish to do something well, you will want to have ways of telling how well you are doing it and whether there is scope for doing it better. Any co-operative endeavour will have purposes (what it is trying to achieve), outcomes (what is actually being achieved) and complementary and co-ordinated processes (what practices are being implemented by the participants). Assuring quality will involve:

- identifying purposes;
- identifying processes;
- finding out outcomes;
- comparing outcomes with purposes;
- reviewing processes for appropriateness to purposes.

If there is any question as to what the purposes are, how they are best to be characterised, or what their relative importance is, then there has to be provision for the purposes to be kept under review and for ensuring that potential contributions to the task of articulating them are not excluded (Maxwell, 1984, pp. 107–10). And, granted that purposes have been provisionally identified and articulated, there has to be provision for monitoring the processes and their appropriateness and success in furthering the purposes and achieving the desired outcomes. It could be said that quality assurance is working when implemented processes lead to outcomes which coincide with the purposes of the organisation. It may be that this cannot always be checked by direct observation and there is a need for a range of indicators. The identification of appropriate indicators then becomes vitally important.

Where selection or prioritisation of an organisation's purposes is a matter of moral dilemma in the public arena, the organisation is morally obliged to make provision for review both of its purposes, and of the activities of its members in relation to those purposes. These obligations to review purposes and processes we may call quality assurance obligations. Thus, just as the efficient functioning of the market and its maintenance of ethical standards require compliance with certain principles of conduct, as above, so certain procedures, quality assurance 'obligations', have to be complied with for the proper functioning of a public institution. A Mental Health Trust is a just such a co-operative, public undertaking, and such Trusts now have programmes for monitoring quality.

Assuring quality: implementation

An industrial model of quality assurance and control has been adopted within the NHS. The origins of this model lie in the teaching and writings of Deming (1982), Juran (1974) and the quality philosophy of the Japanese. Dealing as it does with issues relating to manufacturing, this model may sit uneasily in the people-centred health service. For instance, the industrial quality 'gurus' specify the importance of 'hard data' and of limiting 'process variability' through statistical control. In essence, this entails that standard deviation tests are used to ensure that the processes involved in manufacturing are kept as stable and consistent as possible. The focus is the 'product', and if the quality of the product is assured through an efficient manufacturing process, the company will have more satisfied customers leading to an increased market share and increased profits.

Once you have decided systematically to monitor quality, it is reasonable to seek to learn from any available experience of such monitoring. Thus, it is very natural for NHS managers to look to industry, where such experience is available, for ideas. However, while the analysis of an industrial model of quality assurance may be useful, mental health care need not be committed to mimicking industrial practice. A quality system for the manufacture of widgets may be entirely inappropriate when applied to nursing depressed human beings.

Hard or soft data

There is a trap which has not always been avoided in quality assurance in mental health care, namely the trap of too hastily settling for a certain kind of data because it is handy. The adoption of an industrial model of quality assurance has meant that 'hard', measurable indicators of quality, rather than the 'soft', interpersonal indicators, have been granted credence. This does not take into account the fact that there are many aspects of mental health nursing that cannot easily be measured. For instance, how does one measure emotional coping, or self-esteem? How does one calibrate a therapeutic relationship or dignity?

There are other examples of soft data which are essential components of the caring process but which are conspicuous by their absence within quality assurance initiatives. One could include in these: post-puerperal mother-child bonding; the use of respect, compassion, empathy or tacit knowledge in clinical decision-making; educating clients in health promotion; or simply 'being with' a depressed person. Such 'soft data' are the mainstay of what Barker (1995) would refer to as the 'craft' of psychiatric nursing. Yet most quality auditors show little interest in these issues.

When qualified nurses counsel patients or undertake psychotherapeutic interactions, it may appear to an untrained eye that they are merely talking to the clients. To such an observer, if their agenda were to initiate Quality Assurance, a threshold quality standard could be implemented here. For example, no patient should go an entire day without at least ten minutes of uninterrupted, undivided attention from a registered mental health nurse. It may appear that this could go some way to measuring what could be referred to as soft data. However, there emerges another difficulty in that all one may be measuring is quantity of time, while the actual *quality* of the nurse's 'being with' the patient, her ability to offer 'undivided attention', may be poor! Therefore, in the rush to appraise mental health outcomes, too much emphasis may be paid to superficial factors that are easily measured.

Hard and soft data may be viewed as being at opposite poles of a quality monitoring continuum. Most of the appraisal efforts in mental health have focused on the former. For example, process and outcome studies in mental health have been undertaken on ECT and psycho-pharmacology. The number of ECTs can be calculated, the amount of anaesthetic and muscle relaxant used can be counted and the patient's recovery time, blood pressure and pulse can be quantified. This data is 'hard' in that it allows 'number crunching' to take place. It does not tell you the meaning ECT has for the nurse or what the patient or his family thought of the experience and how hopeless or helpless they may feel. Therefore, when dealing with psychosocial issues, hard data has obvious limitations. Focusing only on hard data misses out much of what is important to the patient, family and nurse in the situation.

None the less, because of the ease of measurement that drug and electro treatments allow, it is possible that they may get better support from purchasers than less easily quantifiable psychosocial treatments (whose invisibility means that they are mostly ignored when it comes to quality assurance). There is an inherent danger here. If mental health nurses begin to focus on those areas that purchasers, caught in the hard data trap, see as significant, it is possible that fundamental psychosocial care interventions could be relegated to secondary status. The implementation of quality assurance schemes that are overly reliant on hard data may thus produce an imbalance in forms of care.

But why do many purchasers of mental health care focus on hard data? It may be that since these are easily quantified and already exist within the organisation, a great deal of money need not be spent on data collection. There is another reason, however, and this may be related to recent political health care ideology. The last government was on record as wishing to contain costs in mental health care. If purchasers place credence on soft indicators of quality, it is possible that this will mean putting more resources into intensive interpersonal approaches to care. This would be costly in terms of increased qualified staffing requirements and longer waiting lists for therapy. An emphasis on rapid patient turnover, fewer admissions, and the closure of beds enables interpersonal therapy costs and waiting lists to be reduced, with more people apparently treated using fewer staff and fewer beds in fewer hospitals. Thus efficiency gains can be claimed, at least in the short term.

Let us now recall the previous discussion on the purposes of the organisation. If these purposes are merely to have early discharges, short lengths of stay and low levels of readmission, then the processes undertaken by mental health nurses can be refined to maximise achievement of these purposes and to eliminate activity that is not directed at achieving them. Quality assurance activities would therefore be directed towards seeing if these purposes were achieved by the staff undertaking the processes. If, however, the purposes of the organisation are to enable clients to gain emotional fulfilment, self-esteem and self-worth, the more invisible processes will have to be granted greater credence and the quality assurance emphasis would be different. The first point to make is that, clearly, the organisational obligation to identify, articulate and review purposes is vitally important here.

Second, to whatever extent the latter purposes of a mental health organisation are prioritised (i.e. quality care rather than fast throughput), the relationship of data collected to meaningful assessment of the quality of care delivered needs examining. Unfortunately, however, quality auditors appear to be saying 'We shall deem the quality of care delivered to correspond to the levels of these "hard" indicators even though we know that such levels may fail to be correlated with the quality of care'. Rather than deciding on what is quality in mental health and then seeking indicators to appraise this, most developers of quality assurance tools select the indicators first and then simply assert that these measure quality! (see Goldstone and Doggett, 1989; Balogh et al., 1993). The result is that in most cases quantifiable data are used as quality indicators and are thus given a high profile in quality assurance reports.

Certainly, it is easy to see why quality auditors prefer indicators based on easily observed or measured 'hard' data, in contrast to indicators of clinical standards and outcomes that are based on apparently less empirical data. But the case for thinking that readily measurable hard data are indicators for what caring purchasers are really looking for or what mental health nurses are really trying to achieve or what patients need, has still to be made.

The community shift: use of outcome data

In the current paradigm shift towards community care the 'hard' outcome indicators referred to above have become particularly relevant to purchasers and providers of mental health care. Policy-makers are being put under pressure to provide hard evidence to indicate whether or not community care is working. Qualitative data may 'not cut any ice' with politicians and so readmission rates, discharge rates, length of stay, bed closures, re-housing figures, etc. are the statistics most often quoted in government reports. However, readmission rates may be a poor indicator of quality since people may stop coming when they are dissatisfied with the service. Furthermore, high discharge rates are hardly a valid pointer to quality if ex-patients are joining the homeless or the prison population. McAulcy and McKenna (1995) noted that 25 per cent of those registered as homeless in the greater Belfast area had recently been discharged from psychiatric hospitals. Therefore, rather than representing an improvement in quality of care, the discharge experience may represent a crisis point for many patients (Robertson, 1992) and staff (Pawlicki, 1992).

Questions such as whether it is right on moral grounds to 'shift' patients into the community without the necessary social and financial support continue to be asked. Decreased length of stay is also commonly used as an indicator of high quality mental health care. But reducing length of patient stay inevitably means that hospital and community nurses are faced with a moral dilemma. Hospital nurses have less time to build up a therapeutic relationship with patients and their families. This causes a predicament for many nurses who know they can provide a higher quality of care while the patient is in hospital but are resigned to doing the minimum within the contact time available. It is not being suggested that patients should remain in hospital just so nurses can build up relationships with them. However, unnecessary decreases in lengths of stay inevitably mean that community nurses are dealing with increased numbers of disturbed clients. There are fears that CPNs will be used as 'scapegoats' for community failures.

The preference for the sort of 'hard' outcome indicators described fits well with the ideology of community shift and reinforces the view, held by many, that psychiatric hospital admission is synonymous with quality failure in mental health care, while community placement reflects quality success. The phrase 'Care in the Community' evokes images of succour, belonging and togetherness. There is clearly an ethical, as well as a legal obligation to provide post-discharge, community support in terms of personnel and financial resources, as well as high quality, accessible preventative work in the community. Indeed, where this has been forthcoming, there have been some success stories. For instance, recent statistics from the TAPS Project found very low levels of homelessness and crime among 671 recently discharged patients in England (Warner, 1994) and many community projects offer high quality and innovative preventative work. But there is evidence that local government expenditure on Social Service provision for Care in the Community is being savagely cut back, and in the context of an individualistic ethos, the reality may be that responsibility for providing care has been devolved on to individuals altogether outside institutional settings; no role is assigned to the community as such. Prior (1991) found that without proper mechanisms in place, quality of 'care in the community' can be worse than in hospital. More recently, Kelly and McKenna (1997) noted that many community-based psychiatric patients were suffering repeated bouts of harassment and victimisation. Some were also being taken advantage of in financial terms by neighbours. Other incidents have been reported in the literature which would suggest that the movement out of institutions continues to be problematic and on some occasions patients, staff and members of the public have suffered as a result (Durgahee, 1996; Ritchie et al., 1994).

Ranking quality and cost-containment

Managers of Mental Health Trusts are on the horns of a dilemma: they have an obligation to the public to see that high quality care is delivered at minimal possible cost and they also have an obligation to see that no harm comes from not having enough resources. In addition, they are also aware that introducing an expensive quality improvement programme could result in little or no improvement in the health of people but could dramatically increase the cost of providing health care.

It is worthwhile here to reiterate the Working for Patients (1989) aims of improving the quality of services to users while at the same time making best use of the resources available. These are distinct aims: keeping quality up and keeping costs down. They may not always conflict, but they can be expected to conflict sometimes. So there will be situations where a higher level of achievement with regard to one of them entails a lower level of achievement with regard to the other. Moreover, there can be no guarantee that, if a minimal acceptable level of each is fixed, these levels will be compatible. If you stipulate that costs are never to exceed a specified limit then you have to be ready for the possibility of the standard of care being lower than you are content to accept. If you stipulate that standards of care are never to go below a specified lower limit then you have to be ready for the possibility that the costs will rise above what you planned.

A solution to this problem would be to rank the aims, specify a minimum level of achievement for the first one, and make the achievement of that level a limiting factor on maximising the achievement of the other. There are two ways of doing this. One is to set minimum acceptable standards of care and then seek to keep down costs as far as is possible without dropping below those standards of care. This would amount to a policy of aiming for cost-effectiveness (which is a matter of achieving a specified objective at least cost). The second way would be to set an absolute limit on expenditure and seek to maximise the standard of care achieved within that expenditure limit. If improving the quality of services to users while making the best use of the resources available means keeping quality standards up and costs down, it is important to be clear and frank about how this is to be achieved. If staying within expenditure limits takes precedence over achieving acceptable standards of care, it should be acknowledged that care standards may sometimes sink below acceptable levels.

In periods of financial stringency within Trusts an imbalance between quality attainment and cost containment may lead to human costs. The government's 'Value for Money' unit (1992), suggested that a possible method of achieving cost savings in health care was to decrease the richness of the nursing skill mix. Therefore in some Mental Health Trusts skill substitution through skill mix reviews is an attractive management option. There is some evidence to suggest that this is taking place. In 1991–92 the number of qualified mental health nurses in England and Wales decreased by 24 per cent (*Nursing Times*, 1992). Also, in a mental health unit in Northern Ireland over 40 experienced qualified nurses were made redundant and subsequently offered B grade nursing assistant posts. The findings from many studies would suggest that such tampering with nursing skill mix could lead to a detrimental effect on the quality of care and therefore the morality of this practice is open to question.

Top-down or bottom-up quality assurance

Deming (1982) believes that decisions about quality are best taken in the 'boardroom rather than the shopfloor'. According to him, quality assurance is the responsibility of managers and they must guide the workforce in this endeavour. The justification for this appears to be a laudable one: to ensure that the boardroom does not just leave others to get on with it but is identified and involved with quality assurance. The key idea here is that quality is led by senior managers but fed and driven by front line staff.

However, the implementation of this model in mental health nursing has been selective. In many instances a managerial *imposition* of quality assurance is the norm, systems to improve the quality of service being designed and implemented in a 'top-down' manner. Standards formulated by management and imposed upon others have a short-lived allegiance. This is because clinical staff cannot develop a 'mind set' for quality if they are being judged on standards written by other, perhaps more senior, team members and implemented with little or no participation on their part. This is inimical to good quality service, leading many staff to view quality assurance activities as policing exercises. There is clearly a case for saying that all those whose activities constitute the activities of the organisation, and not just the board of managers, should contribute to thinking on quality assurance.

When things are ethically unsatisfactory it is often because of the shortcomings of an individual. But in an organisation it may be that the shortcomings are in the structures and systems rather than in any individual. Managers have to realise that quality problems are mostly the result of poor process, not incompetent staff. The persons who are best able to identify problems with processes are the front line clinical staff. As a result, they have to be actively involved in quality initiatives. They are closer to the user of the service than members of the management team and therefore need a major input into the decisions relating to quality assurance. If they do not feel that they have at least shared ownership of the quality initiatives they will be reluctant to identify poor processes or alter these processes towards obtaining the desired outcomes. Take the following example: without consultation with shop floor workers, managers in a motor manufacturing plant introduced audit tools to appraise the processes for the construction of car interiors. The following is part of the process: as the vehicle proceeds down the conveyor, one worker attaches the steering wheel; the job of the next worker down the line is attaching the indicator switch. However, this is an inefficient step in the process because in order to attach the switch she must take off the steering wheel. These workers know how the process can be improved and streamlined but the design of the audit tool is such that it does not detect the problem with the processes. In effect, the tool in its current form is telling managers that the processes are fine whereas the front line workers know it is not a valid indicator of what goes on.

Let us apply this analogy to psychiatric nursing: nurse Smith and nurse Jones are working with people who have depression on an acute psychiatric ward. Through interpersonal therapy and relationship building they are seeing positive results. Two auditors arrive on the unit and armed with an audit tool they proceed to collect data. They check how many patients there are, if each patient has a care plan, if an assessment has been carried out, if each patient has a wardrobe, if consultants' rounds take place when they should, etc. The auditors leave the ward with their criteria-based checklists complete and report their findings. To nurses Smith and Jones the audit exercise has been a waste of time. The tool may be sensitive in appraising those quality indicators perceived as important to managers, auditors and its creator, but as far as staff are concerned it is insensitive to those issues which are at the heart of therapeutic patient care. Practically any member of the assembly team in the first example and the nursing team in the second example could have improved the design of the audit tool, the validity of the audit results and hence its power to motivate them to get involved if they had been encouraged to see it as their own.

So it is not enough for managers to want a quality job to be done, the practitioners themselves have to want quality to be a central component of their work. We believe that practitioners are interested in providing high quality, high therapeutic interventions but they do not see imposed audit tools as measuring this quality, i.e. how well their work is being done. Therefore the organisation and the managers have an obligation to actively work with practitioners to ensure shared ownership of the quality initiatives.

An individualism whose working assumption is that when something goes wrong there must be an individual to blame could have the morally undesirable effect of causing poor practices or system failures to go unnoticed. We should rather be awake to the possibility that organisations can have obligations and rights and virtues and vices. Even if the duty to improve an organisation ultimately falls upon individuals, it is a duty that could go unnoticed and remain undone if we insist on not seeing organisations as having obligations. If in our eagerness to identify the ethical shortcomings of individuals we overlook the ethical shortcomings of institutions or systems, this can be unfair on the individuals who are chosen to carry the blame and it can obscure the need to reconsider structures, decision-making procedures, established group understandings, etc. (Brown *et al.*, 1992, pp. 108–9, 119–20, 124).

Let us look at decision-making at the level of an individual person and then see if analogous points can be made about decision-making in an organisation. When an individual deliberates, she is likely not to deliberate well if she excludes a class of relevant considerations to the matter in hand from her attention. There is a greater chance of her arriving at a conclusion different from one best supported by all the relevant reasons.

This parallels how, in a Mental Health Trust, nurses and other health care staff will have knowledge, experience and expertise that differ from the knowledge, experience and expertise of the board of managers and which are almost certain to be relevant to finding out how well the Trust as an organisation carries out its processes and achieves its outcomes. Here, as when an individual person deliberates, the deliberation is less likely to be done well if it does not have that body of knowledge, experience and expertise to draw on.

Unless some serious objection to this case emerges or an equally powerful case can be made for restricting participation in quality assurance deliberation to the board of managers, we have to conclude that mental health nurses and other health care workers should be involved as shared owners in the quality assurance thinking of the organisation. The same argument can be applied to the involvement of patients, families and the public at large.

Quality assurance and consumerism

The International Standards Organisation defines quality as 'the totality of features and characteristics of a service that bear on its ability to satisfy stated or implied needs of consumers' (Robertson, 1992). In spite of its ill fit with the particular needs of a system for providing mental health care, the industrial model of quality assurance, to its credit, firmly emphasises the 'external customers, their needs and expectations'. Whether the recipients of mental health care are best called consumers/customers is open to question but the emphasis on their needs is clearly appropriate.

Consumerism appears to be one aspect of quality assurance that has not always been well developed in mental health care. If they were consumers in any normal meaning of the term, patients and their families might be supposed to enjoy much greater choice about accepting or rejecting a service offered, as well as enjoying far greater possibilities of selecting from a range of possible alternative 'products'. But patients and their representatives are seldom able to effect such choice and are rarely involved in making decisions concerning the indicators to be included in quality assurance exercises. They are conspicuous by their absence from standard-setting groups and organisational quality steering committees. Furthermore, in many cases the hospital 'downsizing' process is driven by political ideology rather than the views of the patients, which are often opposed to such restructuring (McKenna, 1993).

This lack of patient involvement in decisions regarding quality of care is more in keeping with paternalism (at best) or coercion and deception (at worst) than market-style consumer satisfaction/quality initiatives. Mental health patients are particularly vulnerable to violations of the consumerism doctrine. The autonomy required for proper decision-making is often compromised due to their institutionalisation or lack of involvement in treatment. Mental health managers should seek much greater balance between their right to implement government policy and patients' and staff members' rights to respect, protection and quality.

Patient satisfaction

Using the Griffith's Report (1983) and *The Patients' Charter* (1992) as springboards, the government has exhorted health service providers to evaluate the level of satisfaction patients have with the service offered. Patient satisfaction may after all have significant effects on patients' compliance with treatment as well as clinic attendance. However, Anthony Clare (1990) points out that the satisfied patient may be satisfied with very little. He said, 'We all know physicians with substantial private practices and a clientele of adoring patients but to whom we fellow physicians with our insiders' knowledge would not send our dog'. This supports Bond's finding (1992) that patients' expectations in the UK are typically low. Therefore patients' expressed feelings of satisfaction with the service offered may not correspond with a satisfaction of their needs.

Moreover, whether or not patients' expectations are typically low, we need to look at the position of patients who are invited to make a judgement of the quality of the care they are receiving. They may be compromised in their ability to make such a judgement, not only by their illness itself, but as a result of the fact they are undergoing treatment from the very professionals with power over their lives who they are being called on to express dissatisfaction with. They may rightly fear the consequences on their relationship with such carers if their criticisms became known, and there is a risk that they may undermine their own faith in the treatment through being asked to scrutinise it.

The business of assessing the quality of professional work is a complex team undertaking. One might ask what the relation of patients to the team is. Here a possible lead to follow is that of Paul Ramsey (1970), who suggests that the only morally acceptable way to think of an experimental subject is as a co-adventurer in the research quest. This is in line with much recent thinking on health care which promotes the idea of the recipient of health care as a partner in his/her own care. In the same spirit, it is appropriate to think of the patient as someone who is, where possible, to be recruited to the quality assessment team.

Consider what might be appropriate attitudes on the part of people involved in a group endeavour to persons whose activity is important for that endeavour (for example, attitudes of some office workers to the cleaners). They might ignore those other people, treat them as outsiders, take their work for granted. Or they might include them (by suitable use of an inclusive 'we'), integrate them, cherish them, treat them with respect, indicate that their work is valued as providing conditions for the first group's work to be done well. This line of thought supports a view like Ramsey's. Current quality improvement philosophy specifies that quality is about involvement, valuing and teamwork. Key people, by virtue of being patients, should not be excluded.

However, patients are seldom included in the decision-making processes within team discussions. Of course some patients may not wish to be involved and this should be respected. When involved, their lack of technical knowledge or low expectations of care may mean that they have difficulty truly judging what a satisfactory service is. In such instances, patient advocates such as members of the Schizophrenia Fellowship, MIND, SANE or the Alzheimer's Association should be involved.

What emerges from this discussion is that the use of patient satisfaction data as indicators of good quality care requires great caution. Patient satisfaction surveys are better thought of as having an agenda-setting function, not so much showing how well things are going but pointing at possible directions for further efforts. They may also be relevant to the comparison of competing explanations of satisfaction levels. A common sequence in scientific enquiry is the following:

1. You have some data.
2. You consider an explanation for those data.
3. You devise ways of testing the explanation.
4 Your implementation of tests results in your possession of new data.

The reason for going on to 3. may be that more than one explanation suggests itself at 2. Given patient satisfaction, data may have come about because everyone worships the doctor, because the patients' lives have been improved, because the patients did not want to hurt anyone's feelings, or because the patients have had a rough time and this provides a focus for otherwise diffuse cosmic resentment. A new patient satisfaction survey may be the way to discriminate between competing explanations of the original data. It will typically include some different questions so as to make discriminations not made in the collection of the original data.

Quality Assurance and ethical costs

Let us look at some of the ethical costs of quality assurance initiatives themselves. Taking due note of these does not commit us to any particular outcome, but we need to be clear about what these costs are.

Kennedy (1994) argues that better services come through better management which comes through better information. Therefore, there is a moral obligation on a profession to seek knowledge, e.g. regarding 'consumer satisfaction' from patients. But this is never separate from a moral obligation always to consider the rights of subjects who are expected to provide that new knowledge. When patients' needs are in conflict with the requirements of a quality assurance activity, the auditors are in a professional dilemma.

It is possible that the collection of quality assurance data and data relating to patient satisfaction could cause vulnerable patients to experience added anxiety. For some patients the disclosure of information about staff or the patient's perception of the service could raise fears that may be stressful for them, exposing the person to additional psychological risk. As Schrock (1984) points out, being observed, questioned or singled out can provoke a great deal of anxiety in patients. To the extent that this is so, these effects have to be acknowledged as moral costs and consideration has to be given to whether they are costs that have to be borne or whether they can be reduced.

Nurses too may be open to stress and anxiety as a result of being participants in quality assurance activities, especially if the results are incorporated within a staff promotion/appraisal exercise. Other stresses may impinge on staff who single-handedly try to improve the quality of patients' care. To do so they may have to take calculated risks: e.g., encouraging patients to make decisions or accept domestic and social freedoms. The staff may receive criticism for doing this from relatives and be accused of not caring. In some cases Trust managers have penalised staff for taking such risks (Trevelyn, 1994) even though the staff believed they were improving the quality of care.

THE WAY FORWARD

Progressive Quality Assurance

In deciding what sort of data to collect and how to collect data for quality assurance purposes, you hope for high benefit at low cost. The cost is low if the data can be collected easily or quickly or can be collected by lower-paid rather than higher-paid staff. The benefit is high if the data are likely to have a low error-rate and are likely to tell you what you need to know. If the cost is kept low but no benefit is achieved, then the cost-saving is what is commonly called a false economy.

The idea we have been exploring is that a quality assurance tool which involves hard data collected by relatively unskilled staff is a false economy if the data are not relevant to the main purposes of psychiatric nursing care. Emphasis on hard data may be inimical to effective quality assessment.

It may be thought that hard data whose collection does not depend on expertise or personal judgement are capable of having scientific status and are preferable for that reason. However, in a mature science, observation will often require training, expertise, experience and good judgement. The expertise and judgement needed to interpret an EEG tracing in no way count against the science-based practice of using EEG. A scientific approach does not have to confine itself to quantitative data or to data that unqualified persons can collect. Equally, processes which are visible only to a trained expert eye are not for that reason less real or less substantial. A preoccupation with 'hard' data is not especially scientific or hard-headed.

Where factors that are important for good quality care are not such as can be observed by unqualified persons, there are two possibilities: one is to monitor different factors instead; the other is to find another way of monitoring the important factors. We have suggested that some quality assurance practices go for the former option. But then what is being assured is not quality in any sense that counts. The other option should be explored. Picture an experienced nurse playing a game of Scrabble with four or five patients. While playing the game the nurse may be checking to see how a new patient interacts with other patients, what his eye contact is like, does he express humour or competitiveness? The nurse is observing whether the patient uses neologisms while playing the game and noting his psychomotor agility in his movements of the pieces on the board.

Picture a care assistant in an adjacent room who is also playing a game of Scrabble with another group of patients but who is not carrying out therapeutically guided actions and observations. Enter an auditor who is armed with an audit tool that is concerned with measurable data. Unless the audit tool and the auditor are sensitive enough to pick up the differences in the two scenarios she will merely notice that two games of Scrabble were being played. She may even think that the nurse is slothful!

If the tool is not sensitive enough to detect the 'soft' quality processes and outcomes of concern to the experienced nurse and the patient it is of limited usefulness and validity in evaluating the quality of care. Therefore, a more qualitative approach to evaluating the quality of psychiatric nursing is required. Perhaps what is also required is that the auditors of nursing interventions should be psychiatric nurses: if not they will miss the subtle almost imperceptible processes that nurses at their best carry out. This relates back to the ownership issue addressed earlier.

So is quality assurance integral or alien to psychiatric nursing? In the above example, the nurse is seeking to do a good job (processes) to achieve certain therapeutic purposes, and she would like to know if the actual outcomes achieved coincide with these purposes. An appropriate, sensitive, valid and reliable quality assurance approach will give the nurse the answer. Therefore to the extent that it informs nurses if they are being effective, a quality assurance initiative, rather than being at odds with psychiatric nursing practice, is central to it. If such a sensitive quality assurance approach can be found, it will help to detect whether experienced nurses are therapeutic in what they do. The message that quality assurance approaches values the 'soft' caring interventions will help improve staff morale and attitudes towards being involved and taking ownership for such approaches. This would also have implications for other team members in that the worth of experienced nurses would be realised; managers would also realise that a rich skill mix of mostly qualified staff is therapeutically more valuable than smaller numbers of experienced staff seeking to provide care through cheaper unqualified staff. The gain in terms of patient welfare would more than balance additional salary costs. In America Helt and Jellinek (1988) studied 8 million patient days. They found that when the mix of qualified nursing staff was increased relative to other unqualified care staff the added 5 per cent increase in salary costs was offset by a 10 per cent increase in productivity. Obviously we cannot pre-empt what the results of audit will be, but from this and other extant research on the effect of rich staff skill mixes on quality (McKenna, 1995) we would be surprised if it did not come up that way.

Here is an outline of an approach to quality assurance. First, make a list of key activities such that in a good psychiatric ward those activities would be going on a lot of the time and, where they were going on not much of the time, the psychiatric nursing care could be said to be poor. Identify key levels of frequency for those activities, in particular an unsatisfactory level, a barely satisfactory level, a good level and an excellent level. Note how the frequency of occurrence of those activities could be monitored by checks at random times in the week over a longish period. Focus on whether the monitoring could be satisfactorily done by persons without psychiatric nursing expertise. If it can, then the cost of implementing the quality assurance scheme can be kept down by using less well-qualified staff. If it cannot, then using inappropriately qualified staff for data-collection will be a false economy.

A joint management and nursing initiative could make use of an approach like that just sketched:

1. Make the list of key activities; at this stage don't consider observability.
2. Identify the key levels; at this stage cost should not be a factor.
3. Consider whether the key activities could be observed at all by anyone.
4. Consider what qualifications those monitoring those activities would have to have.

Involving both nursing staff and management in these steps could help to ensure ownership. The process of reaching agreement on centrally important activities, if conducted in an appropriate way between persons who show respect for one another's expertise and judgement, could help to build and sustain team morale. The process of reaching agreement on what is required for competent monitoring of key activities could help to develop a shared sense of wise budget management (including the avoidance of false economies).

If, as we suggest, effective quality assurance in psychiatric nursing requires data collection by psychiatric nurses, there are twin dangers against which protection may be needed. It must be stressed here that integrity and honesty are important in auditing. These are the danger of a cosy relationship where by colleagues are unduly indulgent of each other's shortcomings, and the danger of personal enmities, jealousies, etc. distorting the data.

Furthermore, because qualified nurses must continually induct, supervise, teach and direct unqualified staff they are spending less time in direct patient care. They are faced with a conflict of obligations: by meeting the needs of unqualified staff they have less time to spend on what they believe they ought to be doing – meeting the needs of patients and improving the quality of care.

Both at the institutional level and also 'on the shop-floor', at the level of individual nurses making clinical decisions with individual patients, outcome evaluation inevitably requires mental health managers and nurses to make complex ethical decisions. Trade-offs have to be made between competing alternatives. With a single patient an improvement in one outcome may mean a deterioration in another area. For example, a reduction in a patient's anxiety (say through admission to hospital) may mean that they have to take more time off work or have to leave their home. Similarly, a return home from hospital may lead to a divorce or a spouse having to be referred to the mental health services. It seems to us that hard and soft data both have a place in initiatives by staff and management to monitor the quality of care, and efforts need to be made to ensure a much greater balance than evidenced currently in the measures used.

Conclusions

We have seen that quality assurance in an organisation requires provision for identifying, articulating and reviewing the purposes of the organisation, examining the processes that go on, and monitoring the fit between purposes and outcomes. The effectiveness of markets depends on there being some measure of compliance with the ethical norms of truthfulness, non-coercion and fulfilment of undertakings, so too the effectiveness of quality assurance arrangements depends on some measure of compliance with norms of genuine debate about purposes, honesty about data, seriousness in choice of indicators, etc. Just as too much fraud, force or promise-breaking will undermine markets, so will faking of data or misidentification of purposes or selection of inappropriate indicators undermine quality assurance. If it is morally important that the organisation does its work well, then there is a moral obligation to keep in place arrangements for reviewing purposes, processes and outcomes.

The market-place ethos currently permeating mental health services owes part of its impetus to the teachings of industrial management theorists. However, it appears that managers have been very selective in what has been adopted in their Mental Health Trusts. The principles of mission statements, collection of hard data, process variation and risk management have been focused upon; but equally essential principles of empowerment of staff, consumer involvement, teamwork, management commitment, and blaming the system rather than the individual have not always been given the emphasis they require.

Genuine quality improvement in mental health nursing involves taking steps to ensure that all these relevant factors are taken into account. In practice there are risks; among the risks are that undue importance will be attached to factors that are especially easy to see or to measure, and that other factors will be overlooked, neglected or forgotten. The focus on some measurable and politically driven indicators leads to overall quality loss. This is to be put down not to quality improvement but to its abuse.

References

Balogh, R., Bond, S., Simpson, A. and **Quinn, H.** 1993: An analysis of instruments and tools used in psychiatric nursing audit. Newcastle-upon-Tyne: Centre for Health Services Research.

Barker, P.J. 1995: Empowerment in patient care. Unpublished paper presented at the University of Ulster Empowerment Conference (Sept).

Bond, S. 1992: Outcomes of nursing: proceedings of an invitational developmental workshop. Newcastle upon Tyne: Centre for Health Services Research.

Brennan, T.A. 1990: Ethics of confidentiality: the special case of quality assurance research. *Clinical Research* **38**(3), 551–7.

Brown, J.M. Kitson, A.L. and **McKnight, T.J.** 1992: *Challenges in caring*. London: Chapman and Hall.

Clare, A. 1990: Some conclusions. In Hopkins, A., and Costain, D. (eds), *Measuring the outcomes of medical care*. London: The Royal College of Physicians, pp. 105–9.

Deming, W.E. 1982: *Quality, productivity and competitive position*. Cambridge, Mass: MIT Press.

DHSS 1989: *Working for patients*. Government White Paper. London: Her Majesty's Stationery Office.

DHSS 1992: *The patients' charter*. London: Her Majesty's Stationery Office.

Durgahee, T. 1996: Discharge of psychiatric patients into the community: how many more must die? *British Journal of Nursing* **5**(10), 618–21.

General Medical Council 1993: *Professional conduct and fitness to practice*. London: GMC.

Goldstone, L.A. and **Doggett, D.P.** 1989: *Psychiatric nursing monitor: an audit of nursing care in psychiatric wards*. Leeds: Poly Enterprises Ltd.

Griffiths, R. (Chairman) 1983: *(HC84 13) Health service implementation of the NHS Management Enquiry report*. London: HMSO.

Grodin, P., Pearse, I., and **Wilson, I.** 1987: Keeping the customer satisfied. *Nursing Times* **83**(38): 35–7.

Helt, E. and **Jellinek, R.C.** 1988: In the wake of cost cutting, nurse productivity and quality improve. *Nursing Management* **19**(6), 36–48.

Irvine, D. and **Irvine, S.** (eds) 1991: *Making sense of audit*. Oxford: Radcliffe Medical Press.

Juran, J.M. 1974: *Quality control handbook*. New York: McGraw-Hill.

Kelly, ? and McKenna, H. 199?: Victimisation and harassment of people with enduring mental disorders. *Journal of Psychiatric and Oriental Health Nursing* 4 (?) (in press)

Kennedy, I. 1994: Between ourselves. *Journal of Medical Ethics* **20**, 69–70.

McKenna, H.P. 1993: Research and destroy. *Nursing Standard* **8**(12), 50–1.

McKenna, H.P. 1995: Skill mix substitution and quality of care: an exploration of assumptions from the research literature. *Journal of Advanced Nursing* **20** (in press).

McAuley, A. and **McKenna, H.P.** 1995: Mental disorder among the homeless population in Belfast. *Journal of Psychiatric and Mental Health Nursing* **2**(6), 335–42.

Maxwell, N. 1984: *From Knowledge to Wisdom*. Oxford: Blackwell.

O'Neill, O. 1986: *Faces of Hunger*. London: Allen & Unwin, pp. 6–7, 8.

Pawlicki, C. 1992: Staff trauma as units shrink. *Nursing Times* **88**(46), 8.

Prior, L. 1991: *The social worlds of psychiatric and ex-psychiatric patients in Belfast*. Belfast: Health and Health Care Research Unit. Queens University Belfast.

Ramsey, P. 1970: *The patient as person*. New Haven and London: Yale University Press, pp. 5–6.

Ritchie, J., Dick, D. and **Lingham, R.** 1994: *The report of the inquiry into the care and treatment of Christopher Clunis*. London: HMSO.

Robertson, K. 1992: Unconditional discharge. *Nursing Times* **88**(43), 30–2.

Robertson, L. 1992: Quality assurance: the shape of things to come. *British Journal of Nursing* **1**(3), 154–6.

Schrock, R. 1984: Moral issues in nursing research. In Cormack, D.F.S. (ed.), *The research process in nursing*. Oxford: Blackwell, pp. 193–204.

Trevelyn, J. 1994: A matter of trusts. *Nursing Times* **90**(27) 28–30.

UKCC 1992: *Code of professional conduct*. London: UKCC.

Warner, L. 1994: Where are they now? *Nursing Times* **90**(31), 20–21.

World Health Organisation 1985: *The principles of quality assurance*. Copenhagen: Euro Reports and Studies (94).

22

BUYING A SELF: THE ETHICS OF PURCHASING THERAPY

Vincent Deary

Current trends in therapeutic intervention take on a particular light when set against the backdrop of the massive demographic, political and socio-economic changes over the last decade. Not only do brief psychotherapies appear cost-effective in relation to particular outcome criteria in individual clients and local budget constraints, they may also serve to dissipate belief in the state's responsibility in certain areas, by locating the source of clients' problems in their attitudes to life and responsibility for their plight within their individual sphere of influence. Here Vincent Deary examines these and other aspects of the current trend within the NHS of purchasing brief, individually focused therapies.

He considers the three main therapeutic modalities and their development *as ideology*, rather than offering what may be seen as a complete account of all the schools. In this way, this chapter highlights the most crucial point of Part 3, which is to encourage the reader to look at how ideology is influencing their experience and their belief in this or that (apparently) moral principle. It may, after all, not be a *moral* principle at all, but simply ideology that one has been induced to swallow. Vincent does not seek to argue that one is gullible for having done this – after all, there are vast philosophical, scientific, cultural, financial, religious and other interests at play, and at play over a long period of history, in developing the ideology. Particular therapeutic ideologies have almost *become* an *ethical touchstone* for those of us subscribing to them, so that it is possible to blind ourselves to any merits of the alternatives. In this respect, Vincent reveals his own position in the enmeshed hierarchy of interest and professional status, describing his experience as a behavioural nurse psychotherapist, and also the dread that scrutiny of these issues induces in him as one person trying to sort out the chaff of ideology from the wheat of clear judgement about what is right and fitting in the care of the mentally ill.

Picture yourselves in the therapy supermarket. You are the stock manager. Within a particular budget you must decide which therapies to buy. What would be your decision procedure? Efficacy, popularity, comprehensibility, standard brand names, novelty, price? How do you decide? Now you are a customer strolling down the aisle with a list of needs, longings, problems, unease. From magazines and books, from adverts, you know some of the claims, some of the concepts. Some therapies sound new and enticing – but how will they serve up? What will they do for you? How do you decide?

The first is the state's dilemma, the second the individual's. We are somewhere in the middle – we want customers to buy our versions of them, and our remedies for their life, their longings, their unease. We need them to need us. How do we achieve this? In choosing a brand of therapy we, as wholesale purchasers, clients or practitioners, implicitly endorse a particular therapeutic ideology. Every therapeutic ideology covers four broad areas:

1. A set of beliefs and assumptions about what it is to be human, what constitutes the mind, the self and the self's relation to others.
2. An assumption of states that are 'more or less well'. That is, some concept of the good life; the balanced mind; the sane self and the healthy relation. This in turn depends on an idea of the less good; the imbalanced; the insane and the unhealthy.
3. A theory or model to explain how both 'well' and 'less well' states are arrived at.
4. A set of techniques for arriving at a 'more well' state, as defined by the ideology.

In an ideal situation, individuals seeking help or advice would appraise the contents of an ideology and choose the one which best chimed with their own self-concept or current need, choosing a version of their selves, as they currently are and as they wish to be. This ideal state is, of course, financial. Few are in a position to freely choose their therapy. Instead they must rely on the therapy the state purchases and administers through the Health Service structure.

In the new health service the market-place is not a metaphor. In the delicatessen counter you may still find some analysis. Racking the shelves, however, are brief counselling and cognitive behavioural therapy. In buying therapy for users of the NHS, the state is blanketly endorsing a particular self-concept for an entire nation. On what basis has it made this choice? The quick and obvious answer is again financial, for the therapy that the state is currently buying is brief and cheap. It could be inferred that we are participating in the sale of second-rate selves. As providers and potential users of this service, how are we to evaluate the state's choice?

This chapter will attempt to lay the ground for such an evaluation. As the intermingling of therapy and finance is as old as therapy, I will begin by setting the current debate in its historical context, starting with the death of God and the rise of analysis. The brand proliferation that follows focuses on cognitive and behavioural therapies. This may seem exclusive. I do not propose to explore either drug therapy, group therapies or humanistic/existential approaches. Both medicine as a dominant force in mental health treatment and group/collectivist approaches to care have been addressed elsewhere, while the humanistic approach is back, alive and well as cognitive therapy, which I shall address. Following this historical contextualisation, the chapter will appraise the competing therapeutic ideologies to see more clearly exactly what kinds of self are on offer. Having only been to analytic tastings, not being myself an initiate, I am aware some may object to my cheek in attempting such an appraisal. I hope though that my discussing it *as an ideology* may be acceptable none the less. As far as I can, I offer in relation to analytic forms of therapy, no more or less than in relation to the other schools, a free ideological evaluation of the property without inhabiting it. Finally I shall attempt to construct a decision procedure, a universal rational tool to help you, whether you are state, individual or broker, to choose 'Which Therapy'.

THE GROWTH OF THE THERAPY MARKET-PLACE

Nietzsche's announcement of the death of God has become a convenient marker of an historical shift in our way of understanding the world. Briefly, we could say that at that time – the turn of the century – the job of giving meaning to life passed from the hands of the priests into the hands of the doctors. However, this somewhat over-simplifies the historical juncture in which the therapy market begins. If it was simply a matter of replacing religion with science, the soul with the mind, then the subsequent conflicts within the 'science of the mind' arise apparently *ex nihilo.* Nietzsche's pro-clamation has a more complex resonance that we shall briefly examine.

God as an explanatory principle in himself had long quitted the ideological scene. He was, however, still present in principle in the form of Rationality. From Descartes onwards the world becomes comprehensible because, for him and his scientific and philosophic descendants, God has given man a rational mind as a tool with which to understand the world. Between the mind and the world there is now a perfect symbolic correspondence which allowed the world to be represented as it is. Prior to this, God was truth and the world a veil of tears and darkness. With Descartes came the dawn of the era labelled the Enlightenment. From the seventeenth century onwards the now free mind explored, described and explained the world. The scien-tific method was born.

However, from the mid-nineteenth century onwards a shadow falls over this heaven of the mind. Although any attempt to pinpoint its origin is speculative, it can be seen at work in the poetry of the French symbolists, the science of Darwin, the philosophy of Schopenhauer. The shadow grows from an increasing doubt about the central tenet of rationality – the correspondence between the mind and the world. This doubt finds its definitive embodiment in the work of Nietzsche. For Nietzsche God is indeed dead, killed by the work of science and Darwin in particular. But with God gone, so is the given correspondence of the mind and the world. The relationship between mind and world is arbitrary and contingent. Truth is no longer absolute and impersonal but rather the function of a particular culture's evolved way of describing the world. There are many of the latter, the one that predominates will be the one with the most powerful advocates behind it. Truth becomes a function of power and will. Nietzsche describes a kind of ideological Darwinism in which the most powerful ideas define truth, until a more powerful one comes along. The idea of an absolute unques-tionable truth is no longer attainable – there is no longer a place outside this struggle of ideas from which to judge it. Thus in announcing the death of God, Nietzsche not only tolls the bell for religion, but also for truth and rationality. What is to replace it?

Relativity and ideology. Nietzsche's apocalyptic texts have been incorporated into subsequent culture with surprising ease. It is now almost a commonplace that our particular view of the world is relative to our time and culture. Each culture creates and defines its own objects of knowledge in accordance with the particular ideologies that it has happened to evolve. In our culture this phenomenon has become an object of knowledge in itself. Anthropologists compare and encode the ideologies of other cultures; social scientists search out the interests served and oppressed by ideological structures; philosophers deconstruct ideologies to lay bare their hidden assumptions and absolutes; physicists sanguinely admit to the impossibility of separating observer and observed and encode this in their equations.

This is the historical juncture that Nietzsche marks – the move from the absolute to the relative, from truth to ideology. Seen from this perspective, the evolution of the therapy market-place can be understood not as a battle for the true definition of the human condition but rather a struggle between ideologies trying to monopolise and define a limited market-place. Admit it – there is money to be made by intervening in others' lives.

Setting up shop

The first stall in the therapeutic market-place was psychoanalysis. This section will outline some of the ideological and historical factors underpinning its initial success and then chart the rise of its market competitors.

The ideological and professional contexts in which psychoanalysis arose are a key to understanding its success in creating the therapy market. In the former we find the need that therapy met, in the latter the means by which it succeeded in doing so. Freud in 'The uses of illusion' points out how religion previously served as an explanatory framework for everyday life, in that it gave meaning to events which would otherwise be arbitrary. Like Nietzsche, Freud was intent on unmasking the all too human necessities that lay beneath the structure of religion. With the multiple assaults of Darwin, industrialisation, popular science, Nietzsche and Freud himself, religion was singularly unfit to explain or ameliorate (if it ever had) the conditions of modern life. Similarly, the Cartesian tradition of an understanding based on rationality was now in question. The one discourse where it still held sway, science, was unable to comment on the meaning of life. This collateral crumbling of the two founding ideologies of the enlightenment, God and Reason, left a hole at the centre of Being. It was, essentially, a crisis of meaning.

That this loss of meaning formed the site for the therapy market is made explicit in the work of Jung. In his autobiography Jung describes how his father, a pious Christian pastor, ended his life in an insane asylum. Jung characterises his father's madness as a result of the Christian myth having failed to control or account for his inner conflict. In retrospect Jung sees his own life as a successful attempt to replace this myth with a more personally useful one, and his life's mission to spread the capacity for the creation of personally useful myths to the rest of humanity. This went hand in hand with the unseating of the rational as the supreme function of the mind. For Jung society was in crisis not only because Christianity could no longer contain it, it had also become reliant on a rationality which denied and suppressed the creative/destructive mythopoeic forces of the human mind which had created the Christian myth (also the scientific method) in the first place. To overcome this crisis, Jung proposes a utilitarian religious system, in which each individual needs to create his own myths to live by. Thus the loss of universal meaning caused by the death of God is made good by re-inscribing meaning at the level of the individual's life. The end of the reign of reason frees the mythopoetic power of the mind to effect this re-inscription.

Freud's diagnosis is somewhat less happy than Jung's. In many ways he retains the structure of the religion which he was one of the most instrumental in overthrowing. Like Nietzsche, Freud unmasked the 'absolutes' of religion and rationality to show their human roots in the individual's and society's attempt to control their innate destructive drives. For Freud, original sin was a fact, enacted anew by each generation. The incestuous and murderous impulses each child harboured against its parents were held in check only by internalising parental authority, by forging a personal decalogue to keep the inner pagan masses in check. The removal of God did not alter the problem, it personalised it. God had only been, after all, society's externalisation of its need for protection against its own irrationality, its inner dark gods.

In sum, psychoanalysis opened the therapy market in the gap left by the failure of God and reason to give meaning to life. Strategically it conserved the meaning lost in the loss of the grand narrative of God and transmuted it into a doctrine of individual narratives and personal meaning. It incorporated both instinct and rationality into its doctrine by showing human life to be a struggle between (Freud) or a synthesis and transcendence of (Jung) reason and impulse, order and chaos. Thus not only did it give meaning back to life, it also explained why we lost it in the first place.

If psychoanalysis had been only a doctrine, it might have gone the way of many of the early twentieth-century 'systems of thought' such as theosophy, and become merely an interesting piece of esoterica. However, it was also a professional practice and partook of the gravatus of science.

The science of mind formulated by Freud is essentially an extension, rather than an overthrowing, of the medical paradigm. Prior to Freud unexplained physical symptoms, i.e. disease in the absence of pathology, were due either to malingering or as yet undiscovered pathology. Freud legitimised medical colonialism by validating the study of hysteria, a new entity with origins that are psychogenic. This shifted the focus of medical intervention from looking for the cause of a symptom to looking at the meaning of it. The move may seem slight, but this shift of focus was the foundation of the psychoanalytic movement. If physical phenomena can be an indirect and unwitting expression of an inner meaning, then certain things follow. First, at some level the subject must 'know' the meaning of the symptom to be able to express it. Second, since this meaning is not in consciousness, the knowledge of it must lie outside of consciousness. Following from this there has to be an internal mechanics of knowledge suppression to effect this sequestration. Finally, cure of the symptom would be achievable by bringing the banned knowledge back into consciousness, thus obviating the need for the occult expression of it. Freud spent the rest of his life attempting to describe a structure of mind in which such phenomena were possible. Two aspects of this project are crucial.

First, Freud's texts, although not conventionally scientific, employ the metaphors and rhetoric of science and medicine. Psychopathology is pictured as occurring in an abstract body with particular organs – superego, ego, id – with a particular mechanics – repression, projection, sublimation – motivated by a particular set of drives – sex, death, pleasure. Second, the research of this project took place in the clinical situation. Being already a doctor Freud had access to patients with whom he could generate and test his theories. Crucially, he could demonstrate cures.

The combination of these two factors – Freud's access to, and use of, the language and institutions of conventional medicine – results in a new historical phenomenon. The diagnoses and alleviation of mental suffering, ultimately the meaning of an individual's particular existence, pass into the hands of doctors. A new societal institution evolves from this moment – the therapy market-place. Psychoanalysis becomes an expert practice requiring extensive training. For roughly 50 years it monopolises the territory it created. However, come mid-century, it begins to have competitors.

The rise of behaviourism

Analysis has, at least until recently, effectively colonised the lay vocabulary of self-understanding. At the level of the subject explaining his acts to self or others, much of the validity of his claims arise from their congruence with psychoanalytic theories of self. As such, analysis has a street validity, a power base in common consciousness, which ensures its continued functioning as one of our primary sources of meaning. Behaviourism, on the other hand, has a version of the individual which is inherently non-subjective, a vocabulary much more suited to describing 'them' rather than 'I'. As such, its explanatory currency has much more value within state institutions, where the individual is an abstraction whose behaviour needs to be controlled and predicted in the interests of society. Its concomitant lack of street vocabulary often blinds us to the fact that behaviourism is as grand in its ambitions as analysis.

However, after years in the intellectual wilderness, behaviourism, particularly in the guise of cognitive/behavioural therapy, has come to dominate not only the state-purchased therapy market (*The Economist*, 1995), but is also beginning to acquire a media and street credibility, to the extent that the lay vocabulary for self-understanding is now beginning to move from psychoanalytic metaphors to behavioural cognitive ones.[1] In short, it is becoming fashionable. Let us trace the historical development of behavioural ideology from its inception in ethology to its current incarnation as post-modern therapy.

Like individuals and species, ideologies evolve under environmental pressure. Certain ideas survive and others become extinct. I will attempt to trace the evolution of behavioural theory, illustrate its successive 'mutations' and indicate the environmental factors that currently contribute to its unique fitness to survive in the present cultural climate.[2] I shall consider the evolution of this project as an ideology and as an institution, and hopefully show how the factors that precipitated its successful cross-over into therapy in the 1950s, currently maintain its prominence and explain our state's purchase of it.

Behaviourism arose within the larger framework of the nascent psychology, a new science that attempted to apply scientific principles to human being and mental life. Psychology, however, was, and remains, unique in the field of science in that it is historically riven by ideological strife to a degree which brings its status as science into question. In psychology there is little methodological or ideological consensus between the competing schools (Humanist, Cognitive, Structuralist, Constructivist, etc.). As a discipline, psychology seems fragmented. In short, within psychology we

---

[1] See *Wired*/other hip magazines, 'cyberpunk' novels, and other cultural expressions of the new Zeitgeist. For a more academic discussion see e.g. Dennet's 'Consciousness Explained'.

[2] For a fuller development of the concept of the Darwinian evolution of ideas, a concept already explicit in the epistemology of Skinner as early as the 1940s, see Dawkins (1988).

have several competing ideologies, each with their own language and claims upon truth, its acquisition and verification.

Psychology is born in a time of ideological turmoil. Criticism of the methodology of analysis pre-dates its establishment as a practice. As early as 1840, Comte had pointed out that introspection was logically impossible. The medium of self-examination – consciousness – could not be simultaneously the object of that examination. A microscope cannot magnify itself. Also, the reliability of the data achieved from introspection had been undermined by nineteenth-century studies in hypnotism. From these it emerged that human behaviour was often generated by automatic, non-volitional processes which consciousness could only give a retrospective and erroneous gloss upon. Thus Watson and Pavlov explicitly repudiated the data derivable from introspection as unscientific since it was neither observable or verifiable. Indeed, Comte had rejected this as a scientific procedure in 1842: 'The thinker cannot divide himself in two, of whom one reasons whilst the other observes him reason. The organ observed and the organ observing being, in this case, identical, how could observation take place?' Thus from early on both the means – introspection – and the object – mind – of the psychoanalytic project were of suspect value to those attempting to establish a science of the mind.

Analysis has been described as the first post-enlightenment discourse (Du Preez, 1991). This is so because it opened the therapy market in the gap left by the failure of God and reason to give meaning to life. By contrast behaviourism can be seen as the last science of the Enlightenment period. Behaviourism enshrines the confidence of Enlightenment science. Nature is comprehensible, rational and empirically verifiable. This confidence had paid remarkable dividends in physics and chemistry and biology. Darwin had applied the principles of empiricism to the variety of life and deduced a theory of universal applicability. There was every reason to believe that an application of the same methods to the variety of animal behaviour might generate similar findings. Early behaviourists '[were] influenced by the empiricist view that knowledge is dependent on sensory experience and the positivist requirement that science be based on observation, [they] were concerned that any concept postulated should be tied to observations' (Valentine, 1990). The demand that any data be observable and verifiable goes a long way to explaining why behaviourism focused on behaviour as the index of mental life. No other data was allowable to a truly empiricist theory. As such, behaviourism was explicitly at odds with the epistemology of analysis which allowed for empirically unverifiable truth claims. It is worth pointing out that in the post-Enlightenment climate this does not mean that analysis is invalid, the most that one can say is it does not meet empirical criteria and is only at fault if it tries to claim that it does.

The analogy between behaviourist psychology and Darwinian thought is compelling and instructive. Both abstract a feature of being alive – reproduction, behaving – and attempt to establish laws of this feature to which any living thing is subject. Both generate the same repugnance by emphasising human life's biological determinedness above its apparent existential freedom. Both were successful. Using its methods initially on animals, behaviourism seemed to be able to explain, control and predict behaviour without reference to mental states. Behaviour was to be understood with reference not to its inner life but in the context of the environment in which it occurs. Life learns how to act in an environment by reacting to it. Reactions that are more successful in providing survival and comfort within that environment are selected or re-inforced, shaping future behaviour within that environment. This is the theory of evolution by natural selection re-inscribed at the level of the individual life form: Natural selection explains the biological acquisition of knowledge of the world; behaviourism supplements this with an account of how the life form acquires knowledge of the particular environment in which it finds itself. Had behaviourism limited its scope to animals it would have been an ethology, a science of animal life. By applying its laws to human life, it becomes an epistemology, a highly abstract theory of how humans come to know how to be.

Epistemology was traditionally the province of the philosophers. Whilst other disciplines acquired specific knowledge about particular fields, philosophy tackled the problem of how any knowledge was possible and how its truth was to be ascertained. As such, the other sciences were answerable to philosophy for the validation of their truth claims. By establishing a psychological epistemology, behaviourism trumps even the philosophers. For the ideologically minded behaviourist there is no difference in principle between a pigeon pecking seeds and philosophers producing texts. Both instrumental and conceptual knowledge are subject to the principles of selection by their environment. A person learns those responses which maximise his potential for survival and comfort in his lived environment. A culture will evolve knowledge that is efficacious in allowing it to effectively master its environment. At each level – species, individual and culture – the same epistemology applies.

Beginning with the application of rational values to animal behaviour, behaviourism evolves a theory of learning which it generalises to the human and thus, ultimately, purports to explain how rationality itself evolved under the immutable laws of behaviourism. Skinner is quite explicit on this: 'If it turns out that our final view of verbal behaviour invalidates our scientific structure from the point of view of logic and truth, then so much the worse for logic, which will also have been embraced by our analysis' (Skinner, 1945, p. 272.).

As O'Donohue and Smith (1992) point out, the subordination of behaviourism to the doctrines of positivism is a common strategy used by its ideological opponents to discredit it. The argument goes that since positivism is discredited, so is behaviourism. However, there is a fundamental misapprehension of behavioural ideology at work here which completely misses the ideological evolution behaviourism had undergone by 1945. It is amazing that this ideological move has been missed, even by many behaviourists such as Woolfolk quoted above. Behaviourism is subject to no external ideology such as positivism for its truth claims. Rather, it has become, by 1945, a theory of what constitutes truth itself.

In the light of the intellectual climate of the time, the radical empiricism of behaviourism requires some explanation. Behaviourists adopted their position at a time when the other sciences of the Enlightenment, particularly physics, were beginning to acknowledge the subjective nature of their own truth claims.

For an understanding of the behavioural adoption of positivist empiricism we must look to biology. The Darwinian theory of natural selection had a massive cultural effect on its time. Darwin's theory evidently further demoted the position of man, even as regards his humanity. Darwin had come up with a theory of universal impact and applicability, all life subject to its principles. Crucially, this monumental theory arose from classical empirical methods. Darwin had patiently collected data on a variety of species, sat down with the data and constructed his theory from it. Early behaviourists adopted a similar procedure. Behaviour, like reproduction, was a universal trait of all life. If empirically derived laws of behaviour could be found, then there was the potential to create a science of psychological life of similar scope and impact to Darwin's. Such a method would also secure psychology's position as a true science, rather than a speculative art, like analysis.

Such then was the genesis of behaviourism. A classically positivist science in a post-Enlightenment age, an ideological competitor of psychoanalysis and the two of them the only Western theories adequate in scope to explain human life. However, the cold glamour of behaviourism has little in the way of mass appeal. To understand its success in evolving thus we must look at the institutional structures it used to further itself.

Behavioural colonialism and rhetoric

From its inception at the turn of the century, behaviourism in America received massive state funding. Compare this with Germany around the same time. In Germany the academic powers were the chairs of philosophy. Psychology was a subordinate discipline to be kept under metaphysical scrutiny. As such, psychology remained largely speculative. In America, however, institutional philosophy was a fairly minor force and the new psychology encountered little opposition in establishing itself as an empirical science.

More importantly, there was a mutually agreeable relationship between science and state. The explicit goals of behaviourism were the prediction and control of behaviour. The government was more than keen on investing in a science that held out the promise of providing tools for control and reform in areas as diverse as the military, education, advertising, the penal system, delinquency and deviance.

Departments of psychology were founded, research-funded, experts appointed and students enrolled. The entire machinery of academic science was given to behaviourism to further and disseminate its knowledge. By the 1950s, it had turned its attention to the explanation and reform of human behaviour and from its academic power base it mounted a sustained campaign against psychoanalysis. The strategies it used are typical of ideological combat and it may be instructive to list a few.

Revision

A standard strategy of scientific advancement is to explain the same phenomenon as a rival theory and to do so with fewer extraneous concepts and more predictive power. The behavioural models for neurosis appear to do just that. Set beside the cumbersome poetics of analysis, behavioural neurosis is sleek, scientific and modern. Behaviourists in the 1960s went so far as to rewrite analytic case histories in the vocabulary of behaviourism, emphasising the latter's more elegant explanatory power.

Out doing

Behaviourism used techniques derived from its conceptual models on the same neuroses which, until then, analysis had sole provenance of. This is another standard strategy – solve problems better than the rival. Behaviourism quickly took to advertising that it was doing just that. Not content to rest there, it paid for research to show that its rival *wasn't* solving the same problems. Eysenck's evidence which shows no difference in outcome between those receiving psychoanalysis and those waiting for it was the masterstroke of this campaign.

Be absolutely modern

The function of fashion in science is much under-rated as a motive force in its advancement. There was a basic repugnance in response to behavioural theory which, combined with its self-proclaimed validity, gave it an odd glamour. Indeed, this is Kant's definition of the sublime in art, an admiration tinged with horror, an unexpected encounter with our own mortality and contingency. Behaviourism provided just that thrill: In the cold dress of science it announces our lack of freedom and dignity. As spectacle, it is compelling.

No more importantly, but at a more ideologically profound level, behaviourism chimes surprisingly well with current intellectual trends. Its notion of truth as what is most effective in a particular environment has much in common with the philosophic standpoint of the deconstructionists, who similarly admit to no absolutes outside of a given context by which truth can be judged.

Similarly, its theory of knowledge acquisition was a direct progenitor of the current intellectual trend called evolutionary epistemology. The latter has proponents as weighty as Popper and receives its most recent incarnation in Dawkins and his theory of memes – ideas that replicate themselves in the medium of shared human knowledge. There is no essential theoretical difference between this position and behaviourism.

Define the terms of debate

At the risk of sounding like conspiracy theory, let it merely be said that in education reform, in the compiling of the *Diagnostic and Statistical Manual* of the American Psychiatric Association and in an advisory capacity to the state, behavioural theory has no small role.

Having made clearer some of the factors that led to the rapid and remarkable success of behaviourism *qua* therapy, let us move on. To explain the rise of the third movement, cognitive therapy, we must return to the late 1950s. Here we have two ideologies at war, psychoanalysis and behaviourism. On the one hand, we have a poetics of mind and personality, a cure that works by establishing meaning; on the other, a science of behaving and a mechanics of reform, literally mindless. That the gap in the middle would be filled seems almost inevitable.

The Cybermen and the cognitive revolution

The problem of cognitive states mediating the response of the individual to the environment had constantly reared its head in the history of behavioural theory. For the purists such as Skinner mental life was merely a more private realm of environmental re-inforcement, to which the same behavioural laws applied. As such, there was no necessity for a theoretical reworking of behavioural concepts, they only needed to be extended. However, for others the internal encoding of the behavioural repertoire was not explicable in the conventional stimulus–response vocabulary. The advent of cybernetics and theories of machine information processing in the 1950s provided a vocabulary ideally suited to explaining the individual's encoding of responses. Such was the explanatory power of this new language that it rapidly evolved from being an explanatory adjunct to behaviourism and became a school of psychology in its own right – Cognitive Psychology.

This development was mirrored in the therapy market-place where cognitive therapy takes on the territory of behaviourism and accounts for the latter's success with a new explanatory framework. This framework, in turn, gives rise to new therapeutic techniques which appear to qualify cognitive therapy as an independent and efficacious school of therapy. The relationship between cognitive and behavioural therapies remains uneasy. This is partly because they have more in common than they care to admit. The basic therapeutic armoury of both is very similar. Where they differ is in the explanation of its effect. Cognitive therapists are keen to distance themselves from the mechanistic heritage that taints the behavioural image; behaviourists are resentful of the popular glamour of a therapy whose therapeutic effects are basically behavioural. However, a closer inspection of the cognitive lineage reveals key methodological, ideological and ethical differences from both behaviourism and analysis, which must be understood before an ethical comparison can be attempted.

Metaphorical differences

Explanatory systems are only as good as the metaphors they deploy. Ultimately any science has to appeal to a metaphoric structure that has to be taken on faith. As the level of description changes, so does the metaphoric structure. For example, the molecules and bonds of biochemistry, necessary postulates in an effective explanatory framework, dissolve and lose their certainties at the level of nuclear physics. Explanation is a description mapped onto a tautology, and any science, explicitly or implicitly, must invoke a tautological framework, agreed to be useful (if not actually true), on which to assert itself.

The metaphors of the cognitive sciences are derived from computer science. In the invention and study of machines that could process and transform information a new and distinctively modern science evolves. Its object of study – information – was of such a level of abstraction that its applications reached far beyond the machines it was invented to describe. Bateson's (1979) definition of information is instructive – any difference that makes a difference. Blue is blue because it is not red; a hydrogen molecule is a hydrogen molecule because it is not helium. Any system that is sensitive to its environment is so by virtue of being different. The human eye has evolved a chromatic discrimination which can encode minute differences in tone. The eye of a insect is structurally more simple by virtue of its relative lack of sensitivity to difference. Even at the level of encoding of information the principle of difference applies. From the focus on information a new picture of the human condition emerges. Human beings inhabit a universe of information, they actively construct that universe by virtue of the information they are sensitive to and the manner in which they encode and organise it. The manner of its encoding *is* the universe.

Psychology is presented with a new object and a new explanatory framework. Using analogies derived from computer science, it hypothesises inner neuro-cognitive mechanisms for the encoding and transforming of environmentally derived information. This quickly pays dividends in the field of vision, memory, speech production, mental imagery, etc. Behaviourists were unhappy with this state of affairs and responded in two ways. First they claimed that the explanatory and therapeutic success of cognitive concepts is reducible to the conventional behavioural paradigm, in short, nothing of value has been added. Second, they claimed that historically cognitive mediation has always been in behavioural theory and that the difference is merely one of emphasis.

However, behaviourism could not retain its defensive strategy for long. Piaget (1952) characterises ideological adaptation as a two stage process. First *accommodation*: the new idea enters the old ideological framework but remains 'undigested'. Then there is *assimilation* where the new idea is incorporated into the existing framework, producing a new synthesis in which both are transformed. In behaviourism this has produced the modern hybrid Cognitive/Behavioural therapy which has received its most lucid exposition from Rachman (1990). Employing both cognitive concepts, such as Lang's informational theory reworking of anxiety theory, and the traditional behavioural paradigms of stimulus–response theory, he produces a synthesis which has since become a school of therapy in its own right.

In therapy we see a similar revolution. The concept of the Freudian unconscious is reworked by Beck in the 1950s in the language of information processing. The unconscious in no longer an inaccessible and murky realm but is structured like a language – a computer language. Consciously accessible thoughts are the most easily accessible part of the human software. 'Behind' these are more peripheral, automatic thoughts which are the product of more deeply encoded values and assumptions. Underlying these are the core programmes or schemas, relatively innate, bordering on the hard-wired, versions of the world and the self. The links between these various levels of consciousness are analogous to logical inferences, *if* this, *then*, *it follows*, that. Schemas (core programmes, basic stances towards the world, postures, an embodied experience) generate propositions, values, which in turn generate automatic thoughts which, when activated, determine a person's conduct in the world and define their selves. Rationality is reinserted into the human mind. Although the content of a schema or a thought may be irrational in a given context, its form and derivation follow the rational rules of information processing. This gives rise to a new therapeutic methodology.

Methodological differences

Cognitive therapy reinvests introspection with scientific respectability. If the structuring of the human mind is fundamentally rational, then its investigation is subject to rational enquiry. Using standard phenomenological procedures, clients are asked to investigate the contents of their consciousness. Rational questioning leads them to the assumptions from which these thoughts must logically have arisen. These assumptions in turn are the logical products of schemas which can be unearthed by the same procedure. Compare this with psychoanalysis. The latter posits an unconscious that is fundamentally irrational and inaccessible. Knowledge of it can only be arrived at through attributing, somewhat arbitrarily, meaning, by a process as much art as science. By reinventing the unconscious as accessible and rational, Beck creates a scientific analysis which places cognitive therapy in a uniquely powerful position. It rewrites inner mental life – the province of analysis – in the language of science – the province of behaviourism. As such, it appears to better both, preserving the meaning–giving potential of the former whilst retaining the scientific respectability of the latter. In the latter respect, it had access to the same academic superstructures as behaviourism, and could take on the behaviourism on its own terms.

It proceeded to do this in exactly the way behaviourism had taken on analysis. It rewrote behavioural versions of neuroses and cure in the language of cognitions. It was not the feared object *or* the fear behaviour that was important, but rather the meaning of both. If behavioural therapy had any effect, it was by virtue of it changing the meaning of events for an individual. The fact that both therapies initially used identical therapeutic strategies was not the point: Cognitive therapy had the more powerful explanatory framework with which to explain their effects. Latterly it has developed techniques specifically aimed at altering the meaning of events for the individual. Although these still involve 'behavioural tests', the cognitive therapists argue that the meaning change is the effective therapeutic component, one which behavioural ideology cannot explain. The battle continues. Partly in response to the cognitive challenge, behavioural therapy, in the guise of neo-behaviourism, has acquired an explanatory sophistication with which to fight for the explanatory high ground. The mutual irritation generated by the proximity of these two schools of therapy appears to be beneficial for the advancement of both.

Ethical differences

In both behaviourism and analysis there is a pessimistic determinism – one is shaped by the world and must struggle, with the aid of therapy, to overcome the consequences of this. Cognitive therapy is much more optimistic. We shape the world by our encoding of it. So also we shape ourselves. To change our encoding is to change both world and self. This, with the aid of therapy, is entirely achievable. Much is made of the link between cognitive theory and pre-Socratic Greek philosophy. A quote from a Stoic philosopher encapsulates the basic stance of cognitive therapy: 'Man is not troubled by things in themselves but by his thoughts about them'. There are deeper links than this though. As Foucault has illustrated (Dreyfus and Rabina, 1982), the ethical substrate of the pre-Socratics was the self. The Stoics developed a set of techniques for the mastery of the self and its emotions which bear a striking resemblance to the techniques of cognitive therapy. Both embody the belief that the rational mind is the master–function of the human, which, if properly used, can master the emotions and lead to self-contentment. Both even advocate the keeping of diaries as a record and totem of the process of self-mastery. We have in both a politics, or a policing, of the self, with the rational as the juridical body governing the whole for its greater benefit. This essentially hopeful version of human nature – one can change the world by changing one's self – had enormous popular appeal.

Fashion

The importance of fashion and street currency should not be underestimated as an influence on scientific advance. The principles of cognitive therapy and its companion science, information technology, are currently saturating our world. The advent of personal computers and the Internet has furnished individuals with a new set of metaphors with which to describe phenomenon as diverse as community, democracy, mind, identity, reality, etc. Cognitive therapy receives much reflected kudos from this. Mind becomes the brain's software, therapy a re-programming or debugging. The self is a programme that can be changed if it does not run smoothly. More profoundly, cognitive therapy enshrines the idea of reality as a personal/social construct that can be altered by changing the self-programme. This chimes nicely with the neo-mysticism of cyber-culture and its attempts to de-bug itself of the societally transmitted memes which shape and limit our self-understanding.

Although this vocabulary has not quite seeped to the level of that of analysis, a substantial and influential proportion of the media currently employ a language that is entirely congruent with the tenets of cognitive therapy. In terms of marketing potential this accounts for some of the success of the therapy, and much of the envy of its rivals.

In sum

Above we sketched the growth of three ideologies. To bring the narrative up to date we must turn our focus onto the ideological climate in which they are currently obliged to develop. In a climate of economic evaluation a particular kind of scrutiny predominates, certain discursive practices prevail. In the context of health care evaluation we have the relatively novel spectacle of medicine being forced to justify its practices to an externally imposed evaluative system. To seem impartial, this evaluative system employs the full armoury of rationality and impersonal calculation. Its gaze is avowedly scientific. This places a kind of Darwinian pressure on medical practice – the procedures that survive and propagate are the ones which can prove their efficiency and necessity. Same with therapy.

The cool empirical gaze of state evaluation looks kindly on behavioural therapy. They are written in the same dialect. Lacking the glamour of psychoanalysis, behaviourism sold itself on its efficiency, employing from the beginning the language of outcome, evaluation and therapeutic expenditure. Cognitive therapy, growing in the same institutional milieu, partakes of the same language. More speculative, it yet remains scientific enough to look good in this light. Psychoanalysis, by contrast, operates on a different set of truth criteria – of individual narratives and personal meaning. This leaves the empirical gaze little to go on and psychoanalysis with little to show. Little wonder that it is the least purchased therapy.

Behavioural and cognitive therapy matured within the state milieu which now chooses them. Compared to analysis they are indigenous, native. What has been the strength of analysis in cultural discourse – its metaphoric richness and flexibility – is here its weakness. It has evolved largely outside of state or scientific scrutiny as an autonomous and distinct ideology. Called to account for itself in a foreign tongue, it can only appear clumsy.

Personal narrative

I find myself justifying behavioural therapy, defending it in pubs and in public. Recent media coverage has made it seem simplistic, mechanistic. I have been able to see, and with frustration see that others would not see, that other issues raised in the media mental health jamboree were all deeply infected with behavioural principles, both in definition and cure. I point this out to friends, I defend my chosen profession. I scorn the flabby inefficiency of analysis, the superficial glamour of the cognitivists. I defend my profession.

At a dinner party I meet two journalists in analysis. They tell me 'you brainwash people'. First of all I ask them what kind of therapy they are having.

'I'm not sure, I think she's eclectic.'

Point 1 to me, my punters know what they are buying from session 1. I give them a formulation of how I see the problem and what I think we could do about it. This is informed choice.

'How long for?'

'Two years so far.'

Point 2 to me, if we weren't getting anywhere after a few weeks we would ask why and then change tack.

Then the speech: 'I'm working with chronic fatigue at the moment, and almost without exception all my clients have said to me that they realise that the point of the therapy is for them not to need to see me anymore'.

The journalists nod with slow revelation as I talk about the ethical comfort I have with this – not only do my clients get better they also don't feel that it's me. Rather, I impart information that allows them to get better. The journalists begin to question their dependence on their therapist, what is she actually doing anyway? We share a laugh at people who are in therapy three nights a week and then go off and teach Lacan and the Signifier at a polytechnic. Don't these people have lives?

Game set and match.

My mentors tell me to abjure calling myself a *cognitive* behavioural therapist. They sneer at the graduates of our behavioural course who now call themselves cognitive therapists. I think that these colleagues know good marketing when they see it. I will have to market myself. 'At least call yourself a behavioural cognitive therapist then – after all, weren't we first on the scene?' In supervision I avoid psychoanalytic terms – however necessary I might find the concepts of transference and counter-transference, I know their currency is devalued here. I save that for elsewhere.

Surprisingly I find that more fashionable friends outside the psyche professions have picked up on the *Zeitgeist* relevance of cognitive therapy, even of behavioural ideology. With them I can wax conceptual, keep up the intellectual engagement I need to keep me interested in my profession.

I see clients get better, I see years of misery fade in twelve weeks. I feel an undirected gratitude to God knows what, a gratitude at being involved in this process. I shun responsibility for healing, conscientiously disengage my vanity from the process. I am a conduit of knowledge, the bringer, but not the agent, of salvation. I like myself. I disgust myself even for liking myself for this. I need therapy. Which one?

WHICH THERAPY?

The first section presented a historical context in which to place the current rise of behavioural and cognitive therapies within the state market. The aim of this section is to look in more detail at each of the therapies as it has evolved.

Since ideologies are essentially closed conceptual networks we must compare structure and function, rather than content alone. Ideologies do not share contents – the morality of the Torah or the Koran is not the morality of the Buddhist Canon, but they share a structure – both have a morality as a functional ideological unit.

Let us begin then by positing a generalised framework for comparing ideologies. An ideology is a framework for conceptualising reality, or parts of it. Let us structure the way ideology does this. Every ideology has:

- An ontology – what is the nature of the reality it describes?
- An epistemology – how we may acquire or appraise knowledge about that reality?
- An ethics and/or aesthetics – what we should do about that reality or with that knowledge?
- A praxis – how do we do what we should do?

Obviously these elements are co-dependent – your definition of reality will in turn dictate the kind of knowledge that is possible about it. In turn, what one should do and how, the ethics and praxis, will be delimited by the kind of reality it is and the nature of knowledge about it prescribed by the ideology. This is why ideologies are relatively closed structures. They are self-contained semantic networks where each term defines and is defined by the other terms of the network. Thus judging one ideology by the standards of another is a futile and aggressive act. Let us look at how this structure fits therapeutic ideologies.

- *Therapeutic ontology*: the therapy's angle on what it is to be human, what constitutes a mind, a self, a self's relation to another.
- *Therapeutic epistemology*: how do we come to know of ourselves and our life world, what is learning, what kind of knowledge is possible of ourselves, our motives and our relation to the life world?
- *Therapeutic ethics/aesthetics*: what constitutes wellness and illness; ease and disease; balance, sanity, health, and imbalance, insanity, ill health? What is it good or bad to be?
- *Therapeutic praxis*: the techniques, the means to define and move from less well to more well. The implementation of the ethics.

Assuming that this structure is useful, let us proceed to a comparison of the therapies. Any framework is ultimately arbitrary but its consistent use may give rise to meaning.

Praxis

Analysis: the hermetic therapist

Hermes, in his capacity of messenger or herald, had access even to the underworld, whither he guided the souls of the departed. In his active role the analyst acts as guide to the underworld, the hidden unconscious he has explored himself. With this unique and hard-won knowledge he guides the client through his own unconscious, discerning the messages of dreams, the hidden impulses of acts.

The transmission of this knowledge is, indeed, hermetic. One must be initiated rather than merely taught. Such a guide must attain the role of The Magician, not only as a conduit of secret knowledge, but also as one who is unknowable, the better to become the *tabula rasa* on which the client can write and thus comprehend his neuroses. The relationship of client and therapist is axial to the client's other relationships, and forms a site in which the problems of the latter can be seen and, perhaps, resolved.

Cognitive therapy: the Socratic philosopher

The cognitivist therapist knows that the mind is ultimately rational. In this he shares the analyst's belief in meaning. The therapist has been trained how to follow thoughts laterally – if that is true then what else would be true?; and vertically – what underlies the presenting belief? He will try not to impose this on the client but will, by skilled questioning, lead the client to unearth their own assumptions. The therapist will then suggest that the client empirically investigates the validity of his beliefs, test them against reality, with a view to disconfirming the more disabling beliefs. He has not, necessarily, done any of this to himself. The client is invited to join the therapist in a relationship of collaborative empiricism. The relationship is where hypotheses are formed to be tested in the rest of the client's life.

Behavioural therapy: the informed technician.

The behavioural therapist is armed with a series of models of how specific problems are established and maintained. He also possesses a range of techniques for overcoming the problems which he will suggest the client should employ. The client is presented with a model of his problem and invited to employ the technique to overcome it. Sessions evaluate the success or otherwise of this and plan accordingly. The therapist may or may not have used the techniques depending on his problems.

Ethics/aesthetics

Analysis: lighting the way

It is a commonplace that we could all 'do with some therapy'. Underlying this is the analytic assumption that no-one is completely well, just less unwell. Wellness is a function of knowledge of unconscious drives. To be free of one's demons, one must first bring them into the light. Consequently a state of complete wellness would be to be without an unconscious, to live a translucent existence.

Frank ill health in analysis is much easier to attain, and is the obverse of one's self-knowledge. Illness is a function of the extent and power of unconscious conflicts which express themselves to the afflicted individual in the rhetoric of a possession. Actions are not as intended; damaging relationships are unknowingly repeated; limbs are paralysed.

Cure in analysis is achieved by bringing unconscious drives into consciousness. This excavation is, perforce, hermeneutic. The unconscious speaks in signs and symbols; the analyst must seek their correct interpretation. Once unearthed, the old deforming forces will play themselves out in the arena of therapy until the high noon of understanding puts the shades to rest.

Cognitive therapy: rational analysis

There are many similarities to the above. However, cognitive therapy imposes a rational structure on the underworld, and interposes thought between the person and their being. To be unwell is to think unwell, to harbour dysfunctional schema rather than demons. Whereas analysis brings in interpretation as salvation via the analyst, cognitive therapy finds interpretation at the core of the problem: one is not troubled by the world/the self, but by how one thinks about them. As such, this stratum of thought is the locus of both illness and cure.

Cognitive cure involves a rational, rather than a hermeneutic, excavation of the source of unease. Its method is deductive rather than interpretive. The therapist is sleuth, not poet, and the client is his assistant. Wellness is achieved by the elimination, via Popperian refutation, of negative thinking and the conscious installation of more useful ways of thinking. The mind is debugged rather than exorcised.

The structural analogies with analysis are striking and not surprising. Beck, the founder, was a conventional analyst until he decided that his patients actually knew what was going on in their head, if their attention was properly directed. The latter is the proper occupation of a cognitive therapist.

Behaviourism: dog and vomit

'Habit', said Becket, 'is what chains the dog to his vomit', his remark being an expansion on Proverbs' 'The fool returns to his folly like the dog to his vomit'. For the behaviourist, to be ill is to be doing something that you don't like and don't actually have to do, but can't seem to stop. To be well is to be free of whatever problem brought you to therapy in the first place.

One could trace a kind of declension of locus of problem through the three therapies. For the analyst the locus is the whole self and thus the whole self requires work. For the cognitive therapist the problem lies in particular assumptions. The behaviourist finds the problem in the problem – the problem is as the problem does. As such, there is no general definition of wellness in behaviourism, only problem specification.

Ontology, epistemology.

I have conflated these two because within ideologies they are often hard to disentangle, e.g. behaviourism has an epistemic ontology.

Analysis: gothic romance

For the analyst being is essentially a tragedy. The most horrific of the classical tragedies are taken as metaphors for the psychic condition of the child. There are no innocents in analysis. If the tragedy is not metaphorical then it is structural. Turning to Lacan we find an image of the child fixating on an image of itself as it is for others. With that fatal awareness comes an inner rift. Henceforth the child is alienated from its self unto death, inhabiting a self that can never know itself; a self that is not itself. As with Adam and Eve, as soon as we attain awareness, we are forever expelled from Eden.

As the self is divided, so is the mind. The mind contains distinct systems, usually at odds with each other. The unconscious deceives us, the superego berates us, the ego barely contains us. The consolation of analysis, and its poetic allure lies in its epistemology. The separated parts all speak, but never directly. They talk to us through the relationships they talk us into, through the behaviours we thought we chose, through the dreams we have. Nothing is meaningless, we inhabit an epistemic treasure house to which analysis offers a key. Here all knowledge is self-knowledge, then at least we can form a truce, again with the help of Hermes, the trickster God, the shape shifter, the god of deception and cunning.

Cognitive therapy: post-modern humanists

The cognitive therapist inhabits a universe of information. He is easy with a lack of absolutes. The tragedy of analysis, the lost and divided self, does not trouble the cognitive therapist because, for him, there was nothing to lose. The self is what the self believes itself to be; to be is to know. If one changes thought one changes self, but there is no loss, no removal, only a new informational structure, the self as it now is.

Ontologically speaking, there is no ontology, not in the classic sense where ontology was an absolute, sometimes barely discernible through the clouds of knowing. In cognitive therapy the knowing is the being, there are as many worlds as there are minds. When, as here, ontology becomes epistemic, then epistemology takes on an ethical, even an aesthethical tone – a matter of what is it good to believe. In these circumstances, the right way to be is a function of what it is useful to know, what kind of knowledge best serves me. If I create the world by construing it, then how can I best construe it? Cognitive therapy teeters on the brink of amorality and only its hidden absolute, rationality, saves it.

Cognitive therapy has often been linked to the Stoic philosophers, and rightly so. The Stoics believed the Rational to be the highest function of mankind, and their highest goal was to bring all his other faculties and passions under the conscious control of the rational, to literally manage oneself, like a business or a child. As such, it is an atheistic version of Enlightenment values. Like humanism, cognitive therapy does not seek the support of God for its values. Reason and rationality are assumed to be free-standing and innate. Cognitive therapy works by assuming that the processes of thought are ultimately explicable. Negative thoughts are syllogistically generated by dysfunctional assumptions, which are propositionally congruent with their underlying schemata. This is a world of information, not tragedy.

Behaviourists: responsible sadists

For the behaviourist, ourselves and our world are a series of acquired responses, a thing entirely of learning. We learn what we are, and we become what we learn – so it is with the world. Although he may abjure explicit information science formulation, the behaviourist is more radically anti-absolutist than the cognitive therapist. Rationality itself is learned, therefore has no more right to stand above the rest of life than any other acquired habit. Pleasure and pain, ease and disease become the sole markers of what is true and what is not. If there were not the emphasis on sociality then we would have a truely Sadean amorality in which nothing was true and everything was permitted. However, behaviourism acknowledges a social framework which shapes our desires and their expression from the start, therefore the radical individualism of De Sade could never get off the ground within this network of mutual control and oppression.

However, Sadean morality flavours radical behaviourism. The most recent formulations see no difference between changing a problem behaviour and changing the context in which the behaviour is problematic. Theoretically, wishing to kill is only problematic because the desire occurs in a context in which it is prohibited. Only the relative lack of killer-friendly contexts would render changing the context an untenable solution to this problem.

It is a charge aimed often at deconstructionism – having outed all absolutes as *contingencies with megalomania* how can one then have any universal values, how can ethics be generated? Being a philosophy, deconstruction is forced to answer. Behaviourism is not required to address this because it does not see a problem.

Summary

I shall now conclude this section with a summary of the content of each of the three competing schools, following which, in the next section, I will outline a framework with which we can closer scrutinise them.

TABLE 22.1 Summary of the three competing schools

	Psychoanalysis	Cognitive therapy	Behavioural therapy
The therapeutic relationship	For analysis the therapeutic relationship is a paradigmatic one in which other relationships are worked through.	One of collaborative empiricism in which the therapist and client enter into a joint testing and reform of the client's self.	A structure in which to provide information and rehearse techniques for the alleviation of disease.
The therapist	Almost shamanic, has been through the process and has a special understanding of himself which allows impartiality in aiding self-understanding. A *tabula rasa* for the client's neuroses.	A thought technician and Socratic philosopher. Employs rational techniques to aid the client in unearthing their assumptions. Not necessarily been through therapy himself.	A vehicle for transmission of knowledge, personal qualities fairly unimportant in that function could be performed by a book or a computer. A source of expertise.
Neuroses	Result of unresolved conflicts from childhood, unconsciously suppressed and played out in daily life. A sign of something deeper.	Result of a less useful way of thinking about the self or the world, generated by implicit dysfunctional assumptions.	Acquired pattern of responding to particular cues which becomes self-maintaining through avoidance of cues. Origins unimportant/unknowable.
Cure	Excavation of meaning and significance and theatrical restaging of conflict in the arena of therapy.	Rational excavation of assumptions and challenging/testing of them, both in and out with therapy.	Gradual confrontation with feared cues leading to reduction in anxiety. Mainly out with therapy.
Mind	Contains distinct systems, largely unconscious and often irrational, which are in varying degrees of conflict. Powered by basic drives and guided by complex transformations as one area impinges insidiously on another.	Essentially rational and propositional. More innate inaccessible beliefs generate the contents of consciousness by transformation through deductive logic.	A more private realm of behaviour whose consequences are less open to reinforcement. Consciousness is to behaviour as the commentary is to the football game. An unreliable and not particularly useful concept.

TABLE 22.1 Continued

	Psychoanalysis	Cognitive therapy	Behavioural therapy
Behaviour	Always meaningful, often symptomatic and dictated by inner drives which consciousness is unaware of. Slippery customer.	The result of beliefs, the confirmation or refutation of mental hypothesis. Secondary to cognitions.	The index of the individual – to be is to do. A repertoire of learned responses to maximise efficacy in the lived environment. Prior to consciousness.
Well/Less Well	Uncovering one's conflicts and being aware of the demons that have driven one's behaviour up to then. This is good. Bad is the continuing re-enactment of old problems in new situations.	A normative hierarchy of cognitions. Good ones are efficacious, make you feel better about yourself and your situation. Bad ones whisper poison in your inner ear and are called 'dysfunctional'.	Having less anxiety is good. Receiving reinforcement from the environment is good. More anxiety is bad. So is not being reinforced.

TOWARDS AN ETHICAL APPRAISAL

In attempting to lay the ground for an ethical appraisal of the therapeutic schools, I am in danger of writing myself into an ideological corner. By adopting a style of exposition which is post-absolutist, which emphasises the cultural contingency of truth creation, I am hard pushed to then defend any standpoint from which an ethical appraisal could be attempted. This ethical impotency is a feature of much discourse labelled as post-modern; by emphasising the relativity of all discursive practices, it cannot allow itself a privileged site from which to choose between them. From this position the most we could say is pick the ideology that best suits you.

I will attempt two strategies to escape this impasse. First, I will contend that there are key concepts and practices that all the therapeutic schools share, and that these can provide us with, at least, a useful standpoint from which to exercise our ethical scrutiny and scepticism. Second, I will contend that all ideology requires a framework of communicative rationality in which to propagate itself, and that we should judge ideology by the degree to which it deforms this framework. The latter standpoint is taken from the work of Habermas.

Talking yourself into a job

The most fundamental shared concept between the therapies is that it is 'good to talk'. This has become such a cultural commonplace that we often mistake it for a given truth. There are few who would argue *for* the non-confession of feeling or for the therapeutic neglect of problems. Although, if we are to maintain our ethical suspicion, we should bear in mind that a shift in culture or time presents us with a more relativised prospect. It is not always believed that we must be free of psychic turmoil, or that we need experts to be so. Perhaps, therefore, the standard in this context by which we should evaluate therapies is not so much the extent to which a therapy helps someone to talk, as the extent to which it helps someone talk appropriately, if, indeed, talking *is* appropriate.

The growth of the therapy market can also be seen as a process of professional colonisation, the creation of a therapeutic workload – therapists need problems. The preceding text has not emphasised the strategies of client procurement that therapy employs, but they are key to its growth. I think we can see this most clearly by placing therapy in the context of the growth of medicine.

The good life

Medicine no longer stops at our skin. It has gradually extended its territory to ever more intimate regions of our body and behaviour. The colonisation of mind begun with psychoanalysis extended the medical paradigm into our most intimate realm – our relation to ourself. This importation disqualifies us as experts about ourselves and consequently, creates a culture of externalised value. Medicine and therapy would have us consult it about our most basic acts – how to breathe, how and what to eat, how to talk to others, how to act towards our children, etc. By claiming this as expert knowledge the therapeutic movement creates the need for itself. It also defines the terms of its own efficiency. As noted above, all therapies have an idea of the better adjusted individual/relationship/family which they suggest to us, thereby creating the need for expert assistance in achieving this adjustment.

Historically we can see the dissemination of this expertise from doctors to psychologists, from psychologists to nurses. We should not let this partial professional democratisation of knowledge blind us to the fact that it is predicated on the idea that you need expert assistance to live the good life. This chapter has not touched upon the bewildering proliferation of alternative therapies, of social work, of self-help manuals or on the juridical colonisation of the private realm. Suffice to say that all function on the same premise that we need to be told how to live the good life.

This dissemination of therapeutic claims, its advertising, also has the effect of decreasing the threshold of intervention for therapy. We are now all relentlessly bombarded with images of attainable mental health, in the same way that women (and now men) have been bombarded with the image of the perfectible body. This creates unease with one's less then perfect state and encourages us to turn to the experts to bring us to the level of perfection that they have insisted we attain. Thus therapy actively solicits clients, manufactures the need for itself.

An example may be illustrative. A study in Canada looked at the psychological treatment of a group of 'somatisers' – people who expressed stress by manifesting physical ailments. Therapy aimed at raising their awareness of this particular coping style had the dubious effect of decreasing their somatic symptoms but increasing their subjective psychological distress. Although an ideological point is proven, a therapy furthered, its benefit is questionable.

Here there may be a useful critical standpoint from which to make an ethical evaluation of therapies. Does the therapy support us taking the stand that it may not be necessary? As practitioners we have a vested interest in procuring clients, in selling our ideological panaceas. As consumers we are well advised to be wary of anyone with something to sell.

Evaluating expert cultures

Habermas has argued that in the twentieth century grand ideological narratives (such as religion) have been superseded by focal expert cultures. Rather than comment on the whole of being, these cultures colonise one of its aspects and attempt to monopolise its understanding. In therapy we see this in the commodification of personal experience. Knowledge of anxiety, interpersonal strife, self-understanding are taken from the individual and sold back to them in the therapy market-place. The proliferation of focal expertise marks our century. More and more areas of our life are defined and dealt with by specific professions.

As individuals we are dis-empowered by this. If our lives require expert assistance, yet we are not experts, then we are beholden to 'those who know'. To re-empower the individual Habermas argues for a public forum of ideological evaluation. To undertake this evaluation we must understand, or believe, two things: 'There's no such things as a private language' and 'Experts mystify'.

'There is no such thing as a private language'

Any idea attempting to sell itself, indeed, any act of intersubjective communication must refer to a context of mutual understanding. In speaking to others, we believe that they will know what we mean. In writing texts we assume that our points can be conveyed more or less well, be understood by the reader. Habermas contends that a meta-structure of communicative rationality is implied in *any* act of communication, that its value as communicative act derives from the founding rationality of all communicative action. This rationality provides our site for ideological evaluation. If we are importuned by a belief or value, its worth is to be decided in rational public debate, in which the assumptions of the belief or value are open to scrutiny, where its validity claims can be tested and judged.

Again an example. Medicine, more than therapy, has become increasingly subject to public and state scrutiny, has had to answer to an external evaluative gaze. There are two key factors behind this. One, the importation of market ideology into medicine has necessitated that its practices be based on empirically validated criteria. Two, the increasing medical literacy of the public has put medical expertise into question. This is particularly pronounced in HIV/AIDS culture where medical impotence has resulted in individuals making their own therapeutic decisions, based on public access to relevant research. The doctor becomes a consultant, rather than a dictator.

Another key theme in evaluating therapies should thus be the extent of public access to information, whether the validity of any expertise is up for public appraisal.

Experts mystify

To retain its position as an expert culture, public access must be limited. By dressing itself in jargon, by locating itself in institutions, by equating understanding with initiation, expert knowledge attempts to keep itself beyond public scrutiny. Only by this sequestration of knowledge can it maintain its ideological and financial position.

This creates the necessity for a class of initiated professionals to acquire and dispense the arcane knowledge, to translate it for the public. If the knowledge was easily accessible, the status of the professions would be undermined. As such ideologies have an interest in keeping their validity claims beyond the public reach, they systematically deform rational communication by withholding from it the criteria by which the ideology stands to be judged. This is a job for experts.

Again, an example, in this case of how dissemination of 'expert' knowledge empowers individual decision. A group of men who had been recommended to have a prostate operation were split into two trial groups. One was given the conventional medical counselling, the other had access to a CD-ROM interactive programme in which all the known facts about prostrate operations were laid out and accessible. The latter group had a significantly higher refusal rate of the operation, thus informed.

If the last evaluative principle related to access to information, the principle here is surely accessibility *of* information. We should be wary of being told you wouldn't understand', particularly when the subject is ourself. Put simply, *anything that can be said, can be said clearly.*

With these four evaluative standards, first, how 'appropriately' the consumer is helped to talk, second, how far they are encouraged to question their need for therapy, third, how much access the therapy allows to information about how it operates, and finally, how accessible is that information once received, we may attempt an informed ethical judgement.

CONCLUSION: EVALUATING THERAPIES

Each therapeutic school has its own internal validation. Psychoanalysis would argue that it dispenses personal meaning, cognitive therapy that it is efficacious, behavioural therapy that its is empirically validated. All maintain their expert strongholds.

The aim of this chapter has been to lay the grounds for an ethical evaluation of therapy and its choosing. In the first section I presented a version of why and how we came to turn to doctors and therapists to seek ourselves in them. I have thus attempted to set the evaluation in a historical/ideological context.

In the second section I outlined the kind of selves we might encounter from three leading brands of therapy. In the final section I have outlined the form of this evaluation. I have suggested a decision procedure by which we could, as individuals, state or broker, begin to choose between therapies, making a rational and public appraisal of the validity claims of the ideologies involved. I presume the consumers of this book will be health professionals, purveyors of ideology, the beneficiaries of disease. The implication of the above for us is simple – *invite scrutiny.*

And if any of our customers should happen upon this book then let them remember – *abuse of power should come as no surprise.*

REFERENCES

Bateson, G. 1979: *Mind and nature*: Unnecessary Unity. London: Wildwood House.
Comte, A. 1842: *Course de philosophie positive*. Paris: Bachelier.

Dawkins, R. 1988: *The extended phenotype*. London: Macmillan.

Dreyfus, H.L. and **Raninov, P.** 1982; *Michel Foucault: Beyond Structuralism and Hermaneutics* (2nd edn). Chicago: University of Chicago Press.

Du Preez, P. 1991: *A science of the mind*. London: Academic Press.

The Economist, May 13–19 1995, pp. 125–6.

Eysenck, H.J. and **Wilson, G.D.** 1973: *The Experimental Study of Freudian Theories*. London.

Freud, S. 1910: *Two Short Accounts of Psychoanalysis*. London: Pelican (1960).

Jung, C. 1935: *Analytic psychology*. London: Ark.

Lang, P. 1977: Imagery and therapy: An information processing analysis of fear. *Behaviour Therapy* 8, 862–86.

O'Donohue, W. and **Smith, L.D.** 1992: Philosophical and psychological epistemologies in behaviourism and behavioural therapy. *Behaviour Therapy* 23, 173–94.

Piaget, J. 1952: *The origins of intelligence in children*. New York: International Universities Press.

Rachmann, S. 1990: *Fear and courage*. New York: W.H. Freeman and Company.

Skinner, B. 1945: The operationalist analysis of psychological terms. *Psychological Review* 52, 270–7.

Skinner, B. 1984: Selection by consequences. *Brain and Behavioural Sciences*. 7, 477–510.

Valentine, E. 1990: *Conceptual issues in psychology*. London: Routledge.

23

REFRAMING THE EXPERIENCE OF AIDS: MARGINALISATION, LIMINALITY AND BEYOND[1]

John Daniel

Here John Daniel offers an account of his experience from both sides of the fence of mental health world. Contrasting the restrictive attitudes of some mental health clinicians with the empowering nature of self-help methods such as the Twelve Step approach, John draws on his own past journey through addiction, depression and other mental health problems to inform and reconstruct his present journey into the unknown territory of a terminal illness through AIDS. The themes endorsed throughout the text reappear in this chapter: the potential for abuse of interpersonal power in professional relationships, the political and spiritual potential of developing an alternative approach to understanding mental distress: the politics and the pilgrimage of breakdown and breakthrough. The point is emphasised that any ideology which can be manipulated, can equally well be used to (ethically) good effect. The theme re-emerges that telling one's story, restructuring creatively one's understanding of oneself (one's 'personal ideology') where appropriate, but always remaining true to one's experience, is essential to the pursuit of integrity and an ethical life.

HIGH

I had felt uncomfortable immediately on walking into the room for the counselling session. Besides the two chairs there were mattresses and lengths of rubber tubing and battered telephone directories. What concerned me, though, was the pot plant, which was having a difficult time staying alive. I remembered a Woody Allen quip: Never trust a doctor with dying pot plants in his consultation rooms. Did that apply to counsellors, I wondered.

'But you must be angry,' said the counsellor, as we got into the session. 'You have just received a positive HIV diagnosis.' I knew the moment I confessed to feelings of

---

[1] This chapter is dedicated to the psychiatrist, Dr Rosanne Varley, at the Royal Free Hospital, London.

anger he would have me beating the shit out of the mattresses with the rubber tubing.

'But I do feel something,' I said. 'I feel exaltation.'

He was beginning to look slightly at sea. The session was not going as planned.

In fact the feeling of exaltation had been my immediate response when the doctor had said, 'I am sorry to tell you that you have a positive result'. That dizziness, almost a feeling of vertigo, hadn't left me. It was a month ago that I had received the diagnosis. I was, though, beginning to feel slightly anxious that I harboured some underlying death wish, which was beginning only now to surface. Wasn't I meant to feel rage? Or despair? Or at least fear? Did I have the same ambition as Quentin Crisp, who, when asked, stated that his only ambition in life was to be a chronic invalid? Is that what I wanted?

'Exaltation,' said the counsellor. 'That's a difficult one,' and crossed his arms and legs.

'Aha,' I thought, 'Body language. He feels threatened.'

Silence filled the room. The counsellor surreptitiously began to look at the clock behind me, then beseechingly at me, willing me to have other, more manageable feelings.

The minutes passed and the session was at an end.

'I can offer you another appointment next week,' he said. He looked relieved when I said I would think about it and give him a ring. The filofax was firmly shut. Clearly, he felt out of depth in relation to my experience.

'Exaltation', said Susan Sonntag, 'was my initial response to my diagnosis of breast cancer. I realised that a very complicated and at times empty life had become somehow simplified and somehow fuller. I really only had one thing to worry about. My illness' (Sontag, 1989). The word 'exaltation' conveys a very powerful feeling. It seems Emily Dickinson had in mind something of a powerfully exalted journey into the unknown when she wrote:

> Exaltation is the going
> Of the inland soul to sea –
> Past the houses past the headlands
> Into deep eternity
>
> Bred as we are among the mountains
> Can the sailor understand –
> The divine intoxication
> Of the first leagues out at sea?

(Dickinson, 1995)

I was certainly in unchartered territory, if not completely at sea.

The counsellor was obviously uncomfortable with my feelings of exaltation. To have accepted them he would have had to redefine his understanding of the initial emotional response to a positive HIV diagnosis. This, he was unprepared or unable to do. The non-verbal and not so non-verbal expectation was that if I could only experience anger, we could start at a point in the emotional landscape that to him was intelligible and non-threatening.

As the next year or two progressed, I tried many self-help, radical therapies. I read literature that questioned the role of HIV in causing AIDS. I went to Scotland on a gay men's week and spent much of the time running through the forest naked, trying to contact nature spirits. And I came back to London with probably the worst bout of flu I have had. I learnt to meditate, to visualise, to practise positive thinking. I danced with the Sufis, chanted with the Buddhists, sang at Christian healing services and sat at the feet of Holy Mothers. But the pathway grew dark.

Low

'Crisis,' said the psychiatrist, 'You're in crisis. We need to intervene to bring the crisis to an end'. That sounded hopeful. I had heard of crisis intervention therapy. It was a few years later. The exaltation had passed and a dark despair threatened to engulf me. My doctor at the HIV clinic had referred me to this psychiatrist when I expressed suicidal thoughts. *Suicidal ideation,* I believe he called it, which made me feel important. Such ideation took the form of a kind of gay Hari Kari, a sort of ritual disembowelling of myself on Hampstead Heath. But I suspected that once there, I would become distracted by other activities.

'I see from your notes that you had two periods of depression in your twenties, one requiring admission to hospital,' said the psychiatrist. That was true. The first had occurred in my mid-twenties, when I began the process of coming to terms with my sexuality. It had been a difficult time. The guilt and the shame provoked by my realisation that I was homosexual were probably due in great part to my earlier involvement in Catholicism. I recall how, much earlier, an episode of induced guilt had occurred when I once went to a rather elderly priest for confession. I confessed the sin of impurity. He suggested that as a young man there would be this tendency to self-abuse, so I should get into the habit of saying the Hail Mary at the point of orgasm. I couldn't do it then and I can't do it now. While struggling to accept my sexuality I did go into a very deep depression and was treated with Parnate, a monoamine oxidase inhibitor. It had a miraculous effect. Within six months I had a job, a flat and I had successfully 'come out'. But the depression returned in my late twenties. At this time I was medicating the depression with alcohol and illegal drugs. I was admitted to hospital and given IV anti-depressant therapy. Anafronil was put into an intra-venous infusion and over a period of two hours it was administered directly into my bloodstream. I remember we had to go to the basement of the hospital to a tiny room, which only reinforced the feelings of powerlessness and shame around the depression. The treatment didn't work. I left as depressed as when I had been admitted. Drinking and drugging still helped to medicate the depression, while sexual addiction, to which I was sailing perilously close, began to provide another elixir.

'I think we need to deal first with the depression, so let's try you on Prozac.' He wrote a prescription, gave it to me and stood up rather purposefully. I realised the session was over. 'I'll see you in a month,' he said.

As I walked along the corridor, following the exit signs, I knew this was not the answer, not this time. I could accept I was in crisis, certainly, at some sort of turning point. But I felt I wasn't getting the understanding to negotiate this difficult terrain.

DANGER AND OPPORTUNITY

The first socio-physiological definition of crisis, attributed to Thomas (1909), defined crisis as a threat, a challenge, a strain on the attention and a call to new action, within which lay the germ of new organisation within the psyche.

The most influential contribution to crisis theory comes from the work of Caplan (1957). This theory is based on the concept of emotional homeostasis. An individual confronted with a hazardous situation, which threatens to upset the balance of his emotional functioning, may find resolution through his usual or characteristic problem-solving skills. If, however, the hazard is of such magnitude or the situation so unrelenting that it cannot be mastered by his customary techniques, his emotional functioning will be disturbed, and so he experiences crisis. Caplan recognised that this state of crisis presents unparalleled opportunities for internal boundary realignment, for the acquisition of new ways of coping, and in so doing he recognised the constructive potential of crisis.

The Chinese symbol for crisis combines two pictographs, one standing for danger and one for opportunity. Crisis consists, in part, in the search for a resolution of such dangerous opportunities. Crisis is not itself a pathological state because it presents the opportunity for personal growth if a constructive resolution is achieved. Present crisis also offers the opportunity for resolution of old conflicts, deriving in turn from the maladaptive solutions of earlier crises.

This attempt to elicit potential meaning and the search for a solution was evidently a force very strong within me. Even within the despair I knew I was being presented with something that had the potential for effecting change and growth. Danger, I realised, lurked within the response that saw my situation as only pathological, and therefore needing treatment. Opportunity, as the Chinese had realised, was also present. I wasn't quite sure what opportunity was hidden within my situation, but it was almost like a response of faith. I knew something was there. I reflected that in medicine up to about thirty years ago, crisis was the turning point in illness: either the patient's own defences would overcome the disease or he would succumb and die. I felt like that patient, but the problem was I also intuited that the physician's expectations were that I would succumb. Cooper (1979) wrote 'many individuals feel that the conventional, and often well developed medical and psychiatric services miss out something important'. This something, I have come to believe, is the presence of opportunity.

I stepped out into the crisp air of an October afternoon, the prescription for Prozac in my hand. I walked to the bus stop. There was a litter bin. Slowly, I tore the prescription up and watched it fall into the bin. I wanted, I knew there must be, another way.

Depression is a major factor in living with a positive diagnosis. I suspect that a large proportion of gay men have had the tendency towards depression prior to an HIV diagnosis, though I would not take quite the gloomy view of researchers at John Hopkins Hospital, Baltimore, in 1993, published in a paper called 'Depressive symptoms as predictors of medical outcome in HIV infection', which states confidently that 'a lifetime history of depression is common in all patients afflicted with HIV'. Research conducted by the Centre of Health Economics team at Hull and York Universities suggests that 55 per cent of all gay men living with HIV are clinically depressed, and this will often rise during bouts of illness to 69 per cent.

When diagnosed, there were two areas that I had to negotiate. First I felt that a hex had been placed on me, rather like a voodoo curse. With the current data then available, HIV meant you first became a victim, then a corpse. This led to a feeling of futility and loss of hope. In his study of helplessness, Seligman (1975) makes the comment that when a person is faced with an outcome that is independent of his responses, he *learns* (experientially) that the outcome is independent of his responses. The trauma of diagnosis and this subsequent learning certainly led in my case to increased feelings of helplessness. Seligman would link this learnt helplessness with unpredictability, and unpredictability is beyond doubt a significant aspect of living with HIV. It is common to develop symptoms and for the medical profession to be unsure as to the cause. As a doctor said to me, 'this virus seems to obey the laws of chaos'. Unpredictability is writ large. Why do some die after only a few years infection, and others are healthy and strong after 15 years? Is it the strength of the virus, tissue type, cognitive factors? It is all very unpredictable. The final outcome, though, is an issue that is somewhat more certain and has to be faced.

In many ways this whole process is a vicious circle. In coming to terms with HIV the individual experiences feelings of helplessness, exacerbated by the sense of unpredictability and maladaptation. This leads to emotional exhaustion and so begins a spiral of learned helplessness. This, according to Seligman, results in depression. The underlying belief is that action is futile. You're going to die anyway, a pretty awful death, after years descending into physical and mental disintegration.

The problem here lies not just with the individual, but also with the professions that are approached for help and support. Much psychiatry and psychotherapy, often seemingly benign, promotes helplessness and dependence. Their unconscious influence is exacerbation of the experience. Such psychological helplessness then increases the risk of death. When animals and men learn that their actions are futile and pointless, death often follows, preceded usually by deep depression. At this stage of my journey with HIV, to have taken the medication would have been, in my opinion, an acceptance of helplessness and a collusion in a sort of psychogenic death.

At the time, though, I began to wonder why I had such a resistance to being helped. In accepting care I would have had a clearly definable role, imposed from without, maybe, but still a role. However, the role available to me was one in which I was denied a self-determining future. It was this that I now know I was rejecting.

As the initial phases of exaltation and then helplessness passed, I began to see my life as a journey. And so I looked at various maps that might help me to understand the terrain in which I found myself. Looking at psychological maps of change I found them complex and detailed, though they tended to agree on two points. First, change is a process, and it is possible to define stages or phases within it. Second, the experience of change is potentially both creative and destructive. The major problem, I found, was this distinction between creative and destructive, that one moved through a period of a rocky territory and eventually arrived at a point of integration, of creativity or reorientation and acceptance. I found that both psychological and spiritual maps tended to point in the same direction: after traversing dark nights of soul and sense, one moves into a unitive state. Or, after a process of purgation, one moves into a state of illumination. It was this expectation of final freedom from conflict that I found disturbing. Although perhaps resonating nicely with my inherent optimism, these approaches evidently fail to take into account fully that HIV leads eventually to increased fragility and loss. The list of physical problems are daunting and overwhelming. When the threat of dementia is added, one can feel completely in the grips of a voracious taker of life. It is a very potent mix. To talk of integration, reorientation or illumination at the end of such a process seemed at best wishful thinking, at worst a cruel joke.

A NEW MAP

In the failure of existing maps, I began to form my own. A concept emerged that I felt might resolve the tension between these two themes. The only word I felt that could express the journey through HIV, particularly its ending, was *chaos*. There had to be a way to live creatively with this chaos. Chaos was what was happening, it was reality and therefore had to be guarded and embraced. If that was possible, then perhaps a new map could be drawn. After all, chaos is by its very nature unpredictable. To accept the chaos is not just to view one's situation as irredeemable disaster, but to actively work within it.

One day while idly searching in the library, I came across a text powerfully entitled *Guard the chaos* (Ward and Wild, 1990), which resonated with my experiences. The book itself was a study of women and the woman's experience of being marginalised, by authors who were apparently well qualified to write on this subject. As a result, two new words entered my vocabulary: marginality and liminality.

Marginality

The concept of marginalisation was something I began to explore. Maybe wrongly at the time I equated marginalisation with victimhood. One of the overpowering feelings when sitting in the HIV clinic was one that we were all victims: victims of a sexuality that was unacceptable; victims of a culture that had been unable to form itself into a community; and now victims of a virus.

However, there had always probably been a degree of marginalisation within my life. Born into a fairly arid, Protestant family, I flamboyantly converted to Catholicism in my late teens. This effectively marginalised me within the family structure. In keeping with the co-dependency implicit in much of what passes as Christianity, I then made a decision that my life from then on would consist of helping others. So with a degree of self-regarding drama, I launched into situations where I was the helper, whether with the homeless, the mentally ill, the alcoholic, or the sick, tending always those on the margins of society. I took with me this same paternalistic philosophy of care into my training as a nurse, RGN and RMN. I maintained a rigid distinction: there were the sick and there were the well. And across the divide I was with the well.

This shaky edifice crumbled, as I have already described, during two significant bouts of depression, the latter unremitting and only alleviated through various forms of addiction. In my early thirties I discovered recovery from alcoholism and drug dependency within the twelve-step movements, movements that operate as a democratic community of brokenness, moving towards a visions of wholeness. Rejecting all outside professional help, one experiences within these movements a process whereby brokenness and marginalisation are effectively transformed. From my earlier philosophy, where I saw myself as one of the well, then as one of the sick, I was now moving within a process where I was both the sick and the well. My experience of living this integrative approach of recovery and taking responsibility contributed greatly to my increasing unease, during the years that followed my HIV diagnosis, with the services on offer.

There is a great deal of talk today about margins and fringes. The margins are said to be the place of the prophet, the victim, the oppressed, the creative and the eccentric. Being on the margins has, for some, become a vocation. The language of marginality has provided a meaningful way of seeing and talking about the experience of not fitting in. There is, however, a negative side to this language and imagery. To define oneself as marginalised is to define oneself in relation to another's definition of the centre. And, as mentioned, it is to have a future defined by others. To be marginalised is also to be the recipient of projections from the centre. These three points I realise were powerfully at work within the psychiatric and psychotherapeutic professions. To keep one safely on the margins is effectively to disempower and violate the capacity for growth. The capacity of the client to initiate and follow through his own healing, in whatsoever form that might take, is discouraged. The abusive potential of therapy in this respect is great, in so far as the prospective client is encouraged to adopt another's definition of his experience. In doing so the interests of the carer and society at large are served. Those in the centre will continue to marginalise and keep marginalised those perceived as a threat. This process was demonstrated recently in a well-known HIV centre when, one afternoon, a group of lads were happily watching television, only to be disturbed by a troupe of volunteers, who had returned from rather a grand funeral, laden with flowers. With suitable solemnity and to the disbelief of the residents, they decorated the sitting room with the funereal bouquets, modifying the atmosphere from that of an enjoyable social space to that of a chapel of rest. Pedestrians four floors below were no doubt mystified a short while later to find themselves showered with carnations, lilies and chrysanthemums.

Redefining, depriving someone of their feelings, as above where the counsellor was apparently compelled to reframe the feelings I was presenting, is one of the first steps in creation of victimhood. Once victims, people can be pitied. And so begins again, with each interpersonal encounter based on such distance, the process of marginalisation, enhanced by the fact that the centre wants to keep you firmly on the edge.

Liminality

I drew on the work of Van Gennep (1979), who coined the term *liminality*. Liminality can best be described as an ambiguous, sacred, social state, in which a person or group of persons are separated for a time from the normal structure of society. The title of his seminal work was *Rites of passage*. Rite was defined as an action which accompanies every change of place, state, social position and age. Rites of passage mark time when structural patterns of society are rattled by movement. One of the key functions of a rite of passage is that it facilitates positive change by giving it a definition and a shape. I realised my HIV diagnosis and the changes that were happening to me were a rite of passage. Unfortunately, there seemed to be an incapacity to manage this change both by myself, among my friends and on the part of professionals. There is evidently no existing rite to mark these changes.

Van Gennep distinguished three phases which mark a rite of passage. First, separation; secondly, marginalisation and liminality; and finally, agreation. The map I am proposing slightly changes and extends this. I put separation and marginality as the first stage; liminality, being on the threshold, as the second stage; and agreation, or as I propose to call it, *active boundary living*, as the final stage.

It is this move into liminality that I believe is discouraged and feared by society and particularly care-givers, as representatives of that society. Why? Liminality is to be on the threshold. It is to be at the doorway. The person at the doorway is weak because he is not part of the social group inside. But he is also powerful, precisely because of his unknown quality. Because of this ambiguity involved in liminality, it is often difficult to relate to someone in this place. They are often a repository of our fears and awe, precisely because now they are neither of the centre nor comfortably marginalised by the centre. They are, effectively, between the structures of society. *Between* would also seem to relate to another characteristic of liminality. Liminality is characterised by disorder and chaos. Mary Douglas explains:

> Granted that disorder spoils pattern, it also provides the materials of pattern. Order implies restriction from all possible materials, a limited selection has been made, and from all possible relations a limited set has been used. So disorder, by implication, is unlimited, no pattern has been realised within it, but its patterning is indefinite. That is why, though we seek to create order, we do not simply condemn disorder. We recognise that it is destructive of existing patterns, but also that it has potentiality. It symbolises both danger and power.
>
> (Douglas, 1984)

The above counsel, to simply accept the chaos as a friend, may sound, like the other maps referred to above, at best abstract and trite, and at worst insulting, particularly when you consider the nature of this chaos in concrete terms. For me it had become a long, slow journey. Probably the most important factor in this journey was (and is) the amount of time spent being ill, staying in and going to bed. Feelings surface again and again of being outside the norm, that there is a society which functions *out there*, of which one has been part, but is no longer. Indeed, currently working to complete this chapter to a deadline at the instruction of my editor, and at the same time experiencing a number of health problems both irritating and fearful, I feel very much more inclined to take to my bed and give up, despite all manner of support, encouragement and other inducement. But there is still the need to be able to put a meaning onto that experience.

The worlds of illness and chronic illness are different from the world of the well. As one gets sicker it is as if a parallel universe starts to develop within one's life. With such a 'niggly' illness as HIV, minor infections and accidents happen which increase this sense of alienation from the norm – like throwing up in a restaurant; or having a virulent attack of diarrhoea in the street, while wearing white trousers; or meeting a group of friends to go to the theatre, well protected with incontinence pads: one feels set apart in this parallel universe. This type of illness is a dirty, messy process, but with the mess one does very slowly and painfully begin to extract meaning, and in so doing create one's own path.

The beginning of my path has been to feel exalted, depressed, emotionally overwhelmed, in crisis. As the days have passed I have felt ever more on the margins. And more recently I have felt increasingly that I am also on the threshold. The place of liminality is the place of change between one thing and another. It can be exciting, but it can also be terrifying. It is an experience of wilderness, a place untamed and uncultivated.

There is great energy here, but chaos is also powerfully represented in the annihilation promised by death. It is precisely within this realisation that death is inevitable, and that we and our world are more disordered and disintegrated than we can possibly imagine or cope with, that we become border people. It is some sort of alchemy, within the wilderness of liminal space, that creates the psychic energy and courage for the shift into active boundary living.

ACTIVE BOUNDARY LIVING

To speak of boundaries is to speak of being contained and of moving on. We have reached the border by travelling from within. Boundaries mark the end of something old and the beginning of something new. At the border we are exposed to two conflicting drives: to return to the safety of marginality; and at the same time to leave. It is said that no one can live permanently on the borders, but I suspect that living with HIV and AIDS, one learns to do just that.

At the border one is asked to account for oneself. What are your assets? How much currency do you have? Do you have a passport? Anything to declare? Do you carry goods? This is to be exposed and vulnerable, to live within the chaos of a destiny out of one's control. Once having gone through, it is also to be undeclared, to live without familiar structures such as currency, passport, visa. It is to pass into new territory with the loss of identity. Until we can establish, build and acknowledge a new identity, the past identity may be clung to, but increasingly seems untenable and unreal. Marking boundaries is at one and the same time an attempt to establish and realise this new identity. It is to turn on its head Seligman's helplessness. Often, when we refuse to be categorised or labelled by others, the centre will say our conduct is beyond the bounds of reason. We are outside and may be acting according to our own reason, indecipherable perhaps to those within the centre. In accepting the energy generated in border country, which involves the full realisation of death and disorder and disintegration, one approaches, I believe, a state of fullness. Fullness of darkness, of misery and persecution, but also fullness of life and joy. All of us find it hard to be confronted by such fullness.

The border is not so much a place; more a moment of awakening and an acceptance of space between worlds, between reality and unreality, between health and sickness, between body and spirit. The Tibetan Buddhist tradition uses the word *bardo* to describe this state, *bardo* literally meaning 'gap' and referring also to the 'in-between' state following death and prior to reincarnation in another life. Border living is about being uprooted, about going beyond the limits of one's previous domain, about making contact with a new source of power beyond the opposites. For this to occur though, reality, including the experience of impermanence, fragility, unpredictability and ostracism, must be fully embraced, an embrace within which we may find the energy we need to burn to have the courage to continue on.

My journey from marginality, through liminality, into active boundary living, has involved the shaping of a role which is different, distinct and separate from the cultural norm. Sometimes one feels that one has been cast out. Border living involves a certain solitariness and this brings to mind Whitehead's (1937) definition of religion as 'what the individual does with his solitariness'. 'If you are never solitary,' he writes,' 'you are never religious' (Leclerc, 1958). The border is a place of revelation, encounter and change. Without identities or other status bestowed from the centre, one can only trust and respond to the impulse that says this is the way.

CONCLUSION

If therapists, psychiatrists and nurses can begin to understand and respect this new map, and those that journey on it, then I believe they can accompany and support a person dealing with the tensions that this undertaking necessarily involves. Psychiatry and psychotherapy could contribute to the process by initiating and creating rites of passage. This might prove to be slightly more affirming than being handed benefits and a washing machine.

In many ways I do now 'know the place from [which I] started, for the first time' (Elliot). At the border we have a chance to validate and recognise professional authority in a new form and guise. I have an excellent analyst with whom I work, a psychiatrist who is supportive, a hospital doctor I trust and respect, and an excellent GP. As a border person I need courage and I need their support. The operative words are 'work with'. We work with each other and in discussion they help me to achieve goals and aims that are realistic. I have no problem now with taking anti-depressant medication if I need it. The view, I feel, from the border, standing alone as an equal, is very, very different to the view from the margins, where one is an outcast. The experience of HIV border people is dwelling in the shadows of the chaos of death. Yet it is also to refuse to act as passive victim and to be treated solely as object of compassion. This is a challenge to the centre and to the professions of care, with their sense of goodness, power and control. As one at times still vibrantly alive, I feel disinclined just passively to ebb away; my life is one of love and reconciliation, alongside fear and destruction. It is said that for the Buddhist the concept of the resurrection after the crucifixion is meaningless, because the crucifixion *is* the resurrection. Fear from the centre manifests subtly.

It was six months ago that I went to a respite unit after a particularly virulent chest infection. On discharge, a very concerned doctor offered me a home help, meals on wheels, a community psychiatric nurse, a social worker, a laundry service, an incontinence service and a bottle of sleeping tablets. I refused all and went on a Buddhist retreat instead.

Finally putting this chapter together and seeing the form it has taken, I realise that I have finished on the fairly upbeat note, taking the bull of HIV and AIDS by the horn, actively creating the role of a *border person*. Since starting this piece, and now, I have been encountering some very serious health difficulties, including a drop in my CD4 count (measuring immunity), a significant and frightening drop. I have developed constant night sweats and an ongoing sense of fatigue, neither of which had troubled me a few months back. My earlier working and living concepts of developing through marginality and liminality into a bright border state have taken a large knock. I have begun to realise that, valid and useful though such ideas are, no amount of intellec-tualising can defend against the grimness and sheer messiness of this disease. Border country or no, the terrain where 10 per cent of those with HIV will probably dement and 40 per cent will totally lose bowel control is a sorrowful and bleak place. I say HIV – this is accurate in terms of UK classification; but if I were resident in America I am aware that the mere fact of a CD4 count below 200 would define my condition as AIDS.

The failure of psychiatric and other maps is the failure of all concerned, including the infected person, to put into context the grimness and the potential of HIV. Psychiatric nurses pride themselves on caring *for* and *about* people, with all manner of problems, including HIV and AIDS. The ethical nettle which they must grasp involves exploring their capacity to care *with* people. Among other things this involves accepting, as I now do, that it just is how it is and will be what it will be. Perhaps the most any of us may dare to hope is that we remain true to our experience.

REFERENCES

Caplan, G. 1957: Influential contribution to the crisis theory. Quoted in *British Journal of Medical Psychology* 1984, **57**, 23–4.

Chester, R. *et al.* 1993. *Social care and HIV/Aids.* London: HMSO.

Cooper, J. 1979: Crisis, admission units and emergency psychiatric services. Quoted in *British Journal of Medical Psychology* 1984, **57**, 23–4.

Dickinson, E. 1995: *Selected poems of Emily Dickinson.* ed. E Hamilton. London: Bloomsbury.

Douglas, M. 1984; *Purity and danger: an analysis of the concepts of pollution and taboo.* London: Ark Books.

Leclerc, I. 1958: *Whitehead's metaphysics: an introductory exposition.* London: Allen & Unwin.

The Multicentre AIDS Cohort Study Group 1993: *Depressive symptoms as predictors of medical outcome in HIV infection.* Baltimore: Dept of Psychiatry and Behavioral Sciences, John Hopkins University.

Seligman, M. 1975: *Helplessness in depression, development and death.* New York: H. Freeman.

Sonntag, S. 1989: Television interview on *After Dark* on Channel Four.

Thomas, W. 1909: *A source book of local origins.* Boston: R. Gadger.

Van Gennep, A. 1979: *Rites of passage.* trans. M. Vizedon. London: Routledge and Kegan Paul.

Ward, and **Wild,** 1990: *Guard the chaos.*

24

THE WOUNDED HEALER AND THE MYTH OF MENTAL WELL-BEING: ETHICAL ISSUES CONCERNING THE MENTAL HEALTH STATUS OF PSYCHIATRIC NURSES

Phil Barker, Ed Manos, Vic Novak and Bill Reynolds

Returning to a theme underlined throughout the text, psychiatric nursing is based upon the development of nurse–patient relationships. Within these relationships, nurses may draw upon past life experiences to help them better understand the experiences of people in their care. In this text a number of nurses have been quite candid in their disclosures about mental health problems they have themselves suffered, and have advocated more disclosure of this sort from nurses and mental health workers generally. The contribution made by the concept of the wounded healer to the helping process within psychiatric nursing is reviewed. The authors consider the extent to which nurses are discouraged within orthodox mental health and psychiatric ideology from acknowledging their human frailties, and details the sort of responses which have been made to some nurses who have admitted to serious psychological or psychiatric problems. Their conclusions leave us with a bleak prospect of any potential for initiatives or progress in this area.

THE WOUNDED HEALER

The concept of the 'wounded healer' is well established in Western medicine. Several Greek myths involve individuals who carried wounds as an essential part of their being. Apollo was the Greek god of, among other things, archery and medicine. It was

Apollo who advised Telephus that his wound – caused by Achilles' spear – could only be healed by the weapon which caused it. Rust from Achilles' spear was applied to the wound which was duly healed. Frazer (1993) described this relationship between a wounded person and the agent of the wound as 'contagious magic' (p.41). The notion of the wounded healer is not, however, peculiar to Greek mythology. Frazer described a wide range of cultures, both ancient and modern, from Australian aborigines to English and German rustics, which possessed superstitions involving the ritualistic manipulation of the 'weapon' to ensure recovery from 'the wound'.

These myths and superstitions have given rise, in modern times, to the notion that within any healer lies a vulnerability which equates with the status of patient; and within any patient lies an equivalent capacity of healer. Theoretical explications of this harmonious relationship range from Jung's modern translation of the age-old notion of the archetype (Jung, 1964; Stevens, 1982) to transactional analysis models of human development and interaction (Zigmond, 1984). Albert Schweitzer suggested that this potential for self-healing might serve as the common ground between orthodox medicine and shamanism:

> the witch doctor succeeds for the same reason all the rest of us succeed. Each patient carries his own doctor inside him. They come to us knowing that truth. We are at our best when we give this doctor who resides within each patient a chance to go to work.
>
> (Cousins, 1979)

All such propositions emphasise the idea that healers can best facilitate the patient's self-healing by consciously recognising their own vulnerability. In keeping with the spirit of the Greek myths, the healer who has experienced pain or suffering – through personal loss, professional difficulties or illness – experiences the 'wound'. Providing that such human frailty and weakness can be accepted in full consciousness, this personal experience of suffering, in whatever form, can assist the healer in the practice of the art. This proposition, however, carries a negative corollary: the healer who fails to recognise, or cannot accept, the presence of an inherent vulnerability (wound) is sorely restricted in the practice of the art.

More recently, advocates within the mental health advocacy movement have developed this theme by suggesting that the direct experience of mental illness can be used, constructively, to facilitate developments in mental health services (Chamberlin, 1984; Fisher, 1992). If one accepts the proposition that human development is dependent upon experience, then the experience of what is called mental illness or mental ill-health may make a significant contribution to human development. Difficult circumstances may not ennoble a person but may reveal the person. This may well be one of the outcomes of the experience of mental ill-health.

If psychiatric nurses are involved in the pursuit of genuine understanding of the experience of mental illness, or are empathic towards the experience of mental distress, then such workers (be they nurses, doctors, psychologists or whatever) might be involved in developing an appreciation of their own 'wounds', if not also the part these wounds might play in the healing process. If mental health professionals believe that those with mental health problems can be distinguished easily from those without such problems, then they may fail to recognise the shadow which lurks within their unconscious. Jung suggested that it takes moral courage to acknowledge the presence of these aspects of human nature within us (the shadow). Failure to acknowledge our inherent weaknesses may serve only to strengthen them, resulting in a potential danger to ourselves and others should such forces be released through social and interpersonal pressures (Bennet, 1966).

Mental distress is often viewed as an experience to be avoided at all costs. Far from being a wholly negative experience, periods of mental distress may serve to render people more insightful and compassionate; better able to identify with the suffering of others. At least part of the nurse's responsibility is to seek to understand the patient's experience of illness and to empathise with that experience. Increasingly nurses emphasise concepts such as 'holism' and 'working in partnership' in relation to their practice. Now might be an appropriate time to consider the extent to which the concept of the wounded healer might be accommodated within the over-arching philosophy of psychiatric nursing practice. Perhaps nurses need to develop an appreciation of their own 'wounds', if not also the part such 'wounds' might play in the healing process. Such self-knowledge may be part of the development of genuine understanding of distress or the expression of empathy. When nurses fail to acknowledge their inherent vulnerability (woundedness) this may serve to strengthen such vulnerabilities, and may undermine further their mental well-being, and the healing relationship which they might develop with those in their care.

THE WOUNDED HEALER AND NURSING: FRAILTIES AND ILLUMINATIONS

A significant body of literature describes and defines the core function of psychiatric nursing within an interpersonal paradigm (Peplau, 1990; Travelbee, 1966, 1969, 1971). Within the context of this interpersonal process Travelbee argued that the psychiatric nurse 'assists an individual, family or community to promote mental health, to prevent or cope with the experience of mental illness and suffering and, if necessary, to find meaning in these experiences' (1969, p. 7). Travelbee's notion of the psychiatric nurse's therapeutic use of self provided a seminal anchor for the definition of the 'proper focus of psychiatric nursing' (Barker and Reynolds, 1994): 'by "therapeutic use of self" is meant the ability to use one's personality consciously and in full awareness to attempt to establish relatedness, and to structure nursing intervention' (Travelbee, 1971, p. 19). 'It is implicit within the context of such awareness that if nurses find no meaning in suffering how can they assist others to face the reality of it, to cope with it, to bear it, and to somehow extract some meaning or good out of such tragic experiences?' (Travelbee, 1971, p. 20). Such propositions have been developed more specifically by other nursing theorists who emphasise the wider implications of this interpersonal process, whereby the patient and the nurse co-create the unique human experience of illness (Parse, 1995). Parse (1992) defines the fundamental focus on human-to-human relating as 'co-creating rhythmical patterns of relating' (p.38). Within the context of such co-creation the inherent meaning of illness or disorder within the person or family becomes clearer and open to change. 'In telling about the meaning, persons share thoughts and feelings with one another, which in itself changes the meaning of a situation by making it more explicit' (Parse, 1987, p. 168).

Given this notion of 'co-creation', the discovery of meaning is not exclusive to the patient. The importance of nurses drawing upon their own past life experiences to help them understand better the person-in-care's world has also been acknowledged as a critical component of the interpersonal process. Robinson cautioned against nurses allowing themselves to experience 'the same degree of barrenness, grief and depression as the families (sic) involved' but proposed that 'if we [nurses] deny the possibility of being in similar straits ourselves, we shut off a useful and spontaneous avenue to understanding' (1983, p.6).

Some people who have been users of mental health services have become aware of nurses who have chosen to 'come out', acknowledging and disclosing their own experiences of mental distress. These nurses will always stand out in their memory as empathic individuals, with a heightened understanding of the people in their care. In our view, far from undermining professional performance, personal experience of mental distress may serve to improve professional nursing practice. The nurse's use of such experiences needs, however, to be developed carefully, arguably within the context of sensitive clinical supervision (Barker, 1992a; Robinson, 1983). Having experienced mental distress, nurses must guard against projecting their own feelings onto the people in their care. This caution might apply equally to service users acting as peer advocates. Everyone's experience of mental distress is unique. Nurses should not presume to tell people in their care how they should feel. Rather, the exercise of compassion requires the nurse to 'walk alongside' the person in care, supporting them in the development of the healing process which is unique to every individual.

THE CONSTRUCTION OF A CRISIS OF FAITH

A recent cause célèbre involving an enrolled nurse in the UK (Dept of Health, 1994a) has led to a moratorium on the potential threat to the welfare of patients from nurses with any history of mental illness. The nurse who was found guilty of the murder of four children in hospital was described as having a history of self-harm, and was diagnosed as suffering from Munchausen's Syndrome by Proxy. Nurses joining the profession, or moving to a new job, after May 1995 will have to undergo 'compulsory health checks' which will focus upon 'history of excessive sick leave, over-use of counselling or medical facilities, self-harming behaviour or any other behaviour which may give cause for concern' (Scott, 1994). These guidelines instituted by the government follow the recommendations of the Clothier Report, and were designed to prevent the repetition of the unfortunate events at Grantham and Kesteven General Hospital. Concern has been expressed that they may already have been used in a discriminatory manner against nurses who have acknowledged publicly their histories of mental illness, or receipt of therapy for mental health problems.

Case I

An English male student nurse who sought help following a minor self-harming incident was subsequently dismissed from his course by college staff who heard of the incident from a consultant psychiatrist to whom the student had been referred by his GP. The student commented that one doctor refused to ask the college to change its mind 'because he said he had known someone like me on another course who is now in prison because she murdered someone'. The student's union representative added 'I think there's been a panic in the light of the Allitt case'. Concern has been expressed that the effect of the recommendations may only be to force such problems under-ground (Cassidy, 1994).

Other nurses have reported their uphill struggle to gain employment after disclosing their history of mental illness honestly in applications. One wrote anonymously to the *Nursing Times* expressing concern that the good intentions of the guidelines may 'spark a witch hunt' (*Anonymous*, 1993). Many of these nurses have suffered from very common forms of mental illness especially depression. Ironically, a consensus exists that detection of Munchausen's Syndrome is difficult, if not impossible. In the letter quoted above the nurse noted, 'could we seriously ask in the "do you suffer" section whether the applicant has Munchausen's Syndrome, with or without proxy?' (*Anonymous*, 1993).

Three years after the Allitt Inquiry nursing still appears to be running scared from the old bogeyman, mental illness. In 1996 a nurse with a criminal record of rape and sexual abuse of patients was readmitted to the nursing register in England. Many nurses were incensed by the nursing council's action, which prompted a letter to a national newspaper by a non-nurse:

> My wife was all set to commence training as a nurse this year. For both of us this represented an achievement which would truly celebrate her personal struggle out of the psychosis precipitated by the birth of our son in 1991. Because of the very small statistical risk of her condition recurring, however, her wish to train as a nurse was denied her, as was working in any similar capacity, though it was always recognised that she presented no threat to her child or anyone else. A sensible precaution by the health authority and regulatory body? No one who knows her would believe a risk existed but would see the denial of potential and vocation. How do we reconcile this zealous caution with the same regulatory body's willingness to permit sex offenders back on to the professional register?'
>
> (*The Guardian*, 1996)

Case 2

The lead author published an article in 1994 which included the suggestion that all mental health staff should 'come out of the closet' and declare any history of mental illness, in an effort to reduce the stigma surrounding mental illness (Barker, 1995). Following its publication a final-year mental health branch student wrote, describing the details of a year-long suspension from her studies, which followed disclosure of experience of psychotherapy during a group exercise led by the course tutor. Ironically, all the students in the class were encouraged to 'disclose' something of personal nature, to 'get a feel' of the process of group therapy, and also to experience directly the therapeutic value of self-disclosure. The personal details of the case are not relevant here. What is significant was the tutor's response to the self-disclosure. The student was suspended without warning and remained under suspension for almost nine months despite the consultant psychiatrist who originally saw the student furnishing a letter indicating his support for the student.

The institution of this severe sanction, without any discussion, can only be viewed as a callous punishment. If the student had still been 'suffering' from the psychological problems which led to the original psychotherapeutic contact, the suspension could have been traumatic, if not disastrous. This single example symbolises how badly nurses – or in this case nurse teachers – deal with mental illness, real or imagined, when it occurs within their own ranks. The public is often taken to task for its inability or unwillingness to 'understand' mental illness. What evidence is there that nursing possesses any better understanding?

An accepted principle of self-help, promoted actively within contemporary health services, is that people should learn to recognise – at the earliest possible stage – signs of ill-health, and should seek treatment or support. This principle carries health benefits for the individual and economic benefits for the nation. If people with a history of mental distress believe that they might be penalised if such experiences become public, will they not try to disguise the experience to avoid discrimination, rather than seek treatment? If our assumption is correct, then consideration needs to be given to the possible continued presence of a stigmatising outlook on mental as distinct from physical health. The aim of screening prospective employees aims to avoid prejudicing the welfare of patients by 'weeding out' prospective nurses who may not be fully mentally healthy. This raises the questions: what do we mean by mentally healthy; and who determines this standard?

We need also to consider the potential hazards of the screening procedure. Will nurses try to disguise any current or past experience of mental illness and, by so doing, might this not result in even greater possible threats to their welfare, as well as to those who may end up in their care? If people are cared for by nurses suffering from an undisclosed mental health problem and who feel the need to hide this fact, will these combined pressures not increase the risks to patient care? A procedure designed to screen out nurses with mental health problems may, ultimately, represent a hazard for patients.

THE FAIRY TALE PRINCESS WITH FEET OF CLAY

We might also consider how honest is our public discourse about mental illness. In 1996 the Princess of Wales admitted, in a televised interview, to her history of bulimia and self-harm which, by her report, had extended over several years and led to extensive use of counselling or therapy. This disclosure – which previously had been the subject of media gossip – attracted world-wide publicity, not least because of the original casting of Princess Diana as the archetypal fairy tale princess.

The Princess of Wales was a popular visitor to hospitals, especially those caring for children. Are we to assume that, should the Princess of Wales wished to have registered an interest in training as a nurse, we would have rejected her on the grounds of this acknowledgement of self-harm, bulimia and 'excessive use of counselling'? Are we to suggest that, given her history, her efforts to 'care' for the sick were inappropriate? In that television interview the Princess of Wales stated that she hoped to become a 'queen of hearts' and, since then, had increased her presence in hospitals and at sites of disasters. This amateur 'vocation' as a caring VIP may have been interpreted as part of her own self-healing process.

We may be in danger of cultivating, again, the false assumption that we can easily separate the mentally 'unhealthy' from the mentally 'well'. When popular figures report their experience of mental ill-health, the public may tend to reframe this as 'less serious' or somehow different from the ordinary madness which most people fear. Such reframing ignores the fact that vast numbers of people move in and out of mental distress every day, presenting no danger to themselves or others. The often silent nature of mental ill-health is such that few of us are aware of who – among our friends, family and colleagues – might be suffering at this very moment. The false expectations of the screening procedures are more likely to keep such private suffering a secret, than to bring it to the surface. After an all too brief period of acceptability of talking openly, mental distress is close to being reframed, again, as a taboo. We are in danger of turning the clock back to a time when we pretended that the 'mentally distressed' were only those with manifest psychiatric diagnoses: the mad. Any strategy which encourages people to suppress, or otherwise hide, evidence of their mental distress, runs the risk of aggravating that distress further.

THE ROOTS OF OUR FEARS: THE 'US' AND 'THEM' MENTALITY

The view that mental health staff are qualitatively different from the people-with-mental-illness whom they care for or treat raises major ethical, if not also theoretical, issues. To what extent do professionals working with the so-called mentally ill experience difficulties (simply) because the patient holds up a metaphorical mirror to the professional? Nurses often talk, for example, about 'liking' or 'disliking' particular patients. To what extent are they recognising features in the patient (good or bad) which echo something within themselves? To what extent are the concerns over the mental health status of nurses (or indeed other professionals) a function of an 'us and them' mentality, bred from inappropriate models of deviance? Such models are uniquely Western in origin. However, with the advent of nurses' interest in concepts such as holism, they may find that the simple rules of 'us' and 'them' no longer apply. They may discover the truth of Sullivan's dictum – framed in terms of people in psychosis – that 'we are all more alike than different' (Sullivan, 1953).

Some people with so-called serious mental illnesses can suffer impairments which interfere with their ability to live and work and, therefore, might require them to take leave from work to allow for recovery. In a small number of cases the nature of the disorder may be such that the person may be unable to return to work. Much of the concern expressed recently over the mental health of nurses, especially by the media, appears to suggest that 'mental health' and 'mental illness' are discrete, fixed states; and that the population at large can be distinguished in terms of 'us' (the 'mentally healthy') and 'them' (the 'mentally ill'). In the context of psychiatric nursing, what exactly are we afraid of when a nurse admits to having had a period (whether brief or extended) of mental distress? The implication arising from the Clothier Report is that any nurse with a history of mental ill-health has a potential for 'dangerousness' which represents a risk to patient care, although the statistical probability is negligible. Are we afraid that 'unstable' nurses might contaminate us? If so, the problem is ours, since the fear of contamination denotes a vulnerability on our part? If we fear that we might be like those we care for, the problem remains ours: we may well be denying legitimate experiences of mental distress, or denying (and suppressing) our potential need to express such distress.

When we consider why people acknowledge a past (or current) history of mental ill-health, we need to consider what such an action denotes. Such honesty requires much courage. Given nursing's commitment (or obligation) to 'promote mental health', such honesty should, in principle, be rewarded. We believe that denial of the past experience of emotional weakness is likely to reflect either insensitivity to one's life experience, or a refusal to confront a natural, human vulnerability. It is of course axiomatic that no-one can assert with any confidence that they will not experience any kind of mental distress in the future.

THE AUTHORS: IN AND OUT OF THE CLOSET

The issues which have been addressed so far are by no means academic as far as the authors are concerned. Our reasons for writing this chapter are diverse but are united by the concern that our validity – both human and professional – might be called into question by the illogical and unbalanced perspective on mental health and illness which we are seeking to address here.

We are a mix of 'providers' and 'users': psychiatric nurses and (former) psychiatric patients. A review of the authors' histories reveals, however, a degree of shared experience. Four of the authors have experienced what is commonly defined as depression in sufficient degree to interfere with their work, relationships and life in general. Three of the authors have experienced what is commonly called mania, although this only interfered with the lifestyles of two of them. Two of the authors have had experience of what are defined as auditory and (especially) visual and tactile hallucinations. This common ground is notable to the extent that all these experiences of so-called psychopathology – mania, depression and hallucinations – cross the nurse–patient divide, and illustrate further that we are all more alike than different. What is more important is that the nature of these shared experiences appear to have fostered a degree of mutual empathy among the authors, which is sadly lacking from the sharply divided relationship (professional and patient) discussed earlier.

MENTAL ILLNESS: FIXTURE OR FITTING?

The prevailing anxiety over the mental health status of nurses (in particular) may derive from a concretised construction of mental illness, if it is assumed that some people have 'it' (the 'mentally ill') whereas others do not (the 'sane'). This view is increasingly reinforced by biological models of mental illness which seek to explain everything from 'hearing voices' to 'attention deficit disorder' in terms of genetic influence or putative biological lesions. When one begins to examine the form and function of many mental illnesses, although the experience of distress may be common, the range of experiences are characterised most by the metaphorical – rather than actual – nature of the 'illness' involved. We believe that the experience of mental distress present in a person defined as suffering from a mental illness has much in common with ordinary emotional experience. Although the experiences described by those sorely affected by mental illness appear alien, they represent only an exaggeration of normal human experience, to which all persons are in some way privy.[1]

Consideration needs to be given, therefore, to the conditions under which mental dysfunction, (of any kind) is defined. Western psychology has promoted the view that a 'perfect' mental state can exist, from which various forms of mental dysfunction exist as 'deviances' from this norm. A similar view was expressed in relation to notions of perfection of the physical body, especially by the ancient Greeks. It is now well accepted that some problems of contemporary living – such as eating disorders – are influenced, at least in part, by stereotypical views concerning the 'perfect-ness', or otherwise, of the body.

Eastern philosophies take a quite different view. In Oriental thought, the Western notion of people comprising a singular, stable, personality type, enjoying a direct correlation with behavioural patterns of adaption or maladaption, is unacceptable if not absurd. Instead, the prevailing 'model of man' in Oriental thought is multi-dimensional, if not mercurial. People possess many personalities, although they may only exhibit one at any one time. Similarly, the idea of emotional distress as a fixed phenomenon is untenable. Instead people's distress can be seen as akin to the weather: presently the sun is shining, but soon it may cloud over and begin to rain. This 'atmospheric' state of affairs will not last. Indeed, a core assumption of oriental psychology is that 'nothing lasts'. The same may be said of human experience.

In the caring context there is good reason to assume that some people, may need support for a time, perhaps at intervals throughout their lives. Indeed, occupational health research suggests that on-the-job stresses of rotating shift patters, team deple-tion, unsocial hours (etc.) are likely to lead to a need for 'counselling', whether or not this is defined specifically as 'emotional support'. Leifer described the suicide of a night sister following a hospital reorganisation. The nurse's sister described her belief that the pressures inherent in the NHS reforms stripped her sister of 'her responsi-bilities, pride and professionalism' (Leifer, 1995, p. 19). There is no reason to assume that people who are not (currently) defined (i.e. diagnosed) as mentally un-healthy will not need support, now or at some time in the future, when their world 'clouds over' or is disturbed by emotional, psychological or psychiatric storms.[2]

We might also care to consider the meaning of any assertion about our mental 'stability'. From the perspective of logic, if a person defines her/himself as 'mentally healthy' what does this say about the person? Given that we can only describe our experience from moment to moment, what is such an assertion worth? Who can say that within minutes of making such an assertion they will not be in need of significant emotional (if not psychiatric) support? Some mental disorders – affective disorders in particular – are characterised by their cyclical nature. They are, in effect, like the weather. At one moment the person is affectively well; but at some point their affective state 'clouds over' denoting the onset of a period of 'depression'.[3] The epidemic of depression which has swept the Western world (Barker, 1992b) has

---

[1] Arguably the most serious form of mental disorder, psychosis, can be characterised by disturbances of perception which are akin to a 'waking dream (or nightmare)'. Given that all people dream, we have some experience of what it is like to be in a psychotic state.

[2] It is interesting to note that meterology uses the same metaphor (depression) for low barometric readings.

[3] Manos suggests that in the US such 'sick time' is increasingly referred to as 'mental health days'.

been described from a number of perspectives. If these estimates are in any way accurate, it is likely that significant numbers of the mental health workforce either are suffering, at present, from active or remitting depressive disorder; or are likely to suffer from an affective disorder at some stage in the future. The assumption that one is currently not 'mentally ill' is a highly provisional form of knowledge indeed. Making predictions about the stability of future experience is often viewed as symptomatic of faulty schema. A belief in the stability of one's own mental state flies in the face of the facts concerning the unpredicability of life experience and, if held strongly enough, might be classed as delusional.

THE MYTH OF THE CRIPPLED CARER

Within the guidelines which derived from the Clothier Report was the concern over 'excessive use of counselling or therapy'. Here we should like to consider some of the implications of making judgements on people who seek or use such services. If the nurse does not disclose their history of mental distress – whether this is diagnosed formally as an 'illness' or not – how will their colleagues become aware of it? If the colleagues, ignorant of this 'past history' assume that the nurse is 'sane' like the rest of the team or workforce, does this not mean that the nurse is, in actuality, sane (or at least not 'mentally unhealthy') within the context of the social construction of mental health/illness?

Given the covert nature of many forms of mental disorder, we might consider also how anyone can develop the 'knowledge' that even those close to them are not mentally ill?, If people either do not declare themselves to be so or do not exhibit manifest signs of mental illness, how can any of us know their mental state?

THE ALIENATION OF THE PATIENT

The idea that people with mental health problems can, realistically, be viewed as qualitatively different from those who care for them, is an outmoded concept. The Report of the Mental Health Nursing Review Team (Dept of Health, 1994b) emphasised the importance of 'working in partnership' for the enhancement of mental health care. The Review Team took advice from several quarters, not least from self-advocacy and self-help groups within the psychiatric arena. The expansion of the self-help market not only suggests the need for such forms of support, but also – given that the views of such groups are sought regularly by political or planning groups – that the views of such organisations can have a positive impact on the design or delivery of health care. If professional and government agencies validate the experience of mental ill-health by involving patients in consultation, how can equivalent authorities penalise nurses for admitting to similar experiences of mental ill-health? How can such a manifest double standard be supported in practice?

THE 'OUTING' OF THE WOUNDED HEALER

We reviewed earlier the concerns provided by the Clothier Report and the Allitt Inquiry. There is little doubt that the recognition that any nurse could kill patients (especially children) touched a raw nerve in the nation's sensibilities. Arguably, much of the rhetoric generated in the press since those tragic events has served only to obfuscate the real issues. At the time of writing yet another senior nursing figure (Cohen, 1995) has echoed the view heard frequently since the publication of the Clothier Report that, on reflection, the events might have been prevented, had the procedure for employing Ms Allitt been more carefully monitored. Whether this is wisdom with hindsight or mere rhetoric is unclear. This view is representative of the belief that health care workers can be policed, through screening interventions. We would rather contend that the health care system should be self-policing. All staff with a mental health problem or history, should be encouraged to 'come out of the closet', on the principle that once colleagues are aware of the need, support may be provided through clinical supervison and guidance, if not friendship – qualities which should be considered fundamental to the collegiate relationship. Given that all health care professionals are trained observers, they should be able to recognise when their colleagues need 'extraordinary support'. Such a supportive milieu would obviate the need for policing tactics which involve negative labelling, criticism and the inevitable exacerbation of the original mental health problem.

No nurse should occupy a position of unaccountable autonomy, a position which by definition risks the welfare of the patient, or even colleagues. The same rule would apply of course to any health care professional who should be accountable, in the final analysis, to the patient who – in an increasingly consumer-oriented health care market – should be seen as the final judge of the quality of the service.

This issue prompts consideration of the means by which nurses might be screened for the mental vulnerabilities which might place patients at risk. The assumption underpinning the notion of 'seeking out' mental ill-health is that such a phenomenon is a stable part of the person's overall human structure. What evidence is there for such an assertion? Those readers with experience of working with people defined as 'psychotic' may acknowledge that such persons, often characterised as representative of the most extreme form of mental disturbance are, for much of the time, as reasonable and rational as those who care for them. Of course the distorting lens of the labelling process can obscure recognition of the inherent ordinariness of the psychiatric patient.

Given that we have been aware of the dangers of the labelling process for at least thirty years, we often assume that we (professionals) have benefited from such experience. Recently, Deegan, a psychologist in the USA, observed from personal experience that:

> you used to feel sad but now you are said to be depressed. You used to disagree sometimes but now you are told you lack insight. You used to act independently but now you are told that your independence means you are uncooperative, noncompliant, and treatment resistant. You used to take risks. You learned from your failures as you were growing and learning. But now that you are labelled with a mental illness the dignity of risk and the right to failure have been taken from you.

(1993, p. 9)

Deegan's personal experience of being described as a 'schizophrenic' illustrates clearly the pervasive failure to appreciate the human context of the person-who-is-patient. The irony of the situation does not escape her:

> Normal people get to make many stupid choices over and over again in their lives. Nobody tells them that they need a case manager. How many times has Elizabeth Taylor been married? At last count it was seven or eight times, I think. The poor woman lacks insight! She exercises poor judgement! She is failing to learn from past experiences! She is making the same dumb choice again! How come they don't get her a case manager?

> (ibid., p.9)

Earlier, we presented an argument concerning the manifest instability of emotional life. Leaving aside organic disorders which generate (sustained) physical/physiological dysfunctions with psychological correlates, most forms of mental ill-health are ephemeral 'conditions' which wax and wane and are characterised by relative unpredictability. Indeed, there is much evidence that psychiatric treatments, in general, are sorely limited in effecting significant and lasting change. The research literature suggests that many people 'get better' despite, or in the absence of, any significant therapy. These findings point to the mercurial nature of mental health. If such fluctuations are so common, what is the validity of trying to measure the 'problem' as if it were a stable trait? In a related vein, we would ask whether or not anyone who would deign to judge another's mental health in this fashion was not, perforce, admitting to their own ignorance of mental illness, thereby rendering them incompetent to offer such a judgement.

THE GRANDFATHER PRINCIPLE

We have illustrated how nurses in training, or nurses seeking employment may be the most susceptible to mental health discriminatory practices. If nurses in training, with a past experience of mental illness, are to be considered for possible dismissal on the grounds of 'unsuitability', should not all staff (qualified and otherwise) be vetted at regular intervals to assess their current mental health status, and suitability for continued employment? If mental health is a measurable concept – and if some nurses are deemed 'in need of assesssment' to determine their mental health status – this should (indeed, must) be extended to all staff at every stage in their careers. The regulations which stemmed from the Clothier Report and the emergent attitudes towards mental illness are, in our view, conceptually flawed.

ASSUMPTION I

There exists an assumption that certain forms of mental disorder – such as Munchausen's Syndrome By Proxy, attributed to Beverly Allitt – which might involve a risk to patients are easily identified. Furthermore, there is an assumption that such disorders can be identified even when the person might seek to disguise their presence. Anecdotal evidence from the clinical psychiatrists who are our colleagues appears to seriously challenge this assumption.

ASSUMPTION 2

It is assumed that other forms of mental disorder also involve a potential threat to the welfare of patients or others. Although schizophrenia is most commonly identified as an example, severe depression also is included in this category. Statistical evidence seriously challenges this assertion. Indeed, patients may be at far greater risk from abusive or incompetent staff – illustrated by the catalogue of abuse in mental hospitals in the UK throughout the 1960s and 1970s or from the effects of economic restrictions imposed on services.

In our view there is no evidence to support these two assumptions as the basis for the process of discriminatory screening. Moreover, if these hypotheses were valid it would be necessary to screen all staff at regular intervals to determine whether or not their mental health status had changed and patients might subsequently be at risk. If one accepted the proposition that nurses entering the service might pose a threat to patients, one would have to accept that significant numbers of nurses exist already in the ranks, who might pose a threat to patients. It would follow that such nurses should be identified, and 'flushed out' of the system. Only by 'grandfathering' the principle of vetting – extending the screening process back through the generations of nurses – could it possess any credibility.

CORE ETHICAL ASSUMPTIONS

The scenario outlined above stimulates consideration of a number of core ethical assumptions.

1. The negative process of vetting the mental health status of nurses is an inappropriate practice, born of fear and ignorance. We believe also that a more pro-active approach to mental health problems is the only way to deal with any such problem effectively. By adopting a 'Big Brother' approach, we may deter people with appropriate helping skills and attitudes from entering nursing. More importantly, we may merely encourage people with limited insight into their own mental life to become the core of the services dedicated to helping others heal their mental lives. Such persons may well be wholly unsuited for the craft of caring.
2. A negative vetting process may encourage the 'closeting' of mental health problems. This may encourage nurses to suppress their experience of mental ill health, thereby compounding their mental health problems. A health service which, through its legislative procedures, aggravates ill health, rather than reduces it, can hardly justify its claim to such a title.
3. When nurses need help to address their mental health problems – whether these are (e.g.) manifestations of stress or symptoms of schizophrenia – they should be offered the same counselling, support and 'sick leave' available to people with forms of physical ill health. Only where the problem is unremitting, or enduring in nature, and significantly impairs the nurse's ability to fulfil professional functions, should consideration be given to any investigation of the nurse's tenure. (This principle would apply, of course, equally to physical ill-health.)
4. Where nurses (or other staff) have a short-term mental health problem, or the recurrence of a problem, appropriate counselling, peer support, and – where

necessary – professional support, should be made available. Organisations which attempt to exclude those with mental health problems might well, given current statistics, have to exclude significant numbers of their workforce, within all health care disciplines. More importantly, the use of policing, rather than internal self-regulation, will exacerbate rather than resolve the problem within the organisation.

5. If the experience of mental ill health is viewed from the 'wounded healer' perspective, people with such experiences will be seen as a valuable resource. Although, everyone has the capacity to capitalise on their own 'wounds' as part of the healing process, those who have already 'come out of the closet' are the most outstanding examples of the democratisation of the principles of mental illness and health.[4]

The naïve efforts to police the health care professions presents a threat to the concept of the 'wounded healer'. Instead of 'weeding out' nurses with a history of mental ill-health, we should be developing the supervisory structures which will allow all nurses to recognise their own 'wounds', allowing them to gain a personal under-standing of how their personal vulnerability might echo the vulnerability of the people in their care.

Every day, nurses, in all sorts of clinical settings, are faced with pressures which might threaten their relationship with vulnerable people in their care. The pressures of caring for people with significant forms of mental distress can confront nurses with their own vulnerability. Providing that nurses receive the appropriate kind of support, that confrontation may open access to the nurses' most powerful resources, allowing them to develop the 'therapeutic use of self' (Travelbee, 1971). Through such experiences nurses may learn that:

> Healing brings with it the experience of compassion. When we understand what is needed to heal ourselves an understanding comes of what may be needed by others, and if other people are suffering we experience the suffering with them. To be compassionate, to understand and suffer with others, is to assist their healing and to relieve them of some of their burden. To heal ourselves requires awareness; to heal others requires compassion.

(Anderton, 1995)

REFERENCES

Anderton, B. 1995: *Meditation for every day.* London: Piatkus.

Anonymous 1993: Allitt's terrible crimes must not spark a witch hunt. Letters *Nursing Times* 89(26), 12.

Barker, P. 1992a: Psychiatric nursing. In Butterworth, C.A. and Faugier, J. (eds), *Clinical supervision and mentorship in nursing.* London: Chapman and Hall.

Barker, P. 1992b: *Severe depression: a practitioner's guide.* London: Chapman and Hall.

---

[4] Manos reports that, in the US, the 'consumer–practitioner' network counts among its members directors of state hospitals, hospital administrators, consultant psychiatrists, as well as nurses – all of whom have capitalised on their experience of mental ill-health to enhance the services with which they are involved.

Barker, P. 1995: Coming out of the closet. *Nursing Times* **90**(31), 59–61.

Barker, P. and Reynolds, W. 1994: A critique of Watson's caring ideology: the proper focus of psychiatric nursing. *Journal of Psychosocial Nursing and Mental Health Services* **32**(5), 17–22.

Bennet, E.A. 1966: *What Jung really said.* London: Macdonald.

Cassidy, J. 1994: Exclusion zone: Clothier Inquiry Report. *Nursing Times* **90**(8), 22–3.

Chamberlin, J. 1984: *On our own: patient-controlled alternatives to the mental health system.* New York. McGraw-Hill.

Cohen, P. 1995: Ward leader pivotal in safe recruitment process. *Nursing Times* **91**(22), 8.

Cousins, N. 1979: *Anatomy of an illness as perceived by the patient: reflections on healing and regeneration* New York: W.W. Norton.

Deegan, P. 1993: Recovering our sense of value after being labeled mentally ill. *Journal of Psychosocial Nursing* **31**(4), 7–11.

Department of Health 1994a: *The Allit inquiry: report of the independent inquiry relating to the deaths and injuries on the Children's Ward at Grantham and Kesteven General Hospital during the period February to April 1991* (the Clothier Report). London: HMSO.

Department of Health 1994b: *Working in partnership: report of the Mental Health Nurses Review Team.* London: HMSO.

Fisher, D. 1992: *Humanising the recovery process.* Holyoke, MA: Human Resource Association of the Northeast.

Frazer, J. 1993: *The golden bough: a study in religion and magic.* Ware, Hertfordshire: Wordsworth Reference.

Jung, C.G. 1964: *Civilisation in transition, vol 10: The Collected Works.* London: Routledge and Kegan Paul.

Leifer, D. 1995: Worried to death. *Nursing Standard* **9**(38), 18–19.

Parse, R.R. 1987: Man-living-health theory of nursing. In Parse, R.R. (ed.), *Nursing science: major paradigms, theories and critiques.* Philadelphia: Saunders.

Parse, R.R. 1992: Human becoming: Parse's theory of nursing. *Nursing Science Quarterly* **5**, 35–42.

Parse, R.R. 1995: The human becoming theory. In Parse, R.R. (ed.), *Illuminations: the shuman becoming theory in practice and research.* New York: National League for Nursing.

Peplau, H.E. 1988: *Interpersonal relations in nursing.* London: Macmillan.

Peplau, H.E. 1990: Interpersonal relations model: theoretical constructs, principles and general applications. In Reynolds, W. and Cormack, D. (eds), *Psychiatric and mental health nursing: theory and practice.* London: Chapman and Hall.

Robinson, L. 1983: *Psychiatric nursing as a human experience.* London: W.B. Saunders and Co.

Stevens. A. 1982: *Archetype: a natural history of the self.* London: Routledge and Kegan Paul.

Sullivan, H.S. 1953: *The interpersonal theory of psychiatry.* New York: W.W. Norton.

Travelbee, J. 1966: *Interpersonal aspects of nursing* Philadelphia: FA Davis.

Travelbee, J. 1969: *Intervention in psychiatric nursing: process in the one-to-one relationship.* Philadelphia: FA Davis.

Travelbee, J. 1971: *Interpersonal aspects of nursing.* 2nd edn. Philadelphia: FA Davis.

Zigmond, D. 1984: Physician heal thyself: the paradox of the wounded healer. *British Journal of Holistic Medicine* **1**, 63–71.

25

EPILOGUE:
THE HEART OF THE ETHICAL
MATTER

Phil Barker and Ben Davidson

A RULE FOR ALL

Most of us act as if we were born with a moral conscience. That very expression – moral conscience – suggests the very 'rightness' of our views: how could anyone disagree with us? Why can't they understand? Many of us spend our entire lives struggling with the morally indignant 'self' secreted – not too deeply – inside of us. We are the victims of our moral opinions; terrorised by our values; and seduced by that sly voice which says 'Well, maybe *they* don't agree with you; but everyone else does. It's obvious!' More than anything else our moral self is a hypnotist: we act out our moral lifestyle *as if* in a dream or trance, blissfully unaware of the motives which propel us from beneath the everyday veneer of our personal or professional selves.

Editing a book is usually a trial: authors rarely value criticism and are even less likely to value criticism which, to the editor's eye, is obviously necessary, appropriate or otherwise deserved. The editor-as-critic sounds too much, perhaps, like the voice from behind the mirror which points out each new grey hair or that extra inch round the midriff. We all fear and instinctively reject those messages from reality.

Editors don't value the author's sparse writing style, or balk at their overfamiliarity with the reader, or they think that they are impersonal and verbose. They complain at the start about authors trying to say too much, then return the script later, asking: 'What point, exactly, if any, are you trying to make?' Editors ask for changes in February and, several drafts later, in November, they are asking for more changes, which appear to be inviting the author to go back to where they first started. Editors start off life as friendly strangers: their invitation to contribute to the book represents another opportunity for authors to shine, to polish their CVs and to communicate with the bigger world of our chosen discipline. If they reach the end of the line – acceptance and submission to the publisher – the editors have grown old but not wise in the authors' eyes. When they were not offering 'helpful guidance' they were criticising; when they hadn't heard from the author in a few weeks they started whinging. Soon the author came to dread the editor's letter or phone call. Over time the editors grew to resemble the worst model of parental authority, and the chapter which once excited the author became a homework assignment, and more and more time was spent sharpening pencils or staring out of windows.

Or, at least, that is what we suspect happens within some editor–author relationships. By no means do we believe that anything like this happened with *all* the authors in this book! Perhaps we are confessing here some of our editorial doubts, neurotic anxieties which may have little substance in fact. The sub-text of the editorial process does, however, appear to be 'How to lose friends by trying to influence people!' Each author was invited to let their moral conscience speak. Few, if any, expected that their little moral voice would elicit such a loud echo: one which begged further questions for each ethical question already asked, or which sometimes seemed to diminish the very substance of their ethical value base.

To a great extent, the production of the book involved an analogue of the process of ethical inquiry. The contributors have taken a view of ethical enquiry in their work similar to the editors: that the right way to care for people's psychiatric problems and their 'mental health' is constantly to scrutinise and cultivate the grounds of the care they are offering. As a gardener does not make his specimens grow, neither does the nurse cure his patient but he may facilitate the creation of a healing, therapeutic environment in which the patient is able to grow towards wholeness. The environment in question is likely to be one in which a human relationship is on offer, providing love and challenge. A great deal of work is required to effect such an environment, and a mainstay of this work is the ongoing scrutiny of one's relationship with the patient: how one felt after (and before) an interaction; why one felt that way; whether this was said in the patient's interests; and, if not, how one's own conflicting agenda has come to predominate; why that form of conduct offered the patient an all-too-familiar no-win situation; and what should be done to avoid it recurring. The nurse offers a safe place and a mirror that the patient can use to grow and is helped in so doing by the provision of external reference points that serve to keep them 'grounded' – these will hopefully be provided by clinical supervision and other forms of support. In the same way as the authors have thus cleared and fertilised the grounds of the care they offer their patients, creating an environment in which growth can take place, the editors have facilitated a forum, in putting together this text, in which a sustained period of thought and consideration of some ethical issue may take place on the part of the author. The editors have acted as sounding boards for the authors, challenged their ideas, encouraged more focus, less breadth, greater clarity, increased candour, reduced narcissism, less polemic, more experience, greater balance, wider referencing, extra potency and, hopefully always, some sense in the author of having their struggle heard and acknowledged in a non-abusive, safe, validating and playful relationship. We have tried to make the experience both developmental and fun.

But where, in all this, have we, as editors, got 'grounding'? What external reference points were available to ensure our interpretations were not too 'off the wall', to ensure that the challenges we made served to help the author grow rather than serving to enable the editor to feel powerful and clever? Has our plea for ethical scrutiny extended to our own relationships? Or are we content simply to have acquired positions of superiority?

The genesis of our relationship is perhaps instructive. A major contemporary academic voice in psychiatric nursing in the UK mentions in passing to a student nurse a text he is being commissioned to write; the student comes back to him three days later with a detailed proposal as to the structure and content of the text, with the request that it be edited by the two of them jointly; the professor takes a gamble and agrees to the joint venture; the outline is refined, the publishers review and finally accept it, a contract is dispatched and the book begins to take shape; disputes arise – we become polarised along various spectrums, one of us more directive in our feedback, to the point of rewriting passages for some of the authors (many of whom are, after all, novice writers, requiring substantial input), the other more hands-off in the guidance he offers, to the point of abandoning authors to find a path out of their confusion (which is, after all, the point of the ethical struggle we have endorsed); when strains in the relationship emerge, around these and other polarities, we seek guidance and support from others outside the dyad to ensure we hold it all together; three years, 29 rejected or resigned contributors, various major life crises and substantial greying of hair later, the text is complete and the two sit around gazing into their (respective) navels, at either end of a modem connection, considering the experience; and here we are. To some extent the 'grounding' we have secured has come from relationships outside the project. To some extent we have elicited views from authors within the project about the way we are conducting ourselves in relation to each other and in relation to the project as a whole. And to a very large extent, we have sounded off about the experience to each other, keeping alive and in full focus our central theme – that in the context of a safe and open relationship, something is created that transcends the conflicts and tensions; by struggling to share and remain true to our experience, the ground is tended and conditions are set up out of which will emerge new life.

THE EXTRAORDINARY NATURE OF EVERYDAY LIFE

Much, if not all, of the subject matter of the book is grounded in everyday experience of psychiatric nursing. Indeed, the very few authors who are not practising psychiatric nurses impressed us with their knowledge – at a heartfelt level – of the complexity and challenge of caring for people, as opposed to being always the agents of their treatment. That traditional core assumption – that psychiatric nurses will, above all else, care for people – is in danger of going out fashion to be replaced by notions of nurses as 24-hour therapists of one kind or another. What little evidence exists suggests that when people become psychiatric patients, they would rather receive care than some sophisticated therapy: they require validation of their experience rather than processing for change; they desire an encounter at a fundamentally human level, rather than a carefully negotiated and delimited consumer–provider contract. Even the most sorely distressed among the psychiatric nurse's clientele require to be met with a degree of openness and empathy which might unnerve even the most confident and competent. To be able to replicate the 'trick of being ordinary' with people in extraordinary circumstances, who are witnessing extraordinary experiences, is a challenge on a towering scale: one which we dare not underestimate.

We have talked here mainly in terms of psychiatric nursing. We are aware that the contemporary parlance favours the expression mental health nursing. For the moment we adopt the simple distinction that psychiatric nursing is focused on the identification of, and response to, the problems of living which brought people into contact with the psychiatric services; whereas mental health nursing involves the facilitation of the day-to-day progress of the individual down their life path – growing and developing as people in the diverse and chaotic ways in which people generally grow and develop as human beings. The ethical issues requiring attention by both psychiatric and mental health nurses are, we suspect, much closer than the above distinction suggests. Mental health nurses are not, after all, a new breed, but perhaps represent, at best, an approach to psychiatric nursing which at some level acknowledges the ethical nuances of attending to someone's health (their whole being) rather than their illness alone. Notwithstanding this distinction, mental health nursing, like psychiatric nursing, is anchored within a tradition imbued with power and authority which – as history so consistently advises us – has controlled, diminished, devalued and invalidated the people described and defined as the mentally ill. Given psychiatric nursing's location within this authoritative and powerful church, the ethical boundaries of nursing's everyday activity are wide indeed.

THE LONG AND THE SHORT OF ETHICAL JOURNEYING

The authors which we finally chose, and the subject matter which we invited them to address, tended to reflect our view of psychiatric nursing: our view of the shape and scale of the ethical canvas, and our view of the horizon, beyond which might lie the moral Shangri-La of our dreams. As one might expect, not all the authors shared our concept of morality, far less our vision of the means by which we might transcend the moral indignities which beset everyday psychiatric nursing. However, that very tension – between the abstract forces of our respective moral consciences and our dreams of ideal and virtue – served as a mirror for the struggles which went on in the minds of the individual authors; struggles with their colleagues, their systems, their policies and protocols and – ultimately – their own consciences. We are comfortable, although unsatisfied, with the outcome of this book which, in many of the chapters involved the editors meeting the author at some ethical cross-roads, exchanging words, and agreeing to go our different ways. We were comfortable with such 'agreements to differ', in the few occasions they arose, since we fully expect to meet up with the issues again, somewhere down our own ethical life path. The ethical world is globe-shaped since it is a conceptual reflection of our living world. As a result the ethical dilemmas which we have addressed criss-cross that globe, like lines of latitude and longitude. We entered this project not with the expectation that we might achieve any great resolution, but that we might illustrate to our readership this simple yet profound fact: that ethical inquiry is often a journey from a to b and back again; that ethical inquiry rarely delivers any satisfying answers but, having returned home largely empty-handed, we set out again on the search for what is 'right and fitting', knowing that the meaning we seek is within the search itself. Having completed our own journey from a to b and back again, we are heady from the experience; drunk with the wisdom we have acquired; but sober in the knowledge that, come tomorrow, new ethical headaches will arise, or yesterday's wisdom will have left a sour taste in our mouths.

Philosophy, Authority and Growing Up

We acknowledged in our introductory chapter that we were not philosophers: or at least we might not pass muster as the kind of philosophers who should be writing about ethics. As we look back on the experience of preparing the book we feel even more philosophical – about the futility of dichotomous reasoning (e.g. you are or are not a philosopher); and the unsatisfactory outcome of our search for the 'right and fitting'. If we have learned anything, it probably involves the reinforcement of a belief with which we began the book: that ethics as a state of being involves confronting our childlike self who is constantly looking for absolute answers. And yet, in spite of this knowledge, we spend much of our time in ethical decision-making looking for an authoritative voice, rarely one which comes from within. As Alan Watts observed:

> This is why human beings find it difficult to learn and difficult to adapt themselves to new situations. Because we are always looking for precedents, for authority from the past for what we are supposed to do now, that gives us the impression that the past is all-important and is the determinative factor in our behaviour.

(Watts, 1977, p.102)

Put simply, when faced with an ethical challenge we turn and ask 'What do I do now, Mummy.'

We have no doubt that we are philosophers, although we would be the first to accept that we may not be very good ones. We are confident also that we have brought together here a disparate band of philosophers who also may not – in some readers' eyes – be very good ones, and that may be why we chose them. However, the reason why we came together in this book was to offer some kind of depiction of ethical-philosophy-in-life. We are well aware that for many psychiatric nurses – like many of their colleagues in the field – philosophy is an expendable commodity, if indeed it has any value at all. However, our vain ambition was to reflect the processes of the ethical mind, at work in the everyday world of everyday life; not poring over dusty tomes; or debating within circumscribed learned circles. And we believe we have realised that ambition.

We often ask ourselves how should we act, but perhaps less often do we ask if we should act at all; whether our action may, ultimately, be contributing to the problem which we seek to address and resolve. We should not lose sight, either, of the fact that, often, when we look for answers – or explanations – what we use to help our decision-making simply is not real. When we talk about explaining something, we mean – quite literally – laying the thing out flat, 'on a plain'. Hence our tendency to take slices of human tissue, or droplets of human blood, slice them flat, or smear them across a glass and say 'there's your problem!' We rarely reflect on the obvious fact that those bits of our physical selves, laid out flat in those different ways, can never be the kind of explanation we seek, for they are out of context. They are not the limbs and organs which move across the earth, or blood which courses through our veins. And so it is with the explanation of moral conduct. We can hardly expect to find an explanation for these riddles by taking ourselves out of the contexts within which these problems exist. So, ethical inquiry needs to go on within the wards in which people called psychiatric patients are cared for and treated; within the homes which community psychiatric nurses visit; within the clinics, day centres, and other settings which people attend, expecting an encounter with a psychiatric nurse. And the intellectual thread which is woven through all those situations is that the body of ethical knowledge will be carried around in the minds of the nurses themselves; being revised and edited *en route*, for ethics is a live thing, not a dust-covered tome. But first and last we need to recognise that rather obvious fact.

As we were completing the editing of this book one of editors invited members of a psychiatric nursing list on the Internet to offer examples of ethical dilemmas encountered in their everyday work. The list comprised several hundred psychiatric nurses from around the world. Often, issues of an ethical nature had been alluded to in passing, when other topics were addressed. After the first request, only five responses were elicited, whereas a deluge of responses was expected. The message was sent out again, to be followed by another handful of replies. After several weeks of waiting it was decided that these were all the responses which were going to appear, and the book was, metaphorically, closed. What was of further interest, however, was that at the same time as these handful of ethical dilemmas were appearing, a very active swapping of messages was going on, verging at times on the sort of 'heated' Internet exchanges known as 'flaming', concerning 'control and restraint' in psychiatric nursing practice. Literally dozens of messages appeared over a couple of weeks describing the use of this or that technique, the abusiveness of restraint, physical or chemical, and alternative, interpersonal methods to deal with various problems of aggression, challenging behaviour, non-compliance, etc. While polarised positions were taken that seemed to fall across an Atlantic divide, some resolution and mutual understanding did finally emerge, contextualising the exchange within historical, cultural and ideological factors. Remarkably, none of these issues were submitted as examples of ethical problems for psychiatric nurses. Indeed, it appeared as if none of the correspondents viewed these as in any way ethical issues. Perhaps they saw themselves as dealing with very practical issues, which had nothing whatsoever to do with ethics in particular, or philosophy in general.

We hope that enough has been said and this simple, but crucial point need be laboured no longer. For our practice to be ethically sound, we need to remain aware first and foremost that ethical problems exist. Without that awareness we shall never even dip our toes into the murky waters of reflection and debate which might help us towards a renewed appreciation of the right way to act. Such ethical problems are neither divorced from ordinary activity, nor the exclusive domain of a professional or academic elite. What we are involved in is an ongoing struggle with forces of creativity and inertia, forces of integration and chaos, played out in the arena of the ordinary, everyday choices we all make. This constant struggle is our ethical life. Such struggle manifests in our conduct – our conduct as a society, as groups within that society and as individuals. In Parts 1 and 3 of this text relationships between large groupings within society were considered (for example between the 'sane' and the 'insane'). Relations were also considered between groupings of people and more abstract influences (for example between clinicians and the drive to conform, or between nurses and individualistic political ideology). Part 2 focused on individuals' experience of quite immediate ethical dilemmas, emphasising the direct experience of confusion and uncertainty about conduct in particular situations. What has appeared to be of the greatest importance in this respect is allowing space for people (both clients and clinicians/authors) to experience their feelings of turmoil in relation to these and other ethical issues. A link has emerged between the experience of moral doubt and growth, and the gap between the two is bridged by the provision of such space, and by encouraging people therein to *tell their stories,* which is what we hope we have done.

THE ETHICAL ROLLER COASTER

We observed earlier that although we often think of our moral values as belonging distinctly to us, they are usually a distillation or complex product of the interaction of many age-old philosophies. As Hampshire noted: 'It would be contrary to the evidence of history to think of conceptions of the good as developing in isolation, uninfluenced by rival conceptions. Moral ideas cross and re-cross imagined moral frontiers, sometimes finally obliterating them' (1989, p.156). We as authors and editors share with our readers the struggle to develop and maintain a consistent picture of the 'right and fitting' way of life and living. Our conceptions of what is 'good' or 'bad' are rarely consistent, and the reasoning which lies behind our shifting conceptions is often even less clear to us. Consequently, most of us settle for a rag-bag of ethical ideas which, if we wish to be less harsh, we call an eclectic ethical standpoint. We know that we need some kind of ethical framework for our lives and if we choose one which has more 'angles' to it, so much the better. This is not necessarily something which we work consciously towards. Rather, it seems reasonable, it seems self-evident; this is not philosophy, this is just how one gets on with the business of life and living. Again, Hampshire observes: 'People may arrive quite naturally at an eclectic position, in which they have come to respect duties and obligations which, if pressed, they would realise are drawn from different conceptions of the good' (1989, p.156). And so we find that often our 'ethics' change in form but remain largely stable in content. The reasoning and argument we employ to justify and shape this or that position may change over time, but the heart of the ethical matter usually remains constant. Just as we may develop more and more novel ways of stimulating the human body, ultimately the same set of processes are employed: the most advanced roller coaster only produces the same kind of pleasing disorientation that we first felt when our parents swung us, as infants, over their heads. And here, in this clumsy analogy, may lie the nub of our ethical searching. We are seeking to clarify our view of some constant of the human condition; a constant feature of human experience which might serve as the essential benchmark for all our ethical strife. If we have achieved something of this sort in the preceding pages, if the reader finds resonance in the accounts we have presented with his or her own sense of ethical striving, it will indeed have been a valuable undertaking.

REFERENCES

Hampshire, S. 1989: *Innocence and experience.* London: Penguin.
Watts, A. 1977: *The essential Alan Watts.* Berkeley, CA: Celestial Arts.

INDEX

progressive 293–6
ranking quality and cost-containment 288
shift to community care 286–8
top-down or bottom-up 289–90

racial discrimination
of black nurses 158–62
challenging 166–7
of patients 162–6
resemblance of psychiatric treament to 162
reality 141–56
definition 141
redemption 83–92
creativity and 91–2
definition 78
metaphor as a bridge 83–6
and the middle way 89–91
through participation 86–9
regression 68–9
religion
codes and relationships 6–7
definition of religious 77–8
ethics and 4–5
psychiatry 21–2
resistance 228
responsibility and liberty 24
role of psychiatric nurse 57–65

Sabbadini, Andrea 73
SANE 294
Schatzman, Dr Morton 69, 70
schizophrenia
in Afro-Caribbeans 163, 166
violence and 30
Schizophrenia Fellowship 292
self-awareness 100
Smail, David 57–60, 64, 65, 128, 264
social distance 45
social iatrogenesis 50, 51
Socrates 5
Soteria House, California 74
spiritual, definition 77–8
spiritual experience 79–80
Stoicism 5
Styron, William 85–6
support frameworks 110–11
Survivors Speak Out 63, 243, 244
Szasz, Dr Thomas 20–5, 67–8, 87, 89

Thatcher, Margaret 282
therapeutic collectivism 267, 269–79
feat of 277–9
therapeutic individualism 270–2
Thoreau, Henry David 121
touch, importance of 152–4
training on race, ethnicity and mental health
168–9
transference 196

uncertainty 45
user
needs of psychiatric services 96–8
patient satisfaction 291–2
user movement 243–5

validation therapy 146–8, 218
violence 27–9
black people and 166
control and 31–2
relationship between mental illness and
29–31

Watkins, Jesse 87–8
White City Project 258, 260
Wilson, Michael 89–91
Wittgenstein 12
women
bias against 174–5
black 182
as carers 176–7
definition and treatment of distress 175–6
difficulty in identifying needs 181
expectations of care 180
groupwork with 177–8
as a problem 181
use of mental health services 174
Women's Action for Mental Health 258
wounded healer
alienation of the patient 343–4
core ethical assumptions 346–7
disclosure of illness 337–9
frailties and illuminations 336–7
myth of 334–6
'outing' of 344–5
'us' and 'them' mentality 340–1

yoga 19